Paediatric Handbook
Sixth Edition

Editor
JOANNE SMART

Associate editor
TERRY NOLAN

**Blackwell
Science**

© 2000 by Blackwell Science Asia Pty Ltd

Published by Blackwell Science Asia Pty Ltd

First printed 2000

Editorial Offices:

54 University Street, Carlton South, Victoria 3053, Australia
Osney Mead, Oxford OX2 OEL, UK
25 John Street, London WC 1N 2BL, UK
23 Ainslie Place, Edinburgh EH3 6AJ, UK
350 Main Street, Malden, MA 02148–5018, USA

Other Editorial Offices:

Blackwell Wissenschafts-Verlag GmbH
Kurfilrstendamm 57
10707 Berlin, Germany
Zehemergasse 6
1140 Wien, Austria

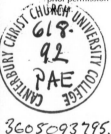

Designed by Stephanie Thompson
Typeset by Graphicraft Ltd, Hong Kong
Edited by Edward Caruso
Production by Limited Edition
Printed in Australia

DISTRIBUTORS

Blackwell Science Pty Ltd
54 University Street,
Carlton South, Victoria 3053, Australia

Orders Tel: 03 9347 0300
Fax: 03 9349 3016
E-mail: info@blacksci-asia.com.au
Internet: www.blackwell-science-asia.com.au

North-America

Blackwell Science, Inc.
Commerce Place, 350 Main Street
Malden, MA 02148–5018

Orders Tel: 617388 8250
              800759 6102
Fax: 617388 8255

Canada

Copp Clark Professional
200 Adelaide Street, West, 3rd Floor,
Toronto, Ontario M5H 1W7

Orders Tel: 416597 1616
              800815 9417
Fax: 416597 1616

United Kingdom

Marston Book Services Ltd
PO Box 87
Oxford, OX2 ODT

Orders Tel: 01865 791155
Fax: ·   01865 791927
Telex: 837515

Cataloguing-in-Publication Data

Royal Children's Hospital (Melbourne, Vic.).
Paediatric handbook.
6th ed.
ISBN 0 86793 011 X.
1. Pediatrics—Handbooks, manuals, etc.   2. Children—Hospital care—Handbooks, manuals, etc.   I. Nolan, Terry.   II. Smart, Joanne, 1965– .   III. Title.

618.92

CONTENTS

CONTRIBUTORS

All authors are staff or associates of the Royal Children's Hospital (RCH) unless otherwise indicated.

Robert Adler
Former Chairman, RCH Mental Health Service
Former Professor, Department of Paediatrics, University of Melbourne

Roger Allen
Paediatrician/Paediatric Rheumatologist, Department of General Paediatrics

Helen Anthony
Former Clinical Specialist Dietitian, Department of Nutrition and Food Services

Peter Barnett
Deputy Director, Department of Emergency Medicine

Robert Berkowitz
Director, Department of Otolaryngology

Julie Bines
Head of Clinical Nutrition
Paediatric Gastroenterologist, Department of Gastroenterology & Clinical Nutrition

Avihu Boneh
Director, Metabolic Services, Victorian Clinical Genetics Services

Barbara Burge
General Practitioner, Visiting Examiner, Department of Paediatrics, University of Melbourne

Fergus Cameron
Endocrinologist, Department of Endocrinology & Diabetes

Tony Catto-Smith
Director, Department of Gastroenterology & Clinical Nutrition

George Chalkiadis
Anaesthetist, Department of Anaesthesia
Co-ordinator, Pain Management

Nigel Curtis	Paediatric Infectious Diseases Physician, Departments of Microbiology & Infectious Diseases and General Paediatrics Senior Lecturer, Department of Paediatrics, University of Melbourne
Lex Doyle	Neonatal Paediatrician, Royal Women's Hospital Associate Professor, Department of Paediatrics, University of Melbourne
James Elder	Director, Department of Ophthalmology
Kay Gibbons	Chief Dietitian, Department of Nutrition and Food Services
Kerr Graham	Director, The Hugh Williamson Gait Laboratory Professor of Orthopaedics, Department of Paediatrics, University of Melbourne
Sonia Grover	Adolescent and Paediatric Gynaecologist, Centre for Adolescent Health Obstetrician and Gynaecologist, Royal Women's Hospital
Simon Harvey	Deputy Director, Department of Neurology Director, Children's Epilepsy Program
John Hutson	Director, Department of General Surgery Professor, Department of Paediatrics, University of Melbourne
David James	Paediatrician, Department of General Paediatrics
Frederick Jarman	Paediatrician, Centre for Community Child Health
Colin Jones	Director, Department of Nephrology, Victorian Paediatric Renal Services Senior Lecturer, Department of Paediatrics, University of Melbourne
Stephen G. Kahler	Clinical Director, Victorian Clinical Genetics Services

CONTRIBUTORS

Andrew Kemp
Director of Clinical Immunology
Paediatrician, Department of General Paediatrics
Professor, Department of Paediatrics, University
of Melbourne

Julian Keogh
Surgeon, Department of General Surgery
Burn Surgeon, Victorian Paediatric Burns Centre

Geoffrey Klug
Senior Neurosurgeon, Department of
Neurosurgery

Margaret Loughnan
Social Worker

Lionel Lubitz
Deputy Director, Department of General
Paediatrics

James Lucas
Deputy Director, Department of Dentistry

Ernest S.L. Luk
Former Psychiatrist, RCH Mental Health Service
Former Associate Professor, Departments of
Psychiatry and Paediatrics, University of
Melbourne

Michael Marks
Paediatrician, Department of General
Paediatrics
Senior Lecturer, Department of Paediatrics,
University of Melbourne

Catherine Marraffa
Paediatrician, Department of Child
Development and Rehabilitation and
Mental Health Service

Peter McDougall
Director, Division of Medicine, Department of
Neonatology

Michelle Meehan
Maternal and Child Health Nurse, Division of
Community Oriented Paediatric and Adolescent
Services

Colin Morley
Director, Neonatal Medicine, Women's and
Children's Healthcare Network
Professor of Neonatal Medicine, University of
Melbourne

Annie Moulden
Paediatrician, Children's Specialist Centre

Margot Nash   Paediatrician, Department of General
Paediatrics
Senior Lecturer, Department of Paediatrics,
University of Melbourne

Terry Nolan   Head, Clinical Epidemiology and Biostatistics
Unit
Paediatrician, Department of General
Paediatrics
Professor, Department of Paediatrics, University
of Melbourne

Anthony Olinsky   Director, Department of Respiratory Medicine

George Patton   Psychiatrist, Mental Health Services for Kids and
Youth
Director, Centre for Adolescent Health
Professor of Adolescent Health, Department of
Paediatrics, University of Melbourne

Rod Phillips   Paediatrician, Department of General
Paediatrics and Centre for Adolescent Health
Senior Lecturer, Department of Paediatrics,
University of Melbourne

Harley Powell   Senior Nephrologist, Victorian Paediatric Renal
Service

Glynis Price   Endocrinologist, Department of Endocrinology
and Diabetes

Philip Ragg   Anaesthetist, Department of Anaesthetics

Dinah Reddihough   Director, Department of Child Development and
Rehabilitation

John Rogers   Senior Medical Geneticist, Victorian Clinical
Genetics Services

Susan Sawyer   Deputy Director, Centre for Adolescent Health
Respiratory Physician, Department of
Respiratory Medicine
Associate Professor, Department of Paediatrics,
University of Melbourne

CONTRIBUTORS

Jill Sewell Deputy Director & Paediatrician, Centre for Community Child Health

Frank Shann Director, Intensive Care Unit
Professor, Department of Paediatrics, University of Melbourne

Lloyd Shield Director, Department of Neurology

Joanne Smart Immunology Fellow, Department of Immunology

Anne Smith Paediatrician, Gatehouse Centre for the Assessment and Treatment of Child Abuse

Peter Smith Stevenson Professor and Chairman, Department of Paediatrics, University of Melbourne
Director, Department of Clinical Haematology and Oncology

Michael South Director, Department of General Paediatrics
Deputy Chairman & Associate Professor, Department of Paediatrics, University of Melbourne

Mike Starr Infection Control Officer/Infectious Diseases Fellow, Department of Microbiology & Infectious Diseases
Paediatrician, Department of General Paediatrics

John Su Dermatologist, Department of Dermatology

Mimi Tang Allergist and Immunologist, Department of Immunology and Allergy
Senior Lecturer, Department of Paediatrics, University of Melbourne

Russell Taylor Surgeon, Department of General Surgery
Burn Surgeon, Victorian Paediatric Burn Centre

James Tibballs Deputy Director, Intensive Care Unit
Resuscitation Officer
Medical Consultant, Poisons Information Centre
Associate Professor, Department of Pharmacology, University of Melbourne

Hubert van Doorn	Co-ordinator, General Practice Education, Department of General Paediatrics
George Varigos	Director, Department of Dermatology
Rowan Walker	Nephrologist, Royal Melbourne Hospital and Royal Children's Hospital Director, Dialysis and Transplantation, Victorian Paediatric Renal Service Associate Professor, Department of Medicine, University of Melbourne
Garry Warne	Endocrinologist, Department of Endocrinology and Diabetes Associate Professor, University of Melbourne
George Werther	Director, Department of Endocrinology and Diabetes Professor, University of Melbourne
James Wilkinson	Director, Department of Cardiology

Acknowledgement of 5th edition contributors

Jennifer Batch (Disorders of Glucose Metabolism)

Glenn Bowes (Adolescent Health)

Doug Bryan (Developmental Delay and Disability)

Neil Campbell (Fluid and Electrolyte Therapy; Infant and Child Nutrition)

Daryl Efron (Procedures)

Keith Grimwood (Infectious Diseases and Microbiology; Respiratory Conditions)

Karen Hogan (Child Abuse and Neglect)

Geoff Hogg (Infectious Diseases and Microbiology)

Jim McGill (Metabolic Conditions)

Frank Oberklaid (Paediatric Health Maintenance)

Peter Phelan (Respiratory Conditions)

Margaret Rowell (Developmental Delay and Disability)

Gerry Silk (The Death of a Child)

John Vorrath (Ear, Nose and Throat Conditions)

EDITORIAL COMMITTEE

FOREWORD

This latest edition of the *Paediatric Handbook* has been revised to take into account changes in medical practice relevant to young people and the handbook's broader role as a pocket-size source of information for both students and practitioners involved in providing care to children and adolescents.

The somewhat artificial distinction between 'medicine' and 'surgery' has been eliminated. Information only of relevance to practitioners in Victoria has been deleted to reflect the broader role of this text as a source of information. The major thrust of this handbook continues to be diagnosis and management of disorders in young people rather than public health or preventive strategies.

Developed countries tend to have low infant and childhood mortality rates with young people composing demographically a declining proportion of the total population. Injuries and cancer are the largest causes of mortality with significant morbidity occurring from disorders such as injury, infection and asthma. The demographic profile of developing countries is quite different with a much larger proportion of young people. In some such countries 40% of the population is under the age of 20 years. In many developing countries there is a significantly higher infant and child mortality rate with significant mortality and morbidity from infection and malnutrition. Those countries that are successfully dealing with issues of infection and malnutrition through public health programs are also being confronted with having to develop strategies for managing diseases in young people, such as asthma, diabetes and cancer without diverting resources away from the important public health area.

The staff of the Royal Children's Hospital has again produced the *Paediatric Handbook* and they are proud of their contribution to the care of young people in Victoria and beyond. They hope that the *Paediatric Handbook* will continue to be a useful adjunct to the diagnosis and treatment of sick children and adolescents both in Australia and in other parts of the world.

Peter J. Smith
Stevenson Professor & Chairman
Department of Paediatrics
University of Melbourne

PREFACE

The *Paediatric Handbook* of the Royal Children's Hospital is intended as a handy reference to be used by a range of medical practitioners, including general practitioners and other primary care providers, as well as hospital residents in secondary and tertiary paediatric centres. Although comprehensive, it is not a textbook—discussion of the finer points of pathogenesis and management of conditions is beyond the scope of a handbook. The emphasis is on a problem-oriented, hands-on approach to common and important clinical conditions encountered in paediatric practice.

The sixth edition of the *Paediatric Handbook* is a substantial revision. All chapters have been improved, and many have been extensively revised and expanded. In addition, several chapters have undergone major rewriting, including Allergy and immunology, Dermatological conditions, Infectious diseases and Metabolic conditions. There is a completely new chapter on immunisation and a new section on chronic pain has been incorporated into the chapter on pain.

The Handbook continues to have a broad base that will ensure its ongoing value to a wide range of community practitioners, dealing with issues such as feeding problems (Infant and child nutrition) and normal variations and common minor problems of newborn infants (Neonatal conditions).

Many new illustrations and diagnostic and management algorithms have been added. These greatly enhance the utility and 'at a glance' accessibility of the information in several chapters, including Procedures, Common surgical conditions, Orthopaedic conditions, Eye conditions and Renal conditions and enuresis.

A new feature is the incorporation of an antibiotic ready reference in the inner back cover and related pages. This will ensure easy and quick access to appropriate first-line therapy, including dosage recommendations, for a comprehensive range of infectious diseases.

The chapter order has been revised to provide a more intuitive structure. Medical emergencies assume a front-line position followed

PREFACE

by practical sections on procedures, pain management, immunisation, fluid therapy and nutrition. These are followed by sections on development and psychosocial problems. The distinction between medical and surgical conditions has been removed and the body system and disease chapters have been incorporated alphabetically into one block.

The appendices have been extended to provide growth charts, laboratory reference ranges, including immunologic parameters, an asthma management plan and the pharmacopoeia.

The index has again been expanded significantly to facilitate easy reference.

Another new feature has been the addition of drug doses, including dosage interval and maximum dosages, whenever a drug is mentioned in the text. While every effort has been made to check drug doses throughout the handbook, it is still possible that errors may have been missed. Furthermore, dosage schedules are constantly being revised and new adverse effects recognised. Therefore, the reader is strongly advised to consult the pharmaceutical company's package insert or other product information before administering any of the drugs recommended in this handbook.

At the beginning of the Handbook we acknowledge the input of previous contributors who for one reason or another have not been directly involved in the production of the sixth edition. Their valuable contributions in previous editions are greatly appreciated.

We would like to acknowledge a number of people for their kind assistance. First, Professor Frank Shann for permission to reprint his booklet, *Drug Doses, 10th Edition*. We are again indebted to Bill Reid for his excellent illustrations and Shirley Green and Catherine Bendeich at Blackwell Science Asia for their support throughout the preparation of the manuscript. Particular thanks are extended to Melbourne artist, Michael Leunig, who generously donated the image that appears on the cover.

Joanne Smart
Editor

Terry Nolan
Associate editor

CHAPTER 1
MEDICAL EMERGENCIES

James Tibballs

CARDIORESPIRATORY ARREST

Cardiorespiratory arrest may occur in a wide variety of conditions that cause hypoxaemia or hypotension, or both. Examples include trauma, drowning, septicaemia, sudden infant death syndrome, asthma, and congenital anomalies of the heart and lung.

The initial cardiac rhythm discovered during early resuscitation is usually severe bradycardia or asystole. The spontaneous onset of ventricular fibrillation in children is uncommon, but it may occur with congenital heart conditions or secondary to poisoning with cardioactive drugs. Respiratory arrest alone may occur.

Diagnosis and initial management

Cardiorespiratory arrest may be suspected when consciousness is lost, or the patient appears pale or cyanosed, or is pulseless or apnoeic.

Assess respiration by observing movement of the chest and by feeling for expired breath while positioning the head and neck to maintain an airway. Movement of the chest without expiration indicates a blocked airway.

Assess circulation by palpation of a carotid, brachial or femoral pulse. Whenever possible, treat in a treatment room. Carry the patient there if necessary. If this is not possible, fetch the resuscitation trolley from a treatment room.

Cardiopulmonary resuscitation (CPR) must commence with basic techniques and be supplemented by advanced techniques.

Airway maintenance and ventilation

If airway obstruction is present, quickly inspect the pharynx. Clear secretions or vomitus by brief suction using a Yankauer sucker. Maintain the airway with backward head tilt, chin lift or forward jaw thrust.

Table 1.1 Table of drugs, fluid volume, endotracheal tubes and direct current shock for paediatric resuscitation

Age	0	2 months	5 months	1 year	2 years	3 years	4 years	5 years	6 years	7 years	8 years	9 years	10 years	11 years	12 years	13 years	14 years
Bodyweight (kg)*	3.5	5	7	10	12	14	16	18	20	22	25	28	32	36	40	46	50
Height (cm)*	50	58	65	75	85	94	102	109	115	121	127	132	138	144	151	157	162
	mL	mL	mL	mL	mL	mL	mL	mL	mL	mL	mL	mL	mL	mL	mL	mL	mL
Adrenaline 1 : 1000																	
10 µg/kg	0.035	0.05	0.07	0.10	0.12	0.14	0.16	0.18	0.2	0.22	0.25	0.28	0.32	0.36	0.4	0.46	0.5
100 µg/kg	0.35	0.5	0.7	1	1.2	1.4	1.6	1.8	2	2.2	2.5	2.8	3.2	3.6	4	4.6	5
Adrenaline 1 : 10 000																	
10 µg/kg	0.35	0.5	0.7	1	1.2	1.4	1.6	1.8	2	2.2	2.5	2.8	3.2	3.6	4	4.6	5
100 µg/kg	3.5	5.0	7.0	10	12	14	16	18	20	22	25	28	32	36	40	46	50
Lignocaine 1% mL																	
1 mg/kg	0.3	0.5	0.7	1.0	1.2	1.4	1.6	1.8	2.0	2.2	2.5	2.8	3.2	3.6	4.0	4.6	5.0
Sodium bicarb. 8.4% mL																	
1 mmol/kg	3.5	5	7	10	12	14	16	18	20	22	25	28	32	36	40	46	50
Fluid volume mL																	
20 mL/kg	70	100	140	200	240	280	320	360	400	440	500	560	640	720	800	920	1000
Endotracheal tube																	
Size (mm) age/4 + 4	3	3.5	3.5	4	4.5	4.5	5	5	5.5	5.5	6	6	6.5	6.5	7	7	7.5
Oral length (cm) age/2 + 12	9.5	11	11.5	12	13	13.5	14	14.5	15	15.5	16	16.5	17	17.5	18	18.5	19
Direct current shock																	
VF; VT 2 J/kg	7	10	20	20	20	30	30	30	50	50	50	50	70	70	70	100	100
VF; VT 4 J/kg	10	20	30	50	50	50	70	70	70	100	100	100	150	150	150	200	200
Unsynchronised																	
SVT 1 J/kg	3	5	7	10	10	14	16	18	20	22	25	28	30	30	50	50	50
Synchronised																	

* 50th percentiles

Source: Oakley, P., Phillips, B., Molyneaux, E. & Mackway-Jones, K. (1993) Updated standard reference chart. *BMJ* 1993; **306**, 1613.

If adequate respiration does not resume, ventilate the lungs with a self-inflating resuscitator (e.g. Laerdal, Ambu, Air-viva) with added oxygen 8–10 L/min. If ventilation cannot be achieved with the resuscitator, use a mouth-to-mask technique.

Whatever technique is used, ensure that ventilation expands the chest adequately.

Intubate the trachea via the mouth if you are able to do this, but do not cause hypoxaemia by prolonged unsuccessful attempts. Select the tube and insert it a depth appropriate to the patient's age in years: for patients over 1 year of age, tube size (internal diameter) is (age/4) + 4 mm and depth of insertion is approximately (age/2) + 12 cm from the lower lip (see Table 1.1).

Secure the tube with cotton tape around the neck or affix it firmly to the face with adhesive tape to avoid endobronchial intubation or accidental extubation.

External cardiac compression (ECC)

Start ECC if a pulse is not palpable within 10 s, or if it is less than 60 b.p.m. in an infant or less than 40 b.p.m. in a child.

Place the patient on a firm surface. Depress the sternum one-third the depth of the chest using two fingers for a newborn infant or an infant (<1 year), the heel of one hand for a small child (1–8 years of age), or the two-handed technique for an older child (>9 years), teenager or adult. The site of ECC is the lower sternum for all age groups.

External cardiac compression in newly born and small infants is better given by a technique in which the hands encircle the chest, the thumbs compress the sternum anteriorly and the fingers stabilise the vertebral column posteriorly. Avoid pressure over the ribs and abdominal viscera whatever technique is used.

Whatever technique is used ensure that compression generates a pulse.

Ideal rates of cardiac compression and ventilation and their ratio have not been determined. The rates and ratios currently recommended by the Australian Resuscitation Council are shown in Table 1.2. Give five initial breaths. Thereafter for newborn infants give successive cycles of three compressions in 1.5 s followed by a breath. For infants

Table 1.2 Recommended rates and ratios for external cardiac compression and ventilation during basic CPR

	Compression rate per min*	Single compression time (s)	Single breath time (max)	Ratio of compressions to breaths	Cycles per min (min)#	Actual compressions per min (min)#	Actual breaths per min (min)#
Newborn infant	120	0.5	0.5	3:1	30	90	30
Infant, small child, large child (1 or 2 rescuers)	100	0.6	2 s	5:1	12	60	12
Large child, adult (1 rescuer, two-handed compression)	100	0.6	3 s	15:2	4	60	8

* Not compressions in 1 min; # determined by breath time (additional cycles recommended if adequate ventilation achievable in less than maximum single breath time).

and all children give successive cycles of five cardiac compressions in 3 s followed by a breath. A single rescuer of a larger child or teenager should give successive cycles of 15 compressions in 9 s followed by two breaths.

If bag-to-mask ventilation or mouth-to-mask ventilation is used, the rescuer giving compressions should count aloud to allow the rescuer giving ventilation to deliver breaths between compressions. If ventilation is given by bag and endotracheal tube, ECC may be continued during ventilation (in the recommended ratios) provided lung expansion can be achieved. This will result in additional cycles of compressions and breaths.

Management of cardiac dysrhythmias

Determine the cardiac rhythm with defibrillator paddles or chest leads. Give DC shock if ventricular fibrillation or hypotensive ventricular tachycardia is present. See Table 1.1 and Fig. 1.1 for energy doses in DC shock. Give adrenaline if any other hypotensive rhythm is present (see Fig. 1.1).

Insert an intravenous cannula. Although this is the preferred access to the circulation, do not waste time with repeated unsuccessful attempts, because access can be achieved with the alternative techniques of bone marrow infusion (intraosseous, see procedures, Chapter 3) or endotracheal administration (ETT).

All drugs and resuscitation fluids can be given via the bone marrow, but only adrenaline, atropine and lignocaine can be given via the endotracheal route. A quick reference guide to drug doses and fluid volume is provided in Table 1.1.

Other drugs
Calcium

This is a useful inotropic and vasopressor agent but it has no place in the management of a dysrhythmia, unless it is caused by hypo-calcaemia, hyperkalaemia or calcium channel blocker toxicity. It is not useful and is probably harmful for asystole, ventricular fibrillation or electromechanical dissociation. The intravenous dose is 0.2 mL/kg of 10% calcium chloride or 0.7 mL/kg of 10% calcium gluconate. Do not administer calcium by endotracheal tube and do not mix it with bicarbonate.

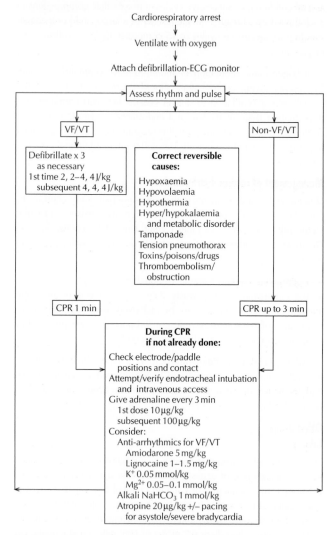

Cardiorespiratory arrest
↓
Ventilate with oxygen
↓
Attach defibrillation-ECG monitor
↓
Assess rhythm and pulse

VF/VT

Non-VF/VT

Defibrillate x 3
  as necessary
  1st time 2, 2–4, 4 J/kg
  subsequent 4, 4, 4 J/kg

Correct reversible causes:

Hypoxaemia
Hypovolaemia
Hypothermia
Hyper/hypokalaemia
  and metabolic disorder
Tamponade
Tension pneumothorax
Toxins/poisons/drugs
Thromboembolism/
  obstruction

CPR 1 min

CPR up to 3 min

**During CPR
if not already done:**

Check electrode/paddle
  positions and contact
Attempt/verify endotracheal intubation
  and intravenous access
Give adrenaline every 3 min
  1st dose 10 μg/kg
  subsequent 100 μg/kg
Consider:
  Anti-arrhythmics for VF/VT
    Amiodarone 5 mg/kg
    Lignocaine 1–1.5 mg/kg
    K^+ 0.05 mmol/kg
    Mg^{2+} 0.05–0.1 mmol/kg
  Alkali $NaHCO_3$ 1 mmol/kg
  Atropine 20 μg/kg +/– pacing
    for asystole/severe bradycardia

Fig. 1.1 Management of cardiorespiratory arrest

Adenosine

This is the preferred drug treatment for supraventricular tachycardia. Administer as a rapid intravenous bolus in an initial dose of 0.1 mg/kg (max 3 mg), increasing by 0.05 mg/kg (max 3 mg) every 2 min to a max 0.3 mg/kg (max 18 mg) if required. Give synchronised direct current shock (0.5–1 J/kg) if a patient with supraventricular tachycardia is pulseless. Adenosine is metabolised too quickly for intraosseous use.

ANAPHYLAXIS

See also Allergy and Immunology, chapter 14.

The life-threatening clinical manifestations are:
- Hypotension due to vasodilatation and loss of plasma volume due to increased capillary permeability.
- Bronchospasm.
- Upper airways obstruction due to laryngeal or pharyngeal oedema.

Immediate treatment

- Vasopressor and bronchodilator therapy. Give adrenaline 0.01 mg/kg; i.e. 0.1 mL/kg of 1 : 10 000 solution by slow intravenous injection (over 10 min) or 0.01 mL/kg of 1 : 1000 solution by intramuscular (i.m.) injection. A continuous infusion (0.1–1.0 µg/kg per min) may be required if manifestations are prolonged.
- Oxygen by mask. Mechanical ventilation may be required.
- Intravenous volume expander. Give colloid or crystalloid solution at 20 mL/kg. Give repeat boluses of 10–20 mL/kg until the blood pressure is restored.
- Bronchodilator therapy with salbutamol – continuous nebulised (0.5%) or i.v. 5 µg/kg per min for 1 h, then 1 µg/kg per min thereafter. Secondary therapy with a steroid, aminophylline and an antihistamine may be helpful for prolonged bronchospasm and capillary leak.
- Relief of upper airways obstruction: mild to moderate oedema may respond to an inhalation of nebulised 1% adrenaline (0.05 mL/kg per dose diluted to 4 mL), but intubation of the trachea may be required.

Anaphylaxis can be biphasic and the patient may deteriorate again over the next few hours. All patients with anaphylaxis should be admitted to hospital and observed carefully for at least 12 h.

HAEMORRHAGIC SHOCK

The normal blood volume is 70–80 mL/kg. A child may lose a substantial volume of blood without developing hypotension. Cardiac output and blood pressure are preserved by tachycardia and vasoconstriction, so hypotension is a late sign of blood loss.

- Control external haemorrhage by direct wound pressure, arterial vessel pressure, or a tourniquet and elevation of the injured area. Investigate or surgically explore internal haemorrhage or both.
- Administer oxygen by mask.
- Insert a large bore intravenous cannula, preferably in the upper limb. Two cannulae may be required.
- Withdraw blood for group and cross-match.
- Infuse rapidly by pressure 20 mL/kg of a colloid solution (e.g. Haemaccel), or a crystalloid solution if colloid is not available. This may also be administered rapidly by syringing with the aid of a three-way tap. Titrate additional volume to the blood pressure and other indices of perfusion.
- If exsanguinating, transfuse urgently with (in order of preference): (i) rapidly cross-matched blood; (ii) uncross-matched blood of the same group as the patient; (iii) uncross-matched O-negative blood.
- Monitor blood pressure, heart rate, oxygenation and urine output. Warm the blood and measure the central venous pressure, serum calcium, and the coagulation and acid–base status if massive transfusion is required. Calcium and fresh frozen plasma are usually needed after 1–2 blood volumes have been transfused.

SEPTICAEMIC SHOCK

Hypotension is due to leakage of fluid from capillary beds and depression of myocardial contractility.

- Collect blood for culture, but do not delay administration of an antibiotic if a blood sample cannot be collected. If no information is available regarding the source of pathogen, give flucloxacillin 50 mg/kg (max 2 g) i.v. 4 hourly and cefotaxime 50 mg/kg (max 2 g) i.v. 6 hourly. For particular circumstances consult Antimicrobial Guidelines. Shock due to meningococcaemia is usually accompanied by a purpuric rash; give cefotaxime 50 mg/kg (max 2 g) i.v. 6 hourly. Give benzyl-penicillin 60 mg/kg (max 3 g) i.v. or i.m. 4 hourly if cefotaxime not available.
- Treat shock with an intravenous colloid or crystalloid solution (20 mL/kg initially – further boluses of 10–20 mL/kg may be needed).
- Commence infusion of an inotropic agent. Dopamine (5–20 µg/kg per min) is preferred. Administration via a central vein is preferred but it may be given via a peripheral vein as a dilute solution (e.g. 15 mg/kg in 500 mL at 10–40 mL/h = 5–20 µg/kg per min). Dobutamine (5–20 µg/kg per min) may be administered into a peripheral vein.
- Give oxygen and monitor blood gases. Mechanical ventilation may be required.

Defer lumbar puncture until the child has been stabilised.

DROWNING

There is a global hypoxic-ischaemic injury often associated with lung damage from aspiration.

- Adequate oxygenation and ventilation are of paramount importance. Mechanical ventilation is required for severe lung involvement, circulatory arrest or loss of consciousness. Lung hypoxic-ischaemic injury is compounded by pulmonary oedema or aspiration of water or gastric contents.
- Decompress the stomach, which is usually distended with air and water.
- Support the circulation with intravenous infusion of colloid or crystalloid solution and infusion of an inotropic agent (e.g. dopamine 5–20 µg/kg per min into a central vein).
- If signs of cerebral oedema are present (i.e. a depressed conscious state) administer mannitol 0.25–0.5 g/kg i.v. once.

- Correct electrolyte disturbances; hypokalaemia is common. The differences between fresh- and salt-water drowning are not usually clinically important.
- Administer benzylpenicillin 60 mg/kg (max 3 g) i.v. 6 hourly (to prevent the complication of pneumococcal pneumonia).

ACUTE LARYNGEAL OBSTRUCTION

The most common cause is laryngotracheobronchitis (croup), and occasional causes are epiglottitis, inhaled foreign body, allergic oedema and trauma. The hallmark of obstruction is stridor, which, when accompanied by a barking cough suggests croup, or when accompanied by dysphagia/drooling suggests epiglottitis. Severe obstruction stimulates forceful diaphragmatic contraction that results in a retraction of the rib cage, tracheal tug and abdominal protrusion on inspiration. Cyanosis and irregular respiratory effort are terminal signs.

Epiglottitis

See also Respiratory Conditions, chapter 32.
- Complete obstruction may occur in just a few hours. In general, tracheal intubation is required. Notify an intensivist or anaesthetist immediately if epiglottitis is suspected.
- Keep the child in a sitting position and administer oxygen by mask. If complete obstruction is imminent, summon immediate help from an intensivist or anaesthetist. If you are inexperienced, do not attempt intubation unless the child becomes comatose. Intubate orally initially with a relatively small endotracheal tube. It may be hard to see the larynx because of secretions in the pharynx and the swollen epiglottis. Be prepared to aspirate the pharynx with a Yankauer sucker. Cricoid pressure is very helpful to visualise the vocal cords.
- If intubation proves to be impossible, attempt to ventilate with bag–valve–mask; a good technique may achieve adequate oxygenation and ventilation. If ventilation is impossible, perform cricothyrotomy or tracheostomy (see below).
- Antibiotic therapy: Ceftriaxone 100 mg/kg (max 2 g) i.v. followed by 50 mg/kg (max 2 g) 24 h later.

Croup

See also Respiratory Conditions, chapter 32.

In severe obstruction, give an inhalation of nebulised 1% adrenaline 0.05 mL/kg per dose diluted to 4 mL to obtain temporary relief, and give dexamethasone 0.6 mg/kg i.v. or i.m. Obtain intensive care or anaesthetic help with a view to endotracheal intubation. If this is not available, intubate when the child is going into respiratory failure. Use an introducing stylet in an endotracheal tube of size 0.5 or 1 mm smaller than usually calculated by age in years; i.e. (age/4) + 4 mm.

Aspirated foreign body

See also Respiratory Conditions, chapter 32.
- Give first-aid (back slaps, Heimlich manoeuvre, lateral chest compressions) if obstruction occurs, otherwise allow the child to cough. Do not instrument the airways if the child is coping, but summon an anaesthetist and ENT surgeon. Give oxygen.
- If complete obstruction occurs, attempt removal of an impacted laryngeal foreign body with forceps – if this is unsuccessful, perform a cricothyrostomy or tracheostomy (see below).
- If respiratory failure is due to a foreign body in the lower trachea or bronchi, attempt ventilation via an endotracheal tube while organising endoscopic removal.

Allergic oedema

Treat with nebulised 1% adrenaline 0.05 mL/kg per dose diluted to 4 mL. Refer to an intensivist or anaesthetist for endotracheal intubation, or an ENT surgeon for tracheostomy.

Emergency relief of a totally obstructed upper airway

- Adequate oxygenation can be obtained by inserting a 14-gauge intravenous cannula percutaneously into the trachea via the cricothyroid membrane (which lies immediately inferior to the thyroid cartilage); the patient should be lying straight, with the cannula in the midline and angled towards the feet. Remove the needle of the intravenous cannula; connect the cannula to a resuscitator or a bagging circuit using a connector from a 3.0 mm endotracheal tube. Ventilate with sustained 100% oxygen inspirations. Alternatively, connect the cannula to the compressed wall oxygen supply via a three-way intravenous tap (to allow expiration) and a length of plastic tubing. A length of plastic tubing that has a side hole cut may also be used to allow expiration. Aid intermittent expiration by lateral chest compression.

- Alternatively, perform cricothyro(s)tomy. Identify and maintain stabilisation of the thyroid–cricoid region with one hand. Incise the skin over the cricothyroid membrane (between the thyroid and cricoid cartilages). Bluntly dissect into the trachea with forceps in the midline or incise vertically with scalpel. Insert a small tracheostomy or endotracheal tube.
- Alternatively, perform percutaneous minitracheostomy.

STATUS ASTHMATICUS

See also Respiratory Conditions, chapter 32.

Severe asthma

Children unresponsive to intermittent inhalation of salbutamol should receive:

- Continuous inhalation of undiluted 0.5% salbutamol solution nebulised with oxygen.
- Methylprednisolone 1 mg/kg i.v. (max 50 mg) 6 hourly.
- Nebulised ipratropium may be added as 250–500 µg/dose 4–6 hourly (beware anticholinergic effects).
- Intravenous salbutamol load 5 µg/kg over 10 min followed by infusion 1–5 µg/kg per min (beware hypokalaemia).
- Aminophylline (subject to prior theophylline use and serum level) 10 mg/kg (max 500 mg) i.v. over 1 h followed by infusion of 1.1 mg/kg per h (age 1–9 years) or 0.7 mg/kg per h (10 years to adult).

Life-threatening asthma – manage in ICU

- Mechanical ventilation.
- Ketamine 1–2 mg/kg then infusion 10–20 µg/kg per min.
- Magnesium sulphate 25–40 mg/kg (max 1.2 g) over 30 min once.
- Halothane inhalation during mechanical ventilation.

STATUS EPILEPTICUS

See also Neurologic Conditions, chapter 29.

A convulsion involving the respiratory musculature and upper airways, and that does not cease within a few min, may cause hypoventilation with hypoxaemia and hypercarbia. Administer oxygen and treat with an intravenous anticonvulsant; be prepared to give mechanical ventilation, particularly if the child has meningitis. Some anticonvulsant choices include:

- Diazepam 0.2–0.4 mg/kg (max 10–20 mg) i.v. May be given per rectum if there is no intravenous access.
- Clonazepam 0.25 mg (<1 year); 0.5 mg (1–5 years); 1 mg (>5 years) i.v.
- Phenobarbitone 20 mg/kg over 30 min; repeat doses 10–15 mg/kg every 15–30 min up to 100 mg/kg in 24 h (beware hypotension) if required.
- Phenytoin 15 mg/kg (max 1.5 g) i.v. over 1 h to avoid negative inotropic effect. Slow onset.
- Thiopentone: titrate dose to effect (usually 2–5 mg/kg). Beware of hypotension.

Prolonged convulsions may require large and repeated doses of anticonvulsant drugs and, consequently, mechanical ventilation. Repeated doses of a single anticonvulsant such as phenobarbitone (where the serum level correlates with the effects) are preferable to using multiple anticonvulsants. Suspect hyponatraemia as the cause of convulsions in meningitis.

RAISED INTRACRANIAL PRESSURE

Acute intracranial hypertension threatens the blood supply of the brain and may cause herniation of the brain. It is recognised by (in approximate sequence):

- Headache, vomiting, papilloedema, deterioration in the conscious state with diminution of spontaneous limb movements.
- Ipsilateral pupillary dilatation and contralateral hemiparesis, limb hypertonicity and spasm if due to uncal herniation into tentorial hiatus with supratentorial lesion. These can be bilateral with an extensive lesion.
- Alteration in pattern of respiration (hyperventilation; irregular respiration), bradycardia and hypertension are near-terminal events due to medullary herniation into the foramen magnum.

Common causes of intracranial hypertension are:

- Acute brain swelling due to cerebral oedema caused by trauma, infection, ischaemia or hypoxaemia.
- Space-occupying lesion, such as an intracerebral haemorrhage, tumour or abscess.
- Obstruction of cerebrospinal fluid circulation.

A neurosurgeon should be contacted immediately where indicated; e.g. in cases of trauma. If it is impossible to treat the cause immediately, reduce the intracranial blood volume by using mechanical hyperventilation to lower the P_aCO_2 and cause cerebral vasoconstriction. (*Note:* prolonged or excessive hyperventilation to P_aCO_2 of <25–35 mmHg may be harmful.) Hypoxaemia and hypotension must be avoided. Mannitol may be used to reduce cerebral oedema (0.25–0.5 g/kg, i.v.). Fluids should be restricted to avoid cerebral oedema, but not at the expense of causing hypotension. Blood pressure may be maintained with a vasopressor (e.g. dopamine up to 10 µg/kg per min).

A guide to the role of lumbar puncture and chemotherapeutic agents is given in Fig. 1.2.

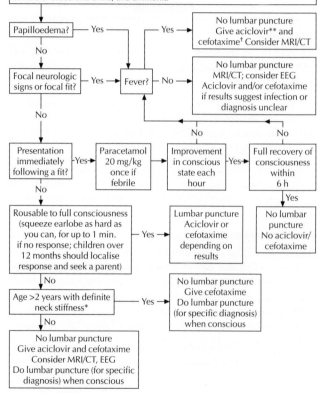

Consider: post-ictal state, infection (meningitis, encephalitis), trauma (including non-accidental injury), poisoning (drugs, toxins), metabolic conditions, hydrocephalus, hypertension, hepatic or renal failure and Reye's syndrome

Look for: bruises, fundal haemorrhages, blood pressure, urinalysis and blood sugar (reagent strip)

Initial investigations may include: full blood examination, urea and electrolytes, glucose, liver function test, arterial blood gas, drug screen, urine antigens, culture of blood and urine, and ammonia

Papilloedema? —Yes→ →Yes→ No lumbar puncture / Give aciclovir** and cefotaxime† Consider MRI/CT

↓No

Focal neurologic signs or focal fit? —Yes→ Fever? —No→ No lumbar puncture / MRI/CT; consider EEG / Aciclovir and/or cefotaxime if results suggest infection or diagnosis unclear

↓No

Presentation immediately following a fit? —Yes→ Paracetamol 20 mg/kg once if febrile → Improvement in conscious state each hour —Yes→ Full recovery of consciousness within 6 h

↓No ↓Yes

Rousable to full consciousness (squeeze earlobe as hard as you can, for up to 1 min. if no response; children over 12 months should localise response and seek a parent) —Yes→ Lumbar puncture / Aciclovir or cefotaxime depending on results

No lumbar puncture / No aciclovir/ cefotaxime

↓No

Age >2 years with definite neck stiffness* —Yes→ No lumbar puncture / Give cefotaxime / Do lumbar puncture (for specific diagnosis) when conscious

↓No

No lumbar puncture / Give aciclovir and cefotaxime / Consider MRI/CT, EEG / Do lumbar puncture (for specific diagnosis) when conscious

* Neck stiffness is not a reliable sign of meningism in children <2 years
** 10 mg/kg i.v. 8 hourly (age 2 weeks–2 years)
   500 mg/m² i.v. 8 hourly (age 2–12 years)
† 50 mg/kg (max 2 g) i.v. 6 hourly

Fig. 1.2 A guide to the role of lumbar puncture and the use of chemotherapeutic agents in the child unconscious due to unknown cause.

CHAPTER 2
POISONING AND ENVENOMATION

James Tibballs

POISONING

Epidemiology

Poisoning during childhood occurs mainly among 1–3 year olds, and tends to follow the ingestion of a wide variety of improperly stored agents in the home.

Other circumstances of poisoning are iatrogenic (particularly in infants), the deliberate self-administration of substances by older children for their recreational use or to manipulate their psychosocial environments. Increasingly, the intention is suicidal.

While poisoning in childhood is frequently minor in severity and mortality is low, serious illness may be caused by prescription and 'over-the-counter' pharmaceutical drugs and non-pharmaceutical products.

General management

The principles of management for all poisonings (see Fig. 2.1) are:
- Resuscitate the patient (airway preservation and protection, assisted ventilation with added oxygen, restoration of blood pressure with intravenous fluid +/– vasopressor-inotropic infusion).
- Remove the poison (if indicated).
- Administer an antidote if one exists (see Table 2.1).

Recovery is expected in the vast majority of cases if vital functions are preserved, and the complications of poisoning and its management are avoided.

A decision to remove the poison from the body should be dependent on the severity of the poisoning and the likelihood of success in removing the poison without further endangering the patient. Most poisonings in childhood are minor, and observation alone or non-invasive treatment is indicated.

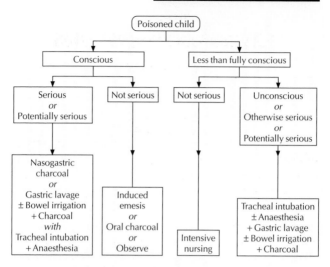

Fig. 2.1 General management of the poisoned child

The severity of poisoning may be assessed by the:
- Quantity of the poison(s)
- Preparation of the poison
- Interval since exposure
- Established and expected effects.

Removal from the body usually involves a technique of gastro-intestinal decontamination but occasionally other methods, such as dialysis, exchange transfusion, charcoal haemoperfusion, plasmapheresis or haemofiltration are required.

If the conscious state is depressed, all methods of gastrointestinal decontamination carry a substantial risk of aspiration pneumonitis. These techniques include induced emesis with syrup of ipecacuanha, gastric lavage, activated charcoal and whole bowel washout. Aspiration pneumonitis is not entirely prevented by endotracheal intubation. The most important factor determining the choice of technique is the conscious state. A guideline for the general management of poisoning using these techniques according to severity of poisoning is shown in Fig. 2.1.

Table 2.1 Antidotes to poisons

Poison	Antidotes and doses	Comments
Amphetamines	Esmolol i.v. 0.5 mg/kg over 1 min, then 25–200 µg/kg per min.	Treatment for tachyarrhythmia.
	Labetalol i.v. 0.15–0.3 mg/kg or phentolamine i.v. 0.05–0.1 mg/kg every 10 min.	Treatments for hypertension.
Benzodiazepines	Flumazenil 3–10 µg/kg repeated at 1 min then 3–10 µg/kg per h by infusion.	Specific antagonist at receptor. Titrate to effect. Caution: may precipitate convulsions or arrhythmia in multi-drug ingestion, especially with tricyclics.
Beta blocker	Glucagon 7 µg/kg then 2–7 µg/kg per min infusion.	Stimulates non-catecholamine cAMP production. Preferred antidote.
	Isoprenaline 0.05–3 µg/kg per min. Beware β₂ hypotension.	
	Noradrenaline 0.05–1 µg/kg per min.	
Calcium blocker	Calcium chloride 10% 0.2 mL/kg.	
Carbon monoxide	Oxygen 100%	Hyperbaric oxygen may be required.
Cyanide	Dicobalt edetate 300 mg over 1 min, then 300 mg at 5 min if no effect (adult dose).	Chelates. Give 50 mL 50% glucose after each dose.
	Amyl nitrite (perles 0.2 mL by inhalation) until sodium nitrite 3% i.v. (0.33 mL/kg over 4 min), *then* sodium thiosulphate 25% i.v. 1.65 mL/kg (max 50 mL) at 3–5 mL/min.	Nitrites form methaemoglobin-cyanide complex (beware excess methaemoglobinaemia – restrict to <20%). Thiosulphate forms non-toxic thiocyanate from methaemoglobin-cyanide.
Digoxin	Digoxin F_ab. Dose: acute ingestion 1 vial/2.5 tablet (0.25 mg); in steady state vials = serum digoxin (ng/mL) × BW (kg)/100.	

Continued overleaf

Table 2.1 Antidotes to poisons *Cont'd*

Poison	Antidotes and doses	Comments
Ergotamine	Sodium nitroprusside infusion 0.5–5 µg/kg per min.	Treats vasoconstriction. Monitor BP continuously.
	Heparin 100 units/kg then 10–30 units/kg per h according to clotting.	Treatment of coagulopathy.
Lead	If symptomatic or blood lead ≥2.9 µmol/L dimercaprol (BAL) 75 mg/m^2 i.m. 4 hourly 6 doses then i.v. calcium disodium edetate (EDTA) 1500 mg/m^2 over 5 days. If asymptomatic and blood lead 2.18–2.9 µmol/L infuse calcium disodium edetate 1000 mg/m^2 per day for 5 days.	
Heparin	Protamine 1 mg/100 units heparin.	Heparin half-life 1–2 h.
Iron	Desferrioxamine 15 mg/kg per h 12–24 h if serum iron >90 µmol/L or >63 µmol/L and symptomatic.	Beware anaphylaxis.
Methanol, ethylene glycol, glycol ethers	Ethanol, infuse loading dose 10 mL/kg 10% diluted in glucose 5% and then 0.15 mL/kg per h to maintain blood level at 0.1% (100 mg/dL).	
Methaemoglobin e.g., 2° to drug treatment	Methylene blue 1–2 mg/kg i.v. over several min.	
Opiates	Naloxone 0.01–0.1 mg/kg i.v., then 0.01/kg per h as needed.	
Organophosphates and carbamates	Atropine 20–50 µg/kg i.v. every 15 min until secretions dry. Pralidoxime 25 mg/kg i.v. over 15–30 min, then 10–20 mg/kg per h for 18 h or more. Not for carbamates.	Restores cholinesterase.
Paracetamol	N-acetylcysteine. i.v.; 150 mg/kg over 60 min, then 10 mg/kg per h for 20–72 h. Oral: 140 mg/kg then 17 doses of 70 mg/kg 4 hourly (total 1330 mg/kg over 68 h).	Give for >72 h if still encephalopathic.
Tricyclic antidepressants	Sodium bicarbonate i.v. 1 mmol/kg to maintain blood pH > 7.45.	

Details of management of specific poisons should be obtained from a Poisons Information Centre, or from appropriate and up-to-date references.

Activated charcoal

Activated charcoal is more efficacious than induced emesis or gastric lavage, and is currently regarded as a 'universal antidote'. It adsorbs most poisons but not metals, corrosives or pesticides. Like other techniques, however, it is contraindicated in the less-than-fully-conscious patient or if ileus is present. If aspirated, charcoal may cause fatal bronchiolitis obliterans. Constipation is relatively common. Addition of a laxative decreases transit time through the gut but does not improve efficacy in preventing drug absorption, and it may upset fluid and electrolyte balance. The initial dose is 1–2 g/kg. Repeated doses of activated charcoal enhance elimination of many drugs, particularly slow-release preparations. A suitable regimen is 0.25 g/kg per h for 12–24 h.

Syrup of ipecacuanha

Syrup of ipecacuanha is useful as a first-aid measure in the home or at hospital with very early presentation after ingestion of a minor poison. Its usefulness in serious poisoning is limited.

Although syrup of ipecacuanha induces vomiting in most children within 30 min of administration, it does not reliably empty the stomach of solids. Moreover, it must be given within 1 h of ingestion to significantly reduce drug absorption. It may cause prolonged vomiting, diarrhoea and drowsiness. The onset of vomiting may be delayed and may mimic the toxic effects of an ingested poison. Contraindications include:

- Impaired conscious state (risk of aspiration pneumonitis).
- Ingestion of a corrosive, hydrocarbon or petrochemical (risks of additional respiratory tract and pulmonary damage).

Gastric lavage

Although gastric lavage appears to be a logical therapy for ingested poisons, it too has a limited place in management. Problems include:

- Poor efficacy in preventing absorption when performed more than 60 min after ingestion.
- Risk of aspiration pneumonitis in the less-than-fully conscious patient, and to a lesser extent in the conscious child.

Gastric lavage is contraindicated after ingestion of corrosives, hydrocarbons or petrochemicals.

In the conscious young child it is psychologically traumatic and difficult to perform, thus predisposing to minor physical trauma.

If undertaken, care should be taken to avoid water intoxication and intrabronchial instillation of lavage fluid.

Gastric lavage is indicated in serious poisoning when a child is already intubated for airways protection and ventilation. The child should be in the lateral position during lavage. If potentially serious effects are expected, gastric lavage should only be performed after rapid sequence induction of anaesthesia and tracheal intubation.

Whole bowel irrigation

Whole bowel irrigation is performed with a solution of polyethylene glycol and electrolytes administered by nasogastric tube. A suitable dosage regimen is 30 mL/kg per h for 4–8 h.

It is useful in delayed presentation; and for the management of poisoning by slow-release drug preparations; substances not adsorbed by activated charcoal, e.g. iron; or which are irretrievable by gastric lavage.

Prevention

Action should be taken according to the circumstance of poisoning to prevent recurrence. Parents should be encouraged to store all medicines in child-proof cabinets and to store toxic substances in places inaccessible to young children.

Urgent psychosocial help should be organised for children who have poisoned themselves intentionally.

Steps should be taken to ensure that iatrogenic poisoning is not repeated.

INDIVIDUAL POISONS

Thousands of poisons exist. The most common poisons in young children that are presented to the Royal Children's Hospital, Melbourne, have been paracetamol, rodenticides, eucalyptus oil, benzodiazepines, tricyclic antidepressants and theophylline.

Only the most common serious poisonings are considered here briefly. Some have antidotes (see Table 2.1). *The general principles of management apply to all individual poisons* (see page 17).

Paracetamol (acetaminophen)

Paracetamol is the most common pharmaceutical poisoning.

Effects

The liver metabolises it to a toxic product, *N*-acetyl-*p*-benzoquinoneimine, which causes hepatic necrosis unless neutralised by the hepatic anti-oxidant glutathione. Multi-organ failure and death may occur after 3–4 days if the ingested quantity exceeds 150 mg/kg or smaller amounts with prior hepatic dysfunction, alcohol or anticonvulsants. Early symptoms are anorexia, nausea and vomiting.

Specific management

An effective antidote given before hepatic necrosis occurs is *N*-acetylcysteine (NAC), but its use is associated with adverse reactions (e.g. rash, bronchospasm and hypotension) that occur more frequently when administered intravenously. If reactions occur, cease NAC temporarily and give promethazine 0.2–0.5 mg/kg i.v. (max 10–25 mg) and recommence the NAC infusion at a reduced rate.

Since the outcome is related to serum levels of paracetamol measured 4–20 h after ingestion, a decision to administer NAC may be made according to time-related plasma levels. Administer if the level exceeds 1000 µmol/L at 4 h, 500 at 8 h, 200 at 12 h, 80 at 16 h, or 40 at 20 h (µmol/L × 0.15 = µg/mL).

- Intravenous NAC: 150 mg/kg in 5 mL/kg of glucose 5% over 60 min, then 10 mg/kg per h for 20 h or longer if the child is encephalopathic, or presentation is 10–36 h after ingestion.
- Oral NAC: 140 mg/kg, then 17 doses of 70 mg/kg – 4 hourly.

Presentation within 1 h after significant ingestion may be treated with gastric lavage (see above). Monitor liver function tests and serum potassium.

Theophylline

Toxicity is related to serum levels and may be delayed with slow-release preparations. The principal effects are:

- Gastrointestinal – nausea, vomiting (protracted), abdominal pain.
- Metabolic – (i) hypokalaemia due to migration into cells, diuresis and vomiting; (ii) metabolic acidosis; (iii) hyperglycaemia and hyperinsulinaemia, hypomagnesaemia.
- Central nervous system – seizures, agitation, coma (uncommon).
- Cardiovascular – atrial and ventricular ectopy, hypotension.

Specific management (in addition to general principles) includes:

- Prolonged observation if a slow-release preparation is ingested.
- Measuring the serum level (anticipate seizures at approximately 300 µmol/L and the need for charcoal haemoperfusion or plasmapheresis at approximately 550 µmol/L or less if there is protracted vomiting).
- Controlling protracted vomiting with metoclopramide 0.12 mg/kg (max 10–15 mg) i.v., i.m. or orally, 6 hourly.
- Monitoring ECG. Beware of early hypokalaemia and late hyperkalaemia when potassium re-enters the blood.

Eucalyptus and essential oils

The principal effects are:

- Initial coughing, choking.
- Rapid onset (30 min, occasionally delayed) central nervous system depression (convulsions and meiosis are rare).
- Vomiting and subsequent aspiration pneumonitis.

Specific management to exclude pneumonitis.

Iron

Small quantities (>20 mg/kg) of elemental iron may be toxic. Ingested usually as iron tablets/capsules, mixtures or multi-vitamin preparations.

The principal effects are:

- Immediate nausea, vomiting, abdominal pain and possible gastric erosion.
- Hypotension, hypovolaemia and metabolic acidosis at 6–24 h.
- Multi-organ failure – gastrointestinal (ileus, gastric erosion), central nervous system, cardiovascular, hepatic and renal at 12–24 h.
- Pyloric stenosis at 4–6 weeks.

Specific management (in addition to general principles, see page 17) includes:

- Obtaining the serum iron level (μg/dL $\times$ 0.1791 = μmol/L). NB: Absorption may be slow.
- An abdominal X-ray, which may reveal the quantity ingested.
- Whole bowel irrigation (not if ileus, obstruction or erosion are present). Activated charcoal is useless.
- An infusion of desferrioxamine no faster than 15 mg/kg per h for 12–24 h if the iron level is greater than 90 μmol/L or greater than 63 μmol/L and symptomatic.

Tricyclic antidepressants

Sudden death may occur.

The principal effects are:

- Central nervous system (CNS) – coma, convulsions.
- Non-cardiogenic pulmonary oedema.
- Cardiac – depression of contractility and hypotension, and sudden dysrhythmias (conduction blocks and ventricular ectopy, including tachycardia/fibrillation).

Specific management (in addition to general principles, see page 17) includes:

- Monitoring ECG – assess heart rate, QRS duration and QT interval.
- Alkalising blood to pH 7.45–7.50 with a sodium bicarbonate infusion or hyperventilation or both.
- Treating convulsions with diazepam 0.2–0.4 mg/kg (max 10–20 mg) intravenous. If dysrhythmia is evident on ECG, give phenytoin slowly (over 30 min). Beware of hypotension.
- Treating hypotension with an α-agonist (noradrenaline 0.01–1 μg/kg per min). Avoid β-agonists and drugs with mixed α and β actions.
- Treating ventricular tachycardia/fibrillation with DC shock, lignocaine (1 mg/kg, then 10–60 μg/kg per min), beta-blocker.
- Treating torsade de pointes with lignocaine as above, or magnesium sulphate.
- Monitoring until there are no convulsions, the conscious state is normal, normotensive, and there is no conduction delay or dysrhythmia.

Salicylates

Toxicity is expected if >150 mg/kg is ingested.

The principal effects are:
- Coma, hyperpyrexia and respiratory alkalosis followed by metabolic acidosis.
- Cardiac depression, pulmonary oedema and hypotension.
- Hepatic encephalopathy (Reye's syndrome) with chronic use.

Specific management (in addition to general principles, see page 17) includes:
- Measuring the serum salicylate level, blood glucose, serum potassium and blood pH.
- Correcting dehydration.
- Correcting acidosis and keeping urine pH >7.5 (with sodium bicarbonate) and correcting hypokalaemia.
- Considering haemodialysis/haemoperfusion if the serum level is >25 mmol/L (μg/mL $\times$ 0.0724 = μmol/L).

Poisoning with unknown agents

Suspect poisoning in any infant or child who presents with convulsions, depression of the conscious state, hypoventilation, hypotension or an illness that is not readily otherwise explained. Multiple poisons may have been ingested. Blood levels of some poisons (paracetamol, iron, salicylate, theophylline, methanol, digoxin and lithium) may influence clinical management.

ENVENOMATION

Snake bite

This section applies to bites by Australian snakes of the family Elapidae. Snake bites by species in other countries cause different effects not outlined in this handbook. Refer to local publications.

Of the many species of snakes in Australia, the principal dangerous species are from the terrestrial genera of Brown, Tiger, Taipan, Death Adder, Copperhead and Black snakes, and from several marine genera.

Venom from these species contains potent neurotoxins and procoagulants (although death adders do not contain significant procoagulant). Neurotoxins cause neuromuscular paralysis with respiratory failure, while procoagulants cause disseminated intravascular coagulation with subsequent haemorrhage due to depletion of clotting factors.

Other less important components are haemolysins, anticoagulants and rhabdomyolysins.

Although not all snakes are venomous and envenomation does not always accompany a bite by a venomous snake, every snake bite should be regarded as potentially lethal.

In young children a history of snake bite is often uncertain.

Symptoms and signs of envenomation

Early clinical evidence of envenomation is headache, vomiting and abdominal pain; these may be experienced within an hour of a bite.

The bite site may be identifiable by fang or scratch marks surrounded by bruising or oedema. It is important to note, however, that a bite site may be undetectable and occasionally unnoticed by a victim.

Early neurotoxic signs are ptosis, diplopia, blurred vision, facial muscle weakness, dysphonia and dysphagia. Later signs are weakness of limb, trunk and respiratory muscles.

Spontaneous haemorrhage may occur from mucous membranes or from needle puncture sites. Hypotension, haemolysis and myoglobinuria may contribute to renal failure, particularly if treatment with antivenom is delayed.

The syndrome culminates in respiratory and cardiovascular failure within several hours after envenomation, but may be accelerated in a small child or after multiple bites.

Suspected envenomation

If there is a history of snake bite but no symptoms or signs, the patient should be admitted for close observation, preferably to an intensive care unit.

A test of coagulation should be performed, as it is both a sensitive and reliable indicator of envenomation by major species (in Victoria).

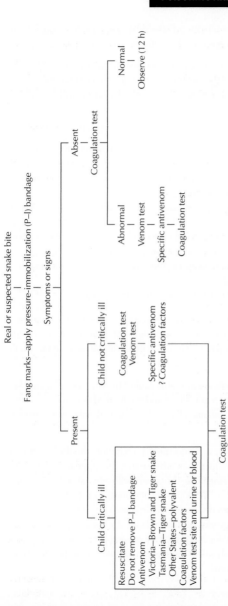

Fig. 2.2 Management of snake bite

If a pressure-immobilisation first-aid bandage has been applied, it can be removed after ensuring that antivenom is available.

The presence of venom can be determined by a venom-detection test. A positive test of the swab from the bite site identifies the snake, and a positive test of a biological sample (blood or urine) confirms envenomation.

Definite envenomation

A number of measures are required, depending on the severity of envenomation:

- Resuscitation with mechanical ventilation, oxygen therapy and fluid volume restoration.
- Application of a first-aid bandage if not already in place. Do not remove an existing first-aid bandage until antivenom has been administered. Cut a hole in the existing bandage to obtain a bite site swab if needed, and reinforce.
- A venom test of urine (preferred), blood or bite site swab or all.
- Antivenom (i.v.).
- Blood and coagulation factors (fresh frozen plasma).

Antivenom therapy

Antivenom is required for clinical signs of envenomation, or for symptomless coagulopathy that may cause a serious (e.g. intracranial) haemorrhage.

Specific antivenoms are available against Brown snake, Tiger snake, Black snake, Taipan, Death Adder and the Beaked Sea snake. A polyvalent preparation contains all the above-named antivenoms except the Beaked Sea snake.

Wherever possible, a monovalent preparation should be infused because of a lower incidence of adverse reaction compared with polyvalent antivenom. Premedicate the patient with adrenaline 0.05 mg/kg; (i.e. 0.05 mL/kg of 1 : 10 000 subcutaneously or 0.005 mL/kg of 1 : 1000 for larger patients) before the first dose of antivenom to prevent or ameliorate the severity of anaphylaxis. A course of prednisolone 1 mg/kg orally, daily for 2–5 days may prevent serum sickness, which may occur after polyvalent antivenom or after multiple doses of monovalent antivenom.

Selection of antivenom should be based on the result of a venom-detection test or on reliable identification of the snake, as there is little cross-reactivity between antivenoms. However, if antivenom therapy is required before identification, administer antivenom according to location. In Victoria give both Brown and Tiger snake antivenom, in Tasmania give Tiger snake antivenom, and elsewhere give polyvalent antivenom. All bites by marine species can be treated with Beaked Sea snake or Tiger snake antivenom. Dilute with crystalloid and infuse over 30 min (faster in life-threatening envenomation).

The dose of antivenom cannot be predetermined because the amount of venom injected and the patient's susceptibility to it are unknown. Initially administer two ampoules of brown snake antivenom or one ampoule of other types (which is sufficient to neutralise the average yield), and titrate additional doses against the clinical and coagulation status. In the treatment of moderate envenomation of children, several ampoules are usually required, while in severe envenomation many ampoules may be required.

Administer antivenom before giving blood or coagulation factors to forestall further disseminated intravascular coagulation.

Spider bites

Red-back spider

The venom of this spider contains a neurotoxin that causes release of neurotransmitters. Although potentially lethal, the syndrome of envenomation (latrodectism) develops slowly over many hours, and no deaths have been recorded since an antivenom has been available. A similar syndrome is caused by many species of the genus *Latrodectus* worldwide (Australia, *L. hasselti*; New Zealand, *L. katipo*, *L. hasselti*).

Symptoms and signs

- The bite is very painful. Many effects have been recorded hours to days after a bite.
- Local immediate effects include erythema, persistent pain, oedema, pruritus, sweating and regional lymphadenopathy.
- Systemic effects may be distal limb and abdominal pain, hypertension, sweating, vomiting, fever and headache.

- Myalgia, spasms, arthralgia, paraesthesia and weakness may last many weeks.

Management

Do not use a pressure immobilisation bandage.

If the effects remain mild and localised up to 24 h after a bite, treatment may be symptomatic only.

Severe local and systemic effects or prolonged mild effects warrant administration of antivenom i.m. (occasionally i.v.). Sometimes several ampoules are needed. Antivenom has been effective even when administered months after envenomation. Premedication with adrenaline 0.05 mg/kg (0.05 mL/kg of 1 : 10 000 subcutaneously (s.c.), or 0.005 mL/kg of 1 : 1000 for larger patients) is recommended.

White-tailed spider

Bites by this spider are not fatal nor always troublesome, but delayed severe local and extended painful skin necrosis may develop over several days and require excision, grafting and parenteral analgesia.

Funnel-web spiders

Several large aggressive species can threaten life by injecting a venom that releases neurotransmitters and catecholamines. Envenomation does not always accompany a bite but it is first indicated by local muscle fasciculation, piloerection, vomiting, abdominal pain, profuse sweating, salivation and lacrimation. Hypertension, tachyarrhythmias and vasoconstriction develop. The syndrome culminates in coma, respiratory failure and terminal hypotension.

Management

- Apply a pressure-immobilisation bandage.
- Administer specific antivenom.
- Provide mechanical ventilation and airway protection as required.

Chironex box jellyfish

This is the world's most venomous animal. It has a cuboid body approximately 30 cm in diameter and numerous trailing tentacles, and inhabits shallow northern Australian coastal waters. Stings are most common from October to May, but have been recorded throughout the year. Contact with the tentacles leads to the discharge of millions of nematocysts that fire barbs through the epidermis and blood vessels, releasing venom that contains myotoxins, haemolysin and dermatonecrotic toxins, and possibly a neurotoxin. The immediate effects are severe pain and possible cardiorespiratory arrest due to direct cardiotoxicity and possible neurological effects causing apnoea. Severity of envenomation is related to the length of tentacles contacting the skin.

Management

- Rescue the victim from water to prevent drowning.
- Cardiopulmonary resuscitation may be required on the beach.
- Dowsing of adherent tentacles with vinegar/acetic acid to inactivate undischarged nematocysts (supplies of vinegar are stocked at popular beaches).
- Application of a pressure-immobilisation bandage (apply over vinegar-inactivated tentacles or after picking off live tentacles).
- Analgesia: parenteral for extensive stings, cold packs for minor stings.
- Intravenous administration of specific antivenom (three ampoules for life-threatening signs, one to two ampoules for analgesia or to prevent skin scarring).

Prevention is most important. Envenomation is prevented by light clothing. Unguarded waters must not be entered when jellyfish are in-shore. Beach warning signs are ignored at one's own peril.

CHAPTER 3
PROCEDURES

Peter Barnett
Joanne Smart

Universal precautions should be used during any procedure (see Infectious Diseases, chapter 26, p. 402). Gloves and protective eye wear should be worn, and a hard plastic container should be within easy reach for the disposal of sharps.

VENEPUNCTURE

Sites
- Cubital fossa.
- The dorsum of the hand.
- Others, as dictated by availability or necessity, or both.

Technique
- In adolescents and older children, blood can be collected through the use of a needle and syringe, as in adults. In infants and small children, a 23-gauge butterfly offers more stability.
- Some visible veins are too small to be used to take blood. A vein that is palpable is more likely to be successful than a non-palpable but visible vein.
- In small children it is often best that the assistant acts as both restrainer and tourniquet.
- An alternative technique is to snap the hub off a 21- or 23-gauge needle, or cut off the tubing of a butterfly. Insert it into a vein on the dorsum of the hand or foot and allow the blood to drip out directly into the tube. Several millilitres can often be collected this way.

INTRAVENOUS CANNULA INSERTION

Sites

- The dorsum of the hand is the preferred site. Use the non-dominant hand whenever possible.
- Alternative sites include the anatomical snuff box, volar aspect of the forearm, dorsum of the foot, great saphenous vein or cubital fossa.
- Using cubital fossa veins has the disadvantage of requiring the elbow to be splinted.
- Scalp veins should only be used when all other possibilities have been exhausted (shaved scalp hair regrows very slowly).

Technique

- Be patient and take time to look carefully for the best option.
- Ensure that the child is warm (especially the extremity in question) and that you have adequate light.
- Unless vascular access is required immediately, topical local anaesthetic cream (e.g. amethocaine or EMLA [lignocaine, prilocaine]) can be used, but must be applied at least 45 min before the procedure to be effective.
- Wrapping small patients in a sheet is often helpful to minimise kicking and wriggling.
- If using the back of the hand in infants, grasp the wrist between your index and middle fingers with your thumb over the fingers, flexing the wrist. This achieves both immobilisation and compression (see Fig. 3.1).
- Insert the cannula just distal to and along the line of the vein at an angle of 10–15°. When a large vein is entered, a 'flash' of blood will enter the hub of the needle. Advance the cannula a further 1–2 mm along the line of the vein, then remove the needle. Continue advancing the cannula to the required depth. If the cannula is in the vein, blood should flow out along the cannula and continue to fill the chamber. When you are trying to cannulate a small vein, you should not expect a flash of blood to enter the hub of the needle. Insert the cannula and, when you think it may be in the vein, remove the needle and watch for

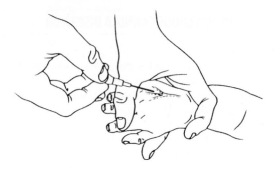

Fig. 3.1 Intravenous cannula insertion

blood moving slowly down the cannula; next advance the cannula along the vein.

- Take blood samples at this stage; strap the cannula securely (using two inverted cross-over straps and another over the top). At this point, flush the cannula with saline to confirm intravenous placement. Connect the intravenous tubing and splint the arm to an appropriately sized board (keeping the thumb free). Wrap the whole distal extremity in a crepe bandage.

LONG LINE INSERTION

Indications
- Prolonged venous access.
- Central venous placement needed to deliver high-concentration dextrose parenteral nutrition.

Sites
Best sites are the basilic, cephalic, axillary or saphenous veins.

Technique
- Measure the distance from the selected site to the approximate level of the right atrium. Cut the catheter to the desired length.
- Strict asepsis should be used.

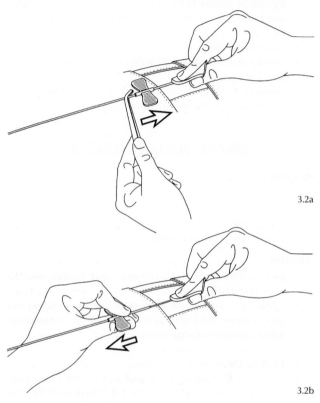

3.2a

3.2b

Fig. 3.2a and b Long line insertion

- Prime catheter with sterile saline. Insert the introducer needle into the vein until free-flowing blood-return is obtained. Release the tourniquet.
- Using smooth forceps, grasp the catheter very close to the tip and feed the catheter through the introducer needle to the desired length. See Fig. 3.2a.
- Slowly withdraw the needle and leave the catheter in position. When the needle clears the skin, secure the catheter by trapping it with a gloved finger at the skin exit site. Keep

the needle parallel to the skin to avoid severing the catheter, and slowly withdraw the introducer needle over the catheter (see Fig. 3.2b).
- Flush the catheter.
- Secure catheter in place with steristrips then a sterile transparent dressing.
- Confirm catheter tip placement radiologically. This may be aided by the injection of 0.3 mL of a contrast agent.

UMBILICAL VEIN CATHETERISATION

Indications

Use in neonates up to 7 days of age for:
- Emergency vascular access for resuscitation.
- Intravenous access for exchange transfusion.
- Central venous pressure monitoring.

Technique

- Measure the distance of a line drawn from the tip of the shoulder to the level of the umbilicus.
- Using Fig. 3.3 determine the catheter length needed to place the tip between the diaphragm and the left atrium. Add length for the height of the umbilical stump.
- Strict asepsis should be used.
- Flush the catheter with sterile saline.
- Loosely tie a sterile umbilical tape around base of the cord. Cut through the cord horizontally 1.5–2.0 cm from the skin; tighten the umbilical tape to prevent bleeding if necessary.
- Identify the large thin-walled vein and smaller thick-walled arteries. Clear any thrombi with forceps, gently dilate the vein with curved iris forceps and insert the catheter. Aim the tip at the right shoulder.
- Gently advance the catheter to the desired distance. Do not force.
- Secure the catheter with both a purse string suture around the cord and a tape bridge. Confirm the position of the catheter tip radiologically.

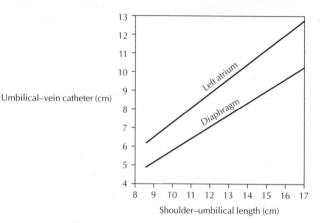

Umbilical–vein catheter (cm)

Shoulder–umbilical length (cm)

Fig. 3.3 Determining umbilical vein catheter length

UMBILICAL ARTERY CATHETERISATION

Indications

- Monitoring blood pressure and arterial blood gases.
- Access and infusion site in low birthweight neonates.

Technique

- Measure the distance of a line drawn from the tip of the shoulder to the level of the umbilicus. Use Fig. 3.4 to determine the catheter length needed for:
  - Low line position: between L3–L5 (below renal and mesenteric arteries); tip just above aortic bifurcation
  - High line position: between T6–T9; tip above the diaphragm.
- Strict asepsis should be used.
- Flush the catheter with sterile saline.
- Stabilise and cut the umbilical stump (see above).
- Identify the artery, clear any thrombi and dilate with curved iris forceps. Insert catheter and advance gently. Aim the tip towards the feet.
- Secure the catheter and confirm tip position (as above).
- Look out for any complications caused by catheter placement, especially blanching or cyanosis of lower extremities.

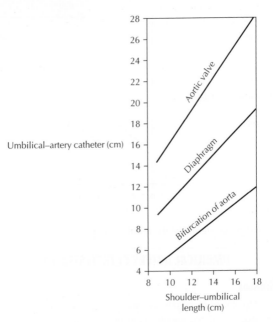

Fig. 3.4 Determining umbilical-artery catheter length

ARTERIAL STAB

Indications

Suspected hypoxaemia, hypercapnia or severe acidosis with poor peripheral perfusion. *Note:* Acid–base status alone can be assessed by a capillary collection.

Sites

Radial or brachial artery. *Note:* The femoral artery is used only in emergencies when no other arteries are palpable. Never use the ulnar artery.

Technique

- Clean the skin with an alcohol swab. Using a pre-heparinised 2 mL syringe and a 23- or 25-gauge needle, pierce the skin at a 15–30° angle directly over the artery.

- On entering the artery, blood will fill the hub; however, gentle aspiration is usually required to fill the syringe. If no blood enters the hub with the needle at its full depth or when the bone is contacted, withdraw the needle very slowly while aspirating because blood will often enter the needle on the way out if the artery has been transfixed.
- Only 0.5 mL of blood is required for arterial blood gas, sodium, potassium and haemoglobin measurements. After obtaining a specimen, quickly remove the needle and apply firm pressure to the puncture site for 3–5 min.

INTRAOSSEOUS INFUSION

Indications

For emergency vascular access when efforts to cannulate a vein are unsuccessful.

Sites

Preferred sites of insertion are:
- Up to 3 years of age: proximal tibia (1–2 cm inferomedial to tibial tuberosity) or distal femur in the midline (approximately 3 cm above the condyles) (see Fig. 3.5).
- Any age: medial malleolus of the tibia (just above the ankle).

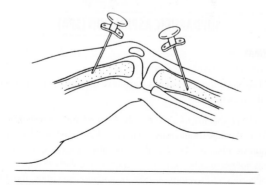

Fig. 3.5 Intraosseous needle insertion sites

Technique

- Prepare the insertion site. Inject 1% lignocaine into the area if the patient is conscious. If an intraosseous needle is not available, a short lumbar puncture needle or bone marrow aspiration needle may be used (intravenous cannulae or venepuncture needles are not appropriate).
- Penetrate the skin and then angle the needle at 10–15° from vertical – caudad for proximal tibial insertion and cephalad for femoral or medial malleolus insertion (see Fig. 3.5). Apply downward pressure with a rotary motion to advance the needle. When the needle passes through the cortex of the bone into the marrow cavity, resistance suddenly decreases. The needle should now stand without support (except in a very young infant).
- Remove the stylet and attach a 5 mL syringe; aspirate to confirm that the needle is in the bone marrow (this is not always possible). Flush the needle with saline to confirm correct placement and connect intravenous tubing. Often fluids will not flow by gravity into the marrow – a three-way tap and syringe or pressure infusion may be needed.
- Watch the infusion site for fluid extravasation. The needle should be removed once intravenous access has been obtained.
- Any fluid or drug that can be given intravenously can be administered through the intraosseous route.

SUPRAPUBIC ASPIRATION (SPA)

Indications

- Fever with no obvious focus.
- The bag urine specimen is suggestive of a urinary tract infection (UTI) on dipstick.

Note: Bag specimens should only be used for a dipstick test to exclude a UTI; they should not be sent for culture (see Renal Conditions and Enuresis, chapter 31). Note that a negative reagent strip screening test does not necessarily exclude infection, particularly in infants under 6 months of age; therefore, an SPA or catheter specimen should be obtained if there is a strong clinical suspicion of UTI.

Contraindications

- Age greater than 2 years (unless the bladder is palpable or percussible).
- Coagulopathy.

Technique

- Wait at least 30 min after the last void. If you are performing a septic work-up, do the SPA first.
- Position the patient with legs either straight or bent in the frog-leg position. In males hold the tip of the penis to prevent voiding. Have a sterile bottle handy for a clean catch in case the child voids.
- The site of entry is the skin crease above the symphysis pubis, in the midline. Prepare the skin with an alcohol swab. Insert a 23-gauge needle attached to a 2- or 5-mL syringe perpendicular to the abdominal wall (see Fig. 3.6). Pass almost to the depth of the needle, and then aspirate as you withdraw. If urine is not obtained do not remove the needle completely. Change the angle of the needle and insert it again, first angling superiorly and then inferiorly.
- In the event of obtaining no urine, either: (i) perform urethral catheterisation; or (ii) wait 30 min, giving the child a drink during this time. Repeat the SPA. It is a good idea to place a urine bag on so that you know whether the child has voided before proceeding with a further SPA.

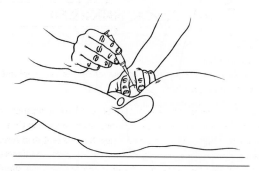

Fig. 3.6 Suprapubic aspiration

URETHRAL CATHETERISATION

Indications
- Suspected UTI.
- Acute urinary retention.

Technique
- An assistant is required to hold the child's legs apart, in the frog-leg position. Prepare the area with a water-based disinfectant solution and drape with sterile towels.
- For diagnostic catheterisation, use a size 5 or 8 feeding tube (depending on the age of the child). For in-dwelling catheters, use a silastic catheter with an inflatable balloon. Lubricants will aid insertion.
- Using a sterile technique, locate the urethral orifice (see Fig. 3.7). In males the foreskin need not be retracted fully for successful urethral catheterisation. Advance the catheter posteriorly with care until urine is obtained.

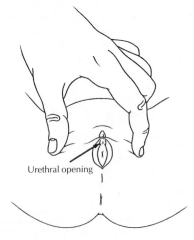

Urethral opening

Fig. 3.7 Urethral orifice

LUMBAR PUNCTURE

Indications

- A febrile, sick infant or toddler with no focus of infection.
- Fever with meningism.
- Prolonged seizure with fever

See also Fig. 1.2, page 15.

Contraindications

- A depressed conscious state, focal neurological signs or coma.
- Thrombocytopenia or clotting defect.

Note: If in doubt, do not proceed to a lumbar puncture.

Technique

- If time permits, local anaesthetic cream should be used. This must be applied at least 45 min before the procedure.
- Positioning of the patient is the key to performing a successful lumbar puncture, and is achieved with the help of an experienced assistant. Restrain the patient in the lateral position. Maximally flex the spine without compromising the airway. Avoid flexing the neck in small babies; this may cause airway obstruction. Flex their shoulders only.
- The iliac crests are at the level of L3–4. Use this space or the space below (see Fig. 3.8). Using a strict aseptic technique, cleanse the skin and drape the patient. Local anaesthetic (1% lignocaine) should be used in children older than 6 months. Anaesthetise the area to near the dura (i.e. about two-thirds the length of your chosen lumbar puncture needle).
- The correct needle size is 30 mm for neonates and infants, 40 mm for 1–4 year olds, 50 mm for 4–10 year olds, and 60 mm for older children. A 22-gauge needle is usually appropriate.
- Grasp the spinal needle with the bevel facing upwards. Ensure that the patient's back is perpendicular to the bed, and that the needle is perpendicular to the back. Insert the needle through the skin slowly, aiming towards the umbilicus (i.e. slightly cephalad). Continue advancing the needle until there is

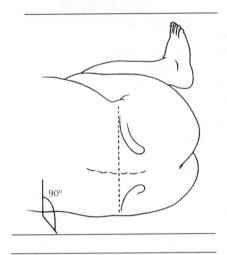

Fig. 3.8 Position for lumbar puncture

decreased resistance (having traversed ligamentum flavum), or the needle has been inserted half its length. Remove the stylet and advance the needle about 1 mm.

- Wait at least 30 s for CSF to appear in the hub. Rotation of the needle 90–180° may allow CSF to flow. Advance 1 mm at a time if no CSF has appeared. If no CSF is obtained when the bone is contacted or the needle is fully inserted, withdraw the needle very slowly until CSF flows, or the needle is almost removed. Reinsert the stylet, recheck the patient's position and needle orientation, and repeat the procedure.
- Collect 0.5–1 mL of CSF in each of two tubes, for microbiological and biochemical analysis. Remove the lumbar puncture needle with one quick motion. Press on the puncture site with a cotton ball for about 30 s. Cover with a light dressing.

NASOGASTRIC TUBE INSERTION

Indications

- Oral rehydration.
- Administration of medications (e.g. charcoal, golytely).
- Decompression of stomach (e.g. bowel obstruction, abdominal trauma).

Technique

- Select the correct tube size (e.g. 8 Fr for newborns, 12 Fr for 1–2 year olds, 16 Fr for adolescents). These sizes may vary depending on the use of the nasogastric.
- If the tube is too pliable, stiffen it by immersing in cold water.
- Spray the nostril with anaesthetic spray (e.g. co-phenylcaine) prior to insertion.
- Measure the correct length of insertion by placing the distal end of the tube at the nostril and running it to the ear and to the xiphisternum. Add a few centimetres. Usually this is the second or third mark on the tube.
- Generous lubrication of the tube with a xylocaine-containing lubricant will facilitate placement and minimise patient discomfort.
- Grasp the tube 5–6 cm from the distal end and insert it posteriorly. Advance it slowly along the floor of the nasal passage (see Fig. 3.9).
- Firm pressure is needed to pass the posterior nasal opening; this may cause some minor bleeding.
- If the child is cooperative, once the tube is in the naso/oropharynx, ask the child to flex their neck and swallow.
- If the child coughs and gags, or their voice becomes hoarse or the tube emerges from the mouth, pull the tube back into the nasopharynx and start again.
- Once the tube has been passed to the measured length, check its position by either: (i) syringing 10 mL of air into the tube and listening over the stomach with a stethoscope for a loud gurgling noise; or (ii) aspirate some fluid from the tube and test with litmus paper to determine its acidity.

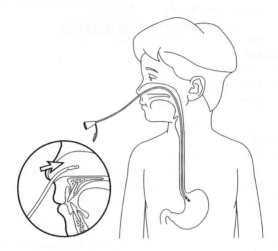

Fig. 3.9 Nasogastric tube insertion

- Secure the tube to the side of the face using adhesive tape (e.g. sleek).

GASTROSTOMY TUBE REPLACEMENT

Indications
- Burst balloon/malfunctioning parts.
- Displacement/extrusion of tube.

Technique
- Check the balloon of the new tube by injecting 3–5 mL of air into the side port. Fully deflate the balloon.
- Slide the skin flange on the new tube to the 8–10 cm mark. Close off the feeding ports and apply a small amount of lubricant to the tube.
- If the old tube is still *in-situ*, attach an empty syringe to the side port and deflate the balloon by removing the water. (*Note:* there is usually less than the expected 4 or 15 mL of water left in the balloon.)

- Gently pull on the tube and rotate it slowly until it is removed.
- Place the tip of the new tube at the opening of the stoma. Hold the distal end of the tube and slowly put pressure on the tube to push it into the hole.
- The new tube should be easily inserted. Insert it to 6–8 cm.
- Inflate the new tube to either 4 or 15 mL (i.e. not to its capacity) with water. Slowly pull back on the tube until resistance is felt.
- Slide the skin flange down until there is a snug fit, but not too tight. This is usually at the 2–4 cm mark.
- In the case of a MIC key, the correct tube for that patient should be inserted to its full depth before inflating the balloon.
- Gastrostomy buttons or Malecot catheters need introducers and should only be replaced by experienced staff.

Note: if there is any difficulty inserting the tube, then a radiographic study (i.e. contrast through the tube) should be performed to check on correct positioning.

WOUND MANAGEMENT

Lacerations

Most are superficial and commonly occur on the face, scalp and extremities.

(i) Local anaesthesia

LAT (lignocaine 4%, adrenaline 1 : 2000 and tetracaine 2%) has been shown to be as effective as TAC (tetracaine 2%, adrenaline 1 : 2000 and cocaine 11.8%) but at 1/10th of the cost, and without the potential complications of cocaine. The dose for LAT is 1 mL per 10 kg bodyweight. It should be applied on to a piece of cotton wool (when wet, and about the size of the wound) that is placed inside the wound. This is held in place with adhesive tape (or by a parent) for at least 15–20 min. An area of blanching approximately 1 cm wide will appear around the wound. The adequacy of anaesthesia should be tested by washing and squeezing the wound. If no pain is elicited, suturing will usually be painless. The sensation of pulling and light touch are preserved and this should be explained to the child and parent. The anaesthesia lasts about 1 hour.

Injectable lignocaine 1% can be used when LAT is contraindicated, or to supplement it if adequate anaesthesia has not been achieved. There are several ways to decrease the pain from injecting local anaesthetic:

- Use topical anaesthesia first.
- Use 27–32-gauge needles.
- Inject slowly.
- Place the needle into the wound through the lacerated surface, and not through intact skin.
- Pass the needle through an anaesthetised area into an unanaesthetised area.
- Use 1% lignocaine rather than 2%.
- Buffer lignocaine with sodium bicarbonate (10 : 1 dilution).

(ii) Wound closure

Tissue glues

Tissue glue is an alternative to suturing a wound in certain circumstances. Ideal wounds for glue are ones that are small, straight, easily approximated and under no tension. To apply tissue glue, the wound is cleaned, the edges held firmly together and a small amount of glue (approximately 0.05 mL) is placed along the line of the laceration. The wound edges are held together for 30 s. Steristrips should then be applied to prevent the child picking the glue off. The wound should be kept dry for 3–4 days. It then can be washed. The scab will come off in 1–2 weeks.

Suturing

Local anaesthesia, occasionally supplemented by sedation or general anaesthesia, will be required for suturing. Using absorbable sutures on areas where the cosmetic advantages of polypropylene or nylon are not required (e.g. scalp or hand) obviates the stress and potential pain of suture removal. Splinting any sutured wound, which is under tension (e.g. across joints or on the hand) for at least 1 week, decreases pain and promotes healing. Deep sutures should be used to close deep tissues; this reduces cavitation and dead space, which increase the risk of infection. The time at which sutures should be removed depends on the area affected: face/scalp 5 days, arm and hand 7 days, and legs 10–14 days. Areas of stress (e.g. over joints) need longer.

Tetanus prophylaxis

See Table 3.1.

Table 3.1 Guide to tetanus prophylaxis in wound management

History of tetanus immunisation		Type of wound	Tetanus toxoid, DT*	Tetanus immunoglobulin
Uncertain, or less than three doses		Clean minor wounds	Yes	No
		All other wounds	Yes	Yes
	If less than 5 years since last doses	Clean minor wounds	No	No
		All other wounds	No	No
Three doses or more	If 5–10 years since last dose	Clean minor wounds	No	No
		All other wounds	Yes	No
	If more than 10 years since last dose	Clean minor wounds	Yes	No
		All other wounds	Yes	No†

* Two different formulations of DT are available, varying in the amount of diphtheria toxoid: 30 Lf for children under 8 years, 2 Lf for adults.

† Tetanus immunoglobulin should be administered for tetanus-prone wounds in this category. Use DT in preference to tetanus toxoid alone.

Source: The Australian Immunisation Procedures Handbook, 5th edn, Australian Government Publishing Service, Canberra, 1994.

For tetanus-prone wounds, if the patient has had a:

- Tetanus course or booster within the past 5 years: no requirement.
- Tetanus course or booster 5–10 years ago: give tetanus toxoid.
- Tetanus course or booster more than 10 years ago: give tetanus toxoid and tetanus immunoglobulin.
- Unimmunised/incomplete/unknown treatment: full three-dose course and tetanus immunoglobulin.

Antibiotics

Antibiotics are not indicated for simple lacerations. They are usually given for bites and wounds with extensive tissue damage, but are of secondary importance to the initial decontamination of the wound.

Recommended antibiotics are amoxycillin/clavulanate 22.5 mg/kg (875 mg) p.o. 12 hourly for 5 days.

FEMORAL NERVE BLOCK

Indication

Pain relief for proximal femur fractures.

Technique

- After skin preparation, palpate the femoral artery below the inguinal ligament. Raise a wheal with local anaesthetic just lateral to the artery.
- Introduce a short bevelled needle (such as a lumbar puncture needle or a 23-gauge needle) through this wheal and advance downwards perpendicular to the skin. A characteristic 'pop' or loss of resistance is felt as the needle goes through the fascia lata and again as it penetrates the fascia iliaca (if using a lumbar puncture needle).
- Aspirate to ensure that the needle is not in a blood vessel. Inject local anaesthetic solution (usually bupivacaine in a dose of 2 mg/kg). The anaesthetic should inject smoothly without subcutaneous swelling. Paraesthesia need not be elicited.

CHAPTER 4
PAIN MANAGEMENT IN CHILDREN

Philip Ragg
George Chalkiadis

GENERAL PRINCIPLES OF PAEDIATRIC ANALGESIA

- Unrelieved pain has negative physiological and emotional consequences, including adverse effects on respiratory, cardiovascular and endocrine systems.
- Premature and term neonates are capable of responding to noxious stimuli and may suffer short- or long-term morbidity if analgesia is inadequate.
- Children's pain is often masked and may present differently from pain in adults. They often will not report pain.
- Paediatric analgesia must be calculated as a dose per kg of bodyweight, and routes of administration must be appropriate for age.
- Children do not like intramuscular injections.
- Parents and children must have realistic expectations of analgesia. It may not be possible to eliminate all pain, but it should be possible to allow normal daily activities.
- Two misconceptions that contribute to undertreatment of paediatric pain are:
  - A belief that all children are 'sensitive' to analgesics.
  - A belief that p.r.n. (or as required) dosing regimens mean 'as little as possible as infrequently as possible'.

PAEDIATRIC PAIN ASSESSMENT

Any assessment of a child's pain must take into account the child's age, cognitive ability and personality. Family traditions, preferences and words used by the child should be considered. Smaller children or those with developmental delay warrant particular attention as they have less mature communication skills.

After eliciting a careful history of the pain (e.g. onset, duration, site and character) and having examined the child, the following are useful assessment tools:

- Behavioural observation: vocalisation, facial expressions, posture, movement, personality, depression, fatigue. Remember that a child lying still and withdrawn may be in severe pain.
- Pain-rating scales: older children can assess their own pain with linear analog scales using a 10 cm line, with '0' meaning no pain and '10' the worst pain ever experienced. For those under 7 years of age similar scales (Wong Baker Faces Pain Rating Scale) are useful.
- Physiological signs: vital signs may add information, especially in smaller children where assessment can be difficult.

GENERAL USE OF ANALGESICS

The three most commonly used analgesics in children are paracetamol, non-steroidal anti-inflammatory drugs and opioids.

Paracetamol

Paracetamol is a very useful analgesic and antipyretic with little anti-inflammatory action.

Note: Paracetamol may reduce the antibody response to infection, prolonging minor illness and possibly increasing mortality in severe infection. It should be used to reduce pain or discomfort, but not simply to treat fever.

The uses are as follows:

- Administration: oral or rectal.
- Dosage: 15 mg/kg 4 hourly, p.r.n. (max 6 doses/day), or 30 mg/kg 8 hourly, p.r.n. Do not exceed 90 mg/kg per day.
- If a child requires continuous pain relief over a 24 h period (i.e. pain is interfering with sleep), a stronger analgesic is indicated.
- A dose of 90 mg/kg per day should *not* be continued beyond 48 h.
- Paracetamol should be used with caution in patients with severe liver disease or jaundice.

Non-steroidal anti-inflammatory drugs (NSAIDs)

NSAIDs have analgesic and anti-inflammatory properties, both of which may be useful in the management of acute pain in children. They have had a long history of use in juvenile rheumatoid arthritis, and indomethacin continues to be beneficial in neonates to promote closure of a patent ductus arteriosus.

The uses are as follows:
- Administration: oral or rectal.
- Dosage:
  Ibuprofen: 5–10 mg/kg (max 600 mg) p.o. 6–8 hourly;
  naproxen: 5–10 mg/kg (max 500 mg) p.o. 12–24 hourly;
  indomethacin: 0.5–1.0 mg/kg (max 50 mg) p.o./p.r. 8 hourly;
  diclofenac: 1 mg/kg (max 50 mg) 8–12 hourly;
  ketoprofen: 1.0–2.0 mg/kg (max 100 mg) p.o./p.r./i.m. 6–12 hourly (max in 24 h is 4 mg/kg or 200 mg).

The advantages of NSAIDs include the avoidance of opioid-related side effects such as vomiting, sedation and respiratory depression. They have several disadvantages, including bronchospasm, and parenteral NSAIDs, such as ketorolac, are not recommended in children. All NSAIDs must be used with caution in patients with bleeding disorders, as they all have antiplatelet effects. Renal dysfunction has been reported in children with NSAIDs, in particular diclofenac and piroxicam. Aspirin has been implicated in Reye's syndrome, and it should not be used as an analgesic in infants and children with suspected viral illness and fever.

Ketamine

Ketamine is a phencyclidine derivative causing dissociative anaesthesia without respiratory depression. It has been a popular general anaesthetic agent in paediatrics. It is an NMDA (N-methyl-D-aspartate) receptor antagonist, relieving neuropathic pain and reducing the development of opioid tolerance.

The uses are as follows:
- It is most usually administered intravenously as an infusion in the dose range of 2–10 µg/kg per min, but it may be infused s.c. or i.m.

- Nasal ketamine 3 mg/kg has been used for premedication and for analgesia in trauma patients. Epidural and intrathecal routes are currently being evaluated.
- Side effects include: hallucinations, hypersalivation and central catecholamine release causing tachycardia and hypertension.

Opioid analgesics
Oral preparations

Most opioids undergo significant metabolism either in the gastrointestinal tract or on first pass through the liver, making their bioavailability low when taken orally.

Codeine

- Codeine is a partial agonist opioid, which is very useful as an oral analgesic.
- Dosage: 0.5–1.0 mg/kg p.o., 4 hourly, p.r.n.

Buprenorphine

- Buprenorphine is a useful partial agonist opioid that can be a very effective analgesic in older children when administered sublingually, thereby avoiding first-pass metabolism.
- Dosage: 5 μg/mg per kg sublingual, 6 hourly, p.r.n.

Fentanyl

- Oral transmucosal fentanyl citrate (OTFC) ('Lollypops') and transcutaneous fentanyl citrate (TCFC) ('Patches') have been evaluated and found to be safe and effective in children.
- Uses include painful diagnostic procedures such as bone marrow aspiration and lumbar puncture.
- Side effects such as nausea, vomiting, itching and desaturation reduce the clinical usefulness of these techniques.

Otycodone: 0.1–0.2 mg/kg (max 10 mg) p.o. 4 hourly.

Morphine

The oral route is approximately 1/5 as bioavailable as parenteral due to first pass metabolism in the liver. Options for chronic pain management include:

Table 4.1 Equipotent doses of opioids for children over 12 months (mg)

	Intravenous (mg)	Recommended maximum dose (mg/kg)
Morphine	1	0.2
Pethidine	0.1	2
Fentanyl	100	0.002
Methadone	1	0.2
Codeine		1 (usually oral 0.5–1.0)

- slow release morphine: 0.6 mg/kg p.o. 12 hourly
- tramadol: a weak opioid with a potency similar to pethidine. 1–2 mg/kg p.o. 4 hourly. It has negligible respiratory depression effects but can cause nausea and dysphasia.

Parenteral opioids

Opioids remain the most powerful parenteral analgesics for children in severe pain (see Table 4.1). These drugs bind to opioid receptors and produce analgesia, as well as respiratory and psychomimetic effects. Infants under 6 months may be more sensitive to opioids. To ensure safe administration in this age group, morphine should be titrated to effect up to a maximum of 50 µg/kg, and the infant should be continually monitored for respiratory depression (e.g. pulse oximetry).

Administration

The administration of parenteral opioids may be as follows:
- Intermittent boluses (i.m., i.v. or s.c.).
- Continuous infusion (i.v. or s.c.).

In general, infusions optimise analgesia by enabling the child to remain in the 'analgesic corridor' without fluctuations in plasma level.

The subcutaneous route is very effective and often convenient in the child with difficult intravenous access. Although absorption is not as predictable as the intravenous route, the deltopectoral groove has been successfully employed for continuous infusions. An intravenous cannula can be safely placed under the skin without risk of trauma.

Parenteral opioids should not be administered without the availability of oxygen, resuscitation equipment and naloxone to reverse the opioid effect.

The common effects of parenteral opioids are:

- Central nervous system: euphoria; sedation; nausea; miosis.
- Respiratory: hypoventilation; bronchospasm.
- Cardiovascular: bradycardia; hypotension.
- Alimentary: constipation; vomiting; biliary colic.
- Skin: histamine release; itch.

Maximum dosage

The maximum doses of intramuscular opioids are:

- Morphine: 0.2 mg/kg (max 10–20 mg), 4 hourly, p.r.n.
- Pethidine: 2 mg/kg (max 25–100 mg), 3 hourly, p.r.n.

Intermittent intravenous opioids

Children dislike intramuscular injections, and intravenous administration is preferred. The following is a suggested protocol to minimise drug calculation error:

- Before boluses are given, ensure:
  - The patient is awake and stable.
  - The intravenous line is patent.
  - The child is older than 12 months.
- Morphine (10 mg) or pethidine (100 mg) is diluted in a 100 mL bottle of normal saline connected to a burette. Final concentration is thus:
  - 100 µg/mL morphine
  - 1 mg/mL pethidine.
- The bolus dose and maximum dose to be given are checked. Only the bolus dose volume should be placed in the burette.
- The bolus dose must be administered over at least 5 min, and administration ceased if the respiratory rate or oxygen saturation decreases.
- Monitoring during administration should be by continuous pulse oximetry, and 5 minutely BP, HR and RR for 20 min.
- After a bolus, allow 15 min before considering another bolus.
- If oxygen saturation falls below 93%, or airways obstruction or respiratory depression is suspected:
  - Cease infusion immediately
  - Administer 100% O_2 by mask
  - Give naloxone 0.01 mg/kg stat, i.v.
  - Resuscitate as necessary.

Continuous opioid infusions

Should a child require ongoing opioid analgesia or more than two intermittent boluses, an infusion should be commenced if practical. A copy of the Royal Children's Hospital Protocol is shown in Fig. 4.1 and may be used for intravenous or subcutaneous infusion. Please note that the volume used may be either 500 mL or 50 mL.

Patient-controlled analgesia (PCA)

PCA usually requires a microprocessor-controlled injector pump. PCA is suitable for children older than 8 years of age who have the ability to understand the concept of pressing a button to relieve pain and the willingness to use it. It has the advantage of involving patients in their own care, and is safe, as children will fall asleep and stop bolusing when plasma levels rise. It also saves nursing time. Indications include postoperative pain, oncology, burns and frequent painful procedures.

Protocol

Dilute 0.5 mg/kg morphine in 50 mL of saline (i.e. 10 µg/kg per mL). Set PCA to: (i) 5 min lockout interval; (ii) 2 mL boluses (20 µg/kg). You may run background infusion (0.5 mL/h or 5 µg/kg per h) concurrently. Fentanyl may be used as an alternative to morphine if nausea or pruritis is problematic. Dose is 15 µg/kg in 50 mL of saline; bolus is 0.3 µg/kg 5 min lockout.

Observations and resuscitation protocols are as per opioid infusions.

LOCAL ANAESTHESIA

Local anaesthesia in children provides very effective analgesia for acute trauma (e.g. fractures), lacerations and postoperative wounds. Although central blocks such as epidurals, spinals and caudals are the domain of anaesthetists in operating theatres, several other applications of local anaesthesia do exist.

Local infiltration

The skin and subcutaneous tissues can be effectively infiltrated with local anaesthetic solutions, as shown in Table 4.2.

OPIATE INFUSION INSTRUCTION

ROYAL CHILDREN'S HOSPITAL, MELBOURNE

OPIATE INFUSION INSTRUCTION
Five hundred (500) mL dilution

AFFIX PATIENT IDENTIFICATION LABEL

Weight

TICK ☐ IF INSTRUCTIONS DIFFER FROM GUIDELINES

GUIDELINES

MORPHINE Add **0.5 mg/kg** to **500 mL** diluent of choice (any i.v. maintenance solution of electrolytes and/or glucose) to make infusion
Infuse at 0–40 mL/h equivalent to 0–40 µg/kg per h. Commonly used 20 mL/h (20 µg/kg/h)
Recommended initial bolus: 50–100 mL (0.05–0.10 mg/kg) of infusion
Recommended bolus for pain or painful procedure 10–20 mL (0.01–0.02 mg/kg) of infusion at intervals of at least 5–10 min

PETHIDINE Add **5.0 mg/kg** to **500 mL** diluent of choice (any i.v. maintenance solution of electrolytes and/or glucose) to make infusion
Infuse at 0–40 mL/h equivalent to 0–400 µg/kg per h. Commonly used 20 mL/h (200 µg/kg per h)
Recommended initial bolus: 50–100 mL (0.5–1.0 mg/kg) of infusion
Recommended bolus for pain or painful procedure 10–20 mL (0.1–0.2 mg/kg) of infusion at intervals of at least 5–10 min

MEDICAL INSTRUCTIONS

1. Add .... **mg** of .... to **500 mL** of ....

2. Infuse at .... **mL/h** to .... **mL/h** as required for analgesia

3. Administer initial bolus .... **mL** of infusion

4. Administer .... **mL** bolus of infusion *pm* for pain or painful procedures, at intervals of no less than .... min

5. Notify doctor if respirations less than .... per min or systolic blood pressure less than .... mmHg

RECORD MR 68 (A) (500 mL)

IF OPIATE TOXICITY SUSPECTED (slow or shallow respirations or hypotension or coma)

- Stop the infusion
- Administer NALOXONE .... i.v. or i.m. (0.01–0.1 mg/kg)
- Call ICU Register (extensions 5211, 6555) and ward HMO

Doctor's signature .... Date .... Printed Name .... ID Number ....

INFUSION RECORD

INFUSION PREPARATION	Time and Date	Registered Nurses' Signatures
Bag 1	....	....
Bag 2	....	....
Bag 3	....	....
Bag 4	....	....
Bag 5	....	....
Bag 6	....	....
INFUSION DISCARDED		
Bag No__	....	....
Bag No__	....	....
INITIAL BOLUS GIVEN		....

Fig. 4.1 Opiate infusions instructions and record

Table 4.2 Local anaesthetic solutions

	Maximum dose (mg/kg)	Duration (h)
Bupivacaine (0.25 or 0.5%)	2	2–3
Lignocaine (1 or 2%)	5	1–2
Ropivacaine (0.2, 0.5, 1.0%)	2	2–3

The addition of adrenaline 1 in 200 000 may increase the duration of action and slow absorption by up to 50%.

Adrenaline should not be used in end organs such as fingers or toes due to the risk of ischaemia.

Topical local anaesthetic cream

The insertion of intravenous drips, lumbar punctures and blood sampling are all potentially distressing for children. Application of local anaesthetic cream 1 h before these procedures ensures an area of analgesia of the skin.

EMLA is a mixture of prilocaine 5% and lignocaine 5%, and often vasoconstricts the area under application. Amethocaine 1% is a topical local anaesthetic with a more rapid onset than EMLA. It has vasodilator properties and may cause a painless erythema of the skin that resolves within a few hours.

NITROUS OXIDE

Increasing use is being made in burns and oncology units of nitrous oxide, which is a very useful inhalational analgesic.

Methods of delivery include:
- Entonox (a mixture of 50% nitrous oxide and 50% oxygen).
- Quantiflex (variable demand delivery system of nitrous oxide and oxygen).

Nitrous oxide provides potent short-term analgesia for painful procedures such as wound dressings and the removal of catheters. It has a rapid onset and offset. Side effects may include sedation, nausea and bone marrow depression with prolonged exposure.

It should not be used in head injuries, pneumothorax, obtunded patients or cardiac patients.

PROCEDURAL PAIN

Everyday events such as blood collection, cannula insertion and suturing are a source of major fear for children. Consideration must be given to the type of procedure, duration, age of the patient, and the emotional and physical condition of the child when any procedure is planned.

Techniques available for the management of these events include:
1 Topical local anaesthetic (EMLA or amethocaine).
2 Anxiolytics and sedatives (Midazolam oral, intranasal or rectal 0.5 mg/kg 30 min prior to treatment).
3 Oral analgesics (paracetamol or codeine).
4 Non-pharmacological techniques (distraction, parental presence, imagery, relaxation, music or aromas).

Occasionally the distress of a child may warrant the presence of an anaesthetist to provide intravenous sedation or general anaesthesia.

ALTERNATIVE TECHNIQUES

Non-pharmacological strategies can be used alone for less painful procedures, or as adjuncts to drugs for better analgesia.

Intervention needs to be tailored to the child and family, as encouragement is often critical to their success. Some suggested techniques are listed below.

Infants
Sensorimotor aids such as pacifiers, feeding, warm blankets, holding and rocking.

Older children
Guided imagery and cognitive techniques such as hypnosis, relaxation, distraction, music, art, play, positive encouragement and rehearsal may be useful. The use of calico dolls to simulate the procedure has been shown to be effective.

Physical techniques

Application of heat or cold, massage, exercise, rest or immobilisation.

CHRONIC PAIN MANAGEMENT

Acute and chronic pain are distinct entities that require vastly different diagnostic and management skills.

Acute pain

- Is tangible and understandable by the patient, family, friends and the treating doctor.
- Is usually brief, evoked by a recognised noxious stimulus and associated with an adaptive biological significance (e.g. protection of injured part to encourage healing).
- Usually improves rapidly and is associated with functional improvement and pain score reduction on a daily basis.
- Is usually related to the nature and extent of tissue damage.
- Responds to pharmacological intervention.

Chronic or persistent pain

- Often nothing to see or minimal evidence of tissue damage.
- Often presents for prolonged duration.
- May be evoked by minor trauma.
- Improves slowly over time with an undulating course. Improvement and deterioration may be linked to life stresses.
- Is not necessarily related simply or directly to the nature and extent of tissue damage.
- Does not always respond to pharmacological intervention.
- Often associated with secondary gains; e.g. school, sport or chore avoidance.

Patient assessment

It is important to assess both physical and psychosocial causes for the child's presentation. Evaluate the contribution of nociception, pain, suffering and pain behaviour by:

- Medical history and examination (nociception and pain).
- Physiotherapy appraisal (posture, muscle deconditioning and mobility).
- Psychological evaluation (situational, behavioural and emotional components).

Who should be involved?

- An anaesthetist, physician, rheumatologist, oncologist, ortho-paedic or neurosurgeon. Not all specialties require direct representation; however, close links are beneficial in facilitating communication and patient treatment.
- A physiotherapist.
- A psychologist with cognitive behavioural therapy (CBT) skills.
- A psychiatrist.
- A social worker.
- Nurses with psychosocial orientation.
- An occupational therapist.

Treatment

The aim of treatment is to eliminate pain. This is not possible in all patients – resuming a more active and fulfilling lifestyle that is less constrained by their pain will become the treatment goal. Therapy is directed at restoring function.

The treatment for each patient will vary according to the cause of their pain and the type of pain that is present. In particular, one can differentiate between nociceptive pain (which arises from the stimulation of superficial or deep tissue nociceptors), neurogenic pain (which may arise at any point from the primary afferent neuron to higher centres in the brain) and psychogenic pain (which occurs in the absence of any identifiable noxious stimulus or injurious process). All can be treated but require different approaches.

Non-pharmacological techniques

Muscle relaxation/distraction techniques

- Muscle relaxation is useful when anxiety facilitates pain. It is based on muscle relaxation and anxiety being mutually exclusive.

- Biofeedback is an aid to teaching relaxation. For example, in tension headaches, the display of electrical activity from the scalp muscles can be used to show patients that they are calm. Hence, patients can teach themselves to relax.
- Guided imagery.
- Art and music therapy.
- Distraction therapy.
- Hypnosis.
- Cognitive behavioural therapy emphasises learning by doing and the use of response–contingent rewards or reinforcement to encourage increases in specific behaviours such as exercises or work-related tasks.

Counselling and Psychotherapy

Treating the family and counselling school teachers may be as important as teaching the individual coping strategies for pain. The following should be considered:

- Counselling – individual and family.
- Assertiveness training – useful in children with low self-esteem, especially when associated with disability or disfigurement.
- Behaviour modification based on modifying the consequences of the patient's pain experience and pain behaviour.
- Emotional support.
- Education.
- Support groups.
- Graded return to school programmes with involvement and education of teachers.

Physical therapy and afferent stimulation

Physiotherapy

- Reconditioning programs (secondary deconditioning occurs rapidly, especially when fear of touch or movement exists).
- Stress loading ('scrub and carry' techniques for the upper limbs, weight bearing for legs).
- Postural exercises.
- Muscle stretches.
- Massage.
- Ultrasound treatment
- Heat/cold treatment.

- Transcutaneous electrical nerve stimulation (TENS) – activates large myelinated primary afferent fibres (A-fibres) that act through inhibitory circuits within the dorsal horn to reduce nociceptive transmission through small unmyelinated fibres (C-fibres). This is more likely to be effective if pain responds to heat or cold.

Hydrotherapy
Acupuncture

Pharmacological techniques

Paracetamol

Limit the dose for long-term administration to 90 mg/kg per day.

Steroids

- Triamcinolone (available as depot preparation) used for joint injections, trigger point injections, tendon sheaths and neuralgias.
- Dexamethasone administered by iontophoresis for soft tissue injuries.
- Methylprednisolone via epidural administration for localised nerve root irritation due to disc herniation without motor weakness.

NSAIDs

- Topical gels (diclofenac).
- Rectal (diclofenac and indomethacin).
- Oral (ibuprofen – comes as a syrup for children).

Capsaicin

Acts by releasing substance P at nerve endings. Applied topically and useful in rheumatic and neuropathic pain.

Tricyclic antidepressants

- Indications include severe unremitting pain, especially if neuropathic, complex regional pain syndrome (CRPS) or associated depression or poor sleep.
- Improve pain even if depression is not present; they suppress pathological neural discharges.
- May take up to 3 weeks to become effective once appropriate dose reached.

- Amitriptyline 0.2 mg/kg increasing over 2 weeks to 2 mg/kg. Administer as a single dose before bed to take advantage of sedative properties. Increase dosage until the side effects become unacceptable; e.g. dry mouth and morning somnolence.

Anticonvulsants

- These include sodium valproate, carbamazepine, gabapentin, vigabatrin, lamotrigine, clonazepam and phenytoin.
- Indicated in neuropathic pain and CRPS.
- Dosage should be used in the therapeutic anticonvulsant range, although there is no evidence of any relationship between analgesic effect and the plasma level. Some recommend increasing the dosage to the point of side effects or analgesia.

Opioids

- These only partially modulate central sensitisation. They are ineffective in controlling neuropathic pain or pain secondary to CRPS.
- Indicated in cancer pain and nociceptive pain.
- They include morphine, fentanyl, pethidine, codeine and oxycodone.

Ketamine

- Reduces primary and secondary hyperalgesia. It is a more potent modulator of central sensitisation than opioids.
- Useful in chronic pain syndromes, especially where pain is neuropathic or where there are escalating doses of opioids; e.g. cancer pain. Can be given as:
  — Subcutaneous continuous infusion
  — Intravenous 0.1–0.3 mg/kg per h.

Sympathetic nerve blocks

- These are useful where pain is present; e.g. CRPS Type I or II.
- Their main function is to facilitate physiotherapy.
- Administer intravenously to the regional upper or lower limb block – guanethidine/bretylium/phentolamine.
- Sympathetic nerve block: bupivacaine or ropivacaine via epidural, lumbar, sympathetic, brachial plexus or stellate ganglion blocks.

Peripheral nerve block

- Bupivacaine +/– steroid.
- Diagnostic: used to identify where the pain is originating; e.g. rectus sheath block for abdominal pain.
- Therapeutic: e.g. in occipital neuralgia and meralgia paraesthetica.

Baclofen

- GABA agonist acting on spinal cord reflex mechanisms.
- It is used to treat spasticity in patients with spinal cord injury or upper motor neuron conditions; e.g. cerebral palsy and post-cerebrovascular accidents.
- It may produce hypotonia, sedation and gastric upset.
- May be used orally or intrathecally.

Clonidine

- Is an α2-agonist useful in neuropathic or sympathetically maintained pain.
- Its side effects include sedation, dry mouth and hypotension.
- May be used orally/transdermally or via epidural.

Anti-arrhythmics

- Lignocaine IV: in neuropathic pain there is reduced ectopic activity associated with A delta and C fibres, in plasma concentrations of 2–10 µg/mL.
- Mexiletine oral: Mechanism is attributed to the abolition of ectopic impulses in primary afferent neurons. The treatment is useful if there is a positive response to lignocaine infusion. Slow introduction over several weeks is necessary, often the treatment is associated with nausea and gastric upset. Plasma levels need to be measured.

Surgical techniques

These measures are reserved for intractable pain not responsive to conventional methods; e.g. neurectomy, sympathectomy, rhizotomy and cordotomy.

COMPLEX REGIONAL PAIN SYNDROME (CRPS) (TYPES I AND II)

The following deserve special mention because the earlier they are identified, the easier they are to treat:

- Type I is formerly known as reflex sympathetic dystrophy (RSD). It often occurs after a noxious stimulus to the affected limb (e.g. trauma or surgery). Symptoms are disproportional to the inciting event.
- Type II is formerly referred to as causalgia. It differs from Type I because it occurs after peripheral nerve injury.

The affected area, usually a limb, manifests autonomic, sensory and motor symptoms:

- Changes in skin blood flow – often red/purple colour change.
- Abnormal sudomotor activity.
- Oedema.
- Loss of function.
- Abnormal hair growth, skin and/or nail atrophy.
- Temperature change.
- Pain.
- Continuous, burning pain in the absence of any visible injury.
- Regional non-dermatomal distribution.
- Allodynia.

NEUROPATHIC PAIN

- This is typified by continuous burning with an intermittent electric shock, stabbing or shooting-type discomfort.
- There is evidence of primary lesion or dysfunction in the nervous system.
- There is associated dysaesthesia; e.g. numbness, pins and needles, allodynia and hyperalgesia.
- Increased sympathetic activity may be present.
- There is a poor response to opioid medication.
- Aetiologies include: CRPS type II, tumour and de-afferentation pain; e.g. post amputation.

CHAPTER 5
IMMUNISATION

Terry Nolan
Margot Nash
Andrew Kemp

WHY IMMUNISE CHILDREN?

Immunisation is one of the most cost-effective public health measures available. Modern vaccines are safe and effective. They prevent clinical manifestations of disease altogether or substantially reduce severity. Health professionals have a responsibility to offer vaccination to those under their care. Every visit to a health-care provider is a valuable opportunity to check the vaccination status of an infant, child or adolescent. Vaccinations should either be brought up to date at that visit, or a firm arrangement made for a follow-up visit. Children admitted to hospital should as a matter of routine be brought up to date with their immunisations. In Australia, the Australian Childhood Immunisation Register (ACIR) now provides a mechanism to check immunisation status at any time should parents not have immunisation records with them. The ACIR can be contacted on 1-800-653-809.

Table 5.1 Vaccine abbreviations

DTP	Diphtheria, tetanus, pertussis vaccine
DTPa	DTP with acellular pertussis vaccine component
DTPw	DTP with whole cell pertussis vaccine component
DT	Child formulation of diphtheria with tetanus vaccine
aDT	Adult formulation diphtheria with tetanus vaccine
HBV	Hepatitis B vaccine
HbOC	Hib vaccine
PRP–OMP	Hib vaccine
OPV	Oral polio vaccine (Sabin)
IPV	Inactivated polio vaccine (Salk)
BCG	Bacille Calmette–Guérin vaccine against tuberculosis

STANDARD IMMUNISATION SCHEDULE IN AUSTRALIA

Table 5.2 Australian NH&MRC standard child and adolescent vaccination schedule (1998)

Age	Disease	Vaccine
2, 4 and 6 months	Diphtheria, tetanus and pertussis	DTP[1]
	Poliomyelitis	OPV – Sabin
	Hib disease	Hib vaccine[2]
		(HbOC)
12 months	Measles, mumps and rubella	MMR
	Hib disease	PRP–OMP only
18 months	Diphtheria, tetanus, and pertussis	DTPa
	Hib disease (HbOC only)	Hib vaccine
		(HbOC)
4–5 years	Diphtheria, tetanus and pertussis	DTPa
	Measles, mumps and rubella	MMR
	Poliomyelitis	OPV – Sabin
10–16 years	Hepatitis B (1st dose)	HBV
1 month later	Hepatitis B (2nd dose)	HBV
6 months later	Hepatitis B (3rd dose)	HBV
15–19 years	Diphtheria and tetanus	aDT
	Poliomyelitis	OPV – Sabin

Note:
1 DTPw or DTPa may be given for the primary course at 2, 4 and 6 months. All of the vaccines in the standard schedule, except OPV, are given by deep injection. OPV is given orally and must never be injected.
2 Hib vaccines – An alternative is PRP–OMP given at 2, 4 and 12 months.

VACCINATION TECHNIQUE

The injection site should be clean. Skin antisepsis is unnecessary. A new, sterile, disposable syringe and needle should be used for each injection. If multidose vials are used, a syringe or needle that has been used to inject a person should never come in contact with the vial. All parenteral vaccines should be injected deep into a muscle except MMR, which is given by deep subcutaneous injection. DTP vaccine may give a much more pronounced local reaction if given sub-cutaneously. The use of a short needle increases the risk of inadvertent subcutaneous injection.

The standard needle for vaccine injections is 23-gauge and 25 mm in length.

The following are exceptions to this rule:

- Preterm babies 2 months or younger and other very small infants – use either a 23-gauge needle 25 mm in length, or a 26-gauge needle 16 mm in length.
- Subcutaneous injections into the upper arm – use a 26-gauge needle 16 mm in length.
- Intradermal injections – for BCG vaccination use a 25- or 27-gauge needle 10 mm in length.

The needle should be inserted at an angle of 45–60° into the anterolateral thigh and pointing towards the knee (<12 months of age), and into the deltoid pointing towards the shoulder (≥ 12 months of age). Never use the buttock for vaccination as the sciatic nerve is vulnerable, and vaccine absorption at this site may be suboptimal.

Vaccine cold chain

Never use a vaccine if there is any doubt about its safe cold chain storage. Vaccines should be kept in a refrigerator reserved for vaccine/medicine storage at 2–8°C, and never frozen.

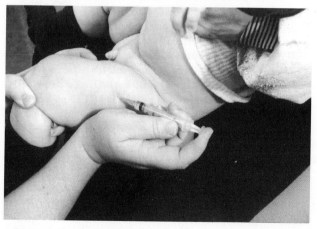

Fig. 5.1
Source: The Australian Immunisation Handbook, 6th edn, National Health and Medical Research Council, 1997.

Vaccination precautions

Children with minor illness (not obviously unwell and temperature <38.5°C) may be vaccinated safely. Major illness or high fever might be confused with vaccine side effects and might increase discomfort to the child, and are therefore a sufficient reason to postpone vaccination for 2–3 days until the child is well. For the same reason, children with unstable neurological disorders should also be deferred until stabilised. A return appointment for vaccination should be made at the time of any deferral.

WHAT TO DO IF SEVERE REACTIONS OCCUR

1   *Encephalopathy* within 7 days of vaccination with DTP (severe acute neurological illness + prolonged seizures ± unconsciousness ± focal signs, but not a simple febrile convulsion). *Action*: DT should be used for subsequent vaccinations instead of DTP.

2   *Immediate severe allergic reaction* (generalised urticaria or bronchospasm, hypotension, collapse; i.e. anaphylactic reaction). *Action*: Do not immunise with the same vaccine again. Refer to a paediatric allergist/immunologist.

3   *Convulsion*, with or without fever, or a temperature of 40.5°C or more. *Action*: Use DTPa subsequently.

4   *Persistent inconsolable screaming* for 3 or more hours, or unusual high-pitched cry. *Action*: Use DTPa subsequently.

5   *Hypotonic–hyporesponsive episode (HHE)* rarely follows DTPw and even less commonly after DTPa and DT vaccines. Irritable and febrile 1–12 h after vaccination, then pale, limp and unresponsive. Shallow respiration and cyanosis. The episode lasts from a few minutes to 36 h. Children with HHE show no long-term neurological or other sequelae. *Action*: Use DTPa subsequently.

6   *Extensive circumferential limb swelling and redness* commences within 48 h of vaccination, it is sometimes followed by a sterile abscess. This is possibly due to inadvertent subcutaneous rather than intramuscular injection. *Action*: Use DTPa subsequently, and ensure deep intramuscular injection.

PREVIOUS INFECTION WITH VACCINE-PREVENTABLE DISEASE

Children who have had culture-positive pertussis after the age of 3 months do not need to receive pertussis vaccine. However, vaccination of previously infected children with pertussis vaccine is not dangerous. If there is any doubt, vaccinate. This also applies to measles, mumps and rubella.

SPECIAL TOPICS

Hepatitis B vaccination before adolescence

HBV should be offered to all infants born to hepatitis B surface antigen-positive (HBsAg+) mothers and to all infants (see next paragraph) and young children from groups with a hepatitis B carrier rate of over 2%. Most countries (including Australia) have endorsed the use of hepatitis B vaccine for all infants. Unless available as a combination vaccine with DTP and/or Hib vaccines, HBV should be administered at birth, 1 month, and 6–12 months of age. Hepatitis B vaccine has not yet been included in the Australian standard infant schedule because it is only available as an additional injection. Parents who express an interest in infant HBV should be encouraged to have their children vaccinated.

Infants of HBsAg-positive mothers

Infants born to HBsAg-positive mothers require 100 IU hepatitis B immunoglobulin (HBIG) on the day of birth to provide immediate passive protection. Active vaccination against hepatitis B should be commenced at the same time. HBIG is not recommended for infants born to HBsAg-negative mothers in families from high-prevalence ethnic groups because there is epidemiological evidence that exposure from non-maternal sources is rare in the first year of life; vaccination alone will suffice in these cases.

Egg allergy

Egg allergy, even anaphylactic egg allergy, is *not* a contraindication to immunisation with measles vaccine or MMR which are not produced in eggs, but in chicken fibroblasts. Children with egg allergy can safely be given MMR vaccine provided this is done under close supervision. Skin testing with small doses of vaccine has been shown to be of no value in management of these cases.

Influenza vaccine

Children who have congenital heart disease or are receiving immuno-suppressive therapy should receive annual influenza vaccination, as should medical and nursing staff who care for them. Children under the age of 9 years need two doses of vaccine given 1 month apart. Subsequent single annual doses will then be required. Children with chronic cardiac and respiratory conditions, including uncorrected congenital heart disease, and cystic fibrosis should be vaccinated against influenza. If influenza vaccine is indicated for children with anaphylactic sensitivity to egg, referral to a paediatric allergist should be undertaken for possible vaccination under controlled conditions because influenza vaccine is produced in eggs.

Pneumococcal vaccine

Polysaccharide pneumococcal vaccine should be given every 5 years to children 2 years and over who have:
- Sickle cell disease.
- Asplenia, either functional or anatomical. The vaccine should be given at least 14 days before splenectomy, but if not possible it should still be administered after splenectomy.

Note: Immunocompromised patients in this age group who are at increased risk of pneumococcal disease (e.g. patients with HIV infection before the development of AIDS) should also be administered this vaccine.

A conjugate 7-valent pneumococcal vaccine has recently been shown to be highly efficacious against invasive disease in young children (including those under 2 years of age), but this vaccine is not yet licensed for general use.

Meningococcal vaccine

Polysaccharide meningococcal vaccine should be given to children 2 years and over who have:
- Asplenia, as for pneumococcal vaccine.
- Complement component deficiency.

Rotavirus vaccine

A rotavirus vaccine is licensed in the United States, and is given at 2, 4, and 6 months of age with the other standard schedule vaccines. Its use has been suspended pending investigation of a possible association with intussusception.

Varicella vaccine

Japanese, American and European monovalent varicella vaccines have been licensed in other countries. Varicella vaccine is now part of the US standard schedule for children at 12–15 months of age. The Japanese and American varicella vaccines must be stored at –15°C. Varicella vaccine is not yet available in Australia.

IMMUNOSUPPRESSED OR IMMUNE-DEFICIENT CHILDREN (INCLUDING TREATMENT FOR MALIGNANCY)

Live vaccines are usually contraindicated in immunosuppressed individuals, including those with malignant disease or those receiving chemotherapy.

Live vaccines should not be administered to:
- Children receiving high-dose oral or injectable corticosteroid (prednisolone 2 mg/kg per day for more than 1 week or 1 mg/kg per day for more than 1 month), or other immunosuppressive treatment, including general irradiation.
- Children with malignant conditions such as lymphoma, leukaemia, Hodgkin's disease or other tumours of the reticuloendothelial system, including those in remission who have received chemotherapy within the last 6 months.
- Children with impaired immunological mechanisms, such as severe combined immunodeficiency, and patients who have had recent bone marrow or other organ transplants.

Children with immunosuppression from disease or chemotherapy should not receive live virus vaccines until at least 6 months after chemotherapy has finished.

For children treated with systemic corticosteroids at high dose (see above), live vaccines (such as MMR, OPV and BCG) should be postponed until at least 3 months after treatment has stopped. Children on lower daily doses of systemic corticosteroids for less than 2 weeks, and those on lower doses on alternate day regimens for longer periods, may be given live virus vaccines (such as MMR and OPV). Inactivated vaccines (such as pertussis and hepatitis A vaccines), modified toxins (such as diphtheria and tetanus vaccines) and subunit vaccines (such as Hib and hepatitis B vaccines) can be given safely to children receiving immunosuppressive therapy, but these may be less effective.

If MMR is indicated, it should be given 3 weeks before or several months after immunoglobulin administration (see below), depending on type, dose and route. This means:

- Packed cell or whole blood transfusion, 6 months.
- Plasma or platelet transfusion, 7 months.
- Humoral immune deficiency (300–400 mg/kg i.v.) 8 months.
- Idiopathic thrombocytopenia purpura (400 mg/kg i.v.), 8 months.
- Idiopathic thrombocytopenia purpura (1000 mg/kg i.v.), 10 months.
- Kawasaki disease (2000 mg/kg i.v.), 11 months.

If the child is at risk of measles, in the interval before vaccination can be administered, further immune globulin may need to be given. Immunocompromised children who are exposed to measles should be given normal immunoglobulin (0.5 mL/kg) regardless of their vaccination status.

Children who have received bone marrow transplants may require booster doses or revaccination, depending on their serological and clinical status.

Household contacts with immune deficiency

Siblings and close contacts of immunosuppressed children should be given MMR as there is no risk of transmission of the vaccine virus, and immunisation will ensure that they have less chance of infecting their immunosuppressed siblings. Because it contains a live virus, OPV should not be given to immunosuppressed individuals or their house-hold contacts. IPV should be given instead.

PRETERM INFANTS

Preterm babies should be immunised according to the recommended schedule, commencing 2 months after birth, provided they are well and that there are no other contraindications.

PREGNANCY

Live vaccines should generally not be administered to pregnant women because of the theoretical possibility of harm to the foetus. However, in cases where there is significant and unavoidable risk of exposure to wild infection, e.g. to poliomyelitis or yellow fever, the need for vaccination outweighs the theoretical risk to the foetus. There is no evidence that rubella vaccine is teratogenic, but women who are to receive rubella vaccine should be advised to avoid pregnancy for 2 months after vaccination.

BREAST-FEEDING AND VACCINATION

There is no evidence of risk to the breast-feeding baby if the mother is vaccinated with any of the live or inactivated vaccines. Conversely, breast-feeding does not adversely affect immunisation and is not a contraindication for the administration of any vaccine to the baby.

SICKLE CELL ANAEMIA

Children with sickle cell anaemia should be immunised with Hib vaccine according to the infant schedule, and should be given pneumococcal vaccine at 2 years of age, with repeat doses every 5 years thereafter. To further reduce the risk of pneumococcal disease, they should also be treated with daily prophylactic doses of phenoxymethylpenicillin, commencing before the age of 4 months (phenoxymethylpenicillin 12.5 mg/kg p.o. b.d.). Penicillin prophylaxis has not been shown to be beneficial in children over 5 years of age with sickle cell anaemia, although the risk of sudden overwhelming pneumococcal sepsis persists at a low level.

FUNCTIONAL OR ANATOMICAL ASPLENIA

Children who have had their spleen removed, or who have a non-functioning spleen, are at increased lifelong risk of fulminant bacteraemia, most notably from pneumococcal and meningococcal infection. All asplenic children aged 2 years and over should receive pneumococcal and meningococcal vaccinations in addition to the vaccinations of the standard schedule (see above). Repeat injections of pneumococcal and meningococcal vaccines should be given every 5 years. In cases of elective splenectomy, the vaccinations should be given 2 weeks before operation, but if not possible they should still be administered after splenectomy. Although the evidence for the use of penicillin prophylaxis in these children is inconclusive it is recommended.

MISSED PERTUSSIS DOSES

Where part or all of the primary vaccination schedule has been given as DT, and where it is subsequently decided to give protection against pertussis, monovalent acellular pertussis vaccine (if available) can be given at any age, at 2-month intervals, up to a total of three or four doses of pertussis vaccine, depending on the age of the recipient and the number of previous doses of DTP or DT.

ANTI-IMMUNISATION CONCERNS

In Australia, only about 1–2% of parents refuse vaccination for their children because they oppose immunisation. A far greater number of children are under-immunised because of health professionals missing opportunities to vaccinate them. Commonly held views about immunisation in the small minority opposed to vaccination include a belief that natural infection is the best way to achieve immunity, that vaccination weakens the immune system, and that homeopathic 'immunisation' is safer and more effective. Some believe that vaccination causes many types of illnesses, including cancer, AIDS, allergic diseases and diabetes. There is abundant evidence to refute these

Table 5.3 Catch-up schedule for DTP vaccination

DTP doses already given	DTP 1	DTP 2	DTP 3	DTP 4	DTP 5
0	Now	1–2 months after first dose	1–2 months after second dose	6 months after third dose or after age 18 months*	Give at age 4–5 years**
1	Not applicable – dose already given	Now	1–2 months after previous dose	6 months after third dose or after age 18 months*	Give at age 4–5 years**
2	Not applicable – dose already given	Not applicable – dose already given	Now	6 months after third dose or after age 18 months*	Give at age 4–5 years**
3	Not applicable – dose already given	Not applicable – dose already given	Not applicable – dose already given	Now*	Give at age 4–5 years**
4	Not applicable – dose already given	Not applicable – dose already given	Not applicable – dose already given	Not applicable – dose already given	Give at age 4–5 years**

Notes: * Omit if DTP3 was given after the 4th birthday.
** Omit if DTP4 was given after the 4th birthday or if DTPw4 was not given.

Table 5.4 Catch-up schedule for Hib vaccination

Vaccine	Age at first Hib vaccination				
	2 months	**3–6 months**	**7–11 months**	**12–14 months**	**15–59 months**
HbOC	2, 4, 6 months; booster 18 months	three doses 2 months apart; booster 18 months	three doses 2 months apart; booster 18 months	one dose; booster 18 months	Single dose
PRP–OMP	2, 4 months; booster 12 months	two doses 2 months apart; booster 18 months	two doses 2 months apart; booster 18 months	one dose; booster 18 months	Single dose

claims, and parent concern should be taken seriously and specifically responded to with the scientific facts. In Australia and elsewhere, authoritative booklets are now available to help parents and practitioners understand why these concerns are ill-founded. Intensive re-examination of several studies has recently confirmed that there is no basis for concern that vaccination has an aetiological role in diabetes mellitus. The same applies to concerns about a possible association between measles vaccination, autism and Crohn's disease, and between hepatitis B vaccination and Guillain–Barré syndrome.

SOME IMPORTANT IMMUNISATION PRACTICE POINTS

- Half doses of vaccine are never indicated.
- Vaccines should not be mixed in the syringe.
- Never use tetanus toxoid alone. Always use DT or aDT (adult formulation DT).
- Pertussis vaccination should not be given to children over the age of 8 years, pending efficacy and safety trials of the newer acellular vaccines in this age group.
- Refer for specialist advice for unusual or complicated reactions, or both.
- Pretreatment with paracetamol (15 mg/kg per dose) in infants receiving DTPw vaccine reduces the incidence of distress and fever.

Reference

1   *The Australian Immunisation Handbook*, 6th edn, National Health and Medical Research Council, 1997.

CHAPTER 6
FLUID AND ELECTROLYTE THERAPY
Frank Shann

There are marked differences between children and adults in fluid and electrolyte composition and maintenance requirements. Maintenance fluid requirements are the daily water needs per kg of bodyweight in a disease-free state. This is high in infancy and gradually decreases throughout childhood.

Table 6.1 Fluid distribution

	Total body water (mL/kg)	Intracellular fluid (mL/kg)	Extracellular fluid (mL/kg)	Blood volume (mL/kg)
Neonate	750	350	450	85
Infant	700	400	300	80
Child	650	400	250	70
Adult	600	400	200	60

Table 6.2 Daily maintenance intravenous fluid requirements

Bodyweight	Requirements
3–10 kg	100 mL/kg per day
10–20 kg	1000 mL + (50 mL/kg per day for each kg over 10 kg)
20 kg and over	1500 mL + (20 mL/kg per day for each kg over 20 kg)

Table 6.3 Hourly maintenance intravenous fluid requirements

Weight (kg)	4	6	8	10	12	14	16	20	30	40	50	60	70
mL/h	16	24	32	40	45	50	55	65	70	80	90	95	100

Table 6.4 Adjustments to maintenance intravenous fluid requirements

Condition	Adjustment to fluid intake
Renal failure	× 0.2 + urine output
Basal state	× 0.7
High ADH (e.g. brain injury, meningitis)	× 0.7
High room humidity	× 0.7
Breathing humidified gas	× 0.75
Fever/hypothermia	± 12% per °C from 37 °C
Burns	
Day 1	+ 4% per 1% burn
Subsequent days	+ 2% per 1% burn

For example, a 6-kg comatose child with meningitis and a temperature of 38°C needs 24 × 0.7 (basal) × 0.7 (high ADH) + 12% (fever) = 13 mL/h for full intake; fluid restriction requires a lower intake (monitor the serum sodium; low levels suggest over-hydration).

DEHYDRATION

Dehydration without shock can usually be managed with oral re-hydration fluid plus food. Children with shock (hypotension and acidosis) caused by hypovolaemia should be given parenteral fluid immediately: administer 20 mL/kg repeatedly until the plasma volume is restored (this may need 20–100 mL/kg). The fluid can be given intravenously or into the bone marrow (see p. 39); nasogastric or intraperitoneal fluid is not effective in shock.

In states of hyponatraemia or hypernatraemia, the correction of serum sodium towards normal should not occur at more than 1–2 mmol/L per h.

HYPOVOLAEMIC SHOCK

In general, 0.9% saline solution is suitable for rehydration in hypo-volaemic shock. If other factors such as septicaemia or blood loss are involved, 5% normal serum albumin solution (NSAS) or blood may be required. Five per cent dextrose with low sodium concentrations (e.g.

5% dextrose in 0.225% saline) must not be used for rapid infusion as severe hyponatraemia with fitting may occur.

REPLACEMENT THERAPY

Three basic aspects are considered:
- Existing deficit.
- Continuing losses during therapy.
- Maintenance requirements.

Existing fluid deficit

This is calculated from the bodyweight according to the degree of dehydration; it is estimated by the following clinical features:
- Decreased peripheral perfusion (pallor or reduced capillary return).
- Deep (acidotic) breathing – not useful in diabetic ketoacidosis.
- Decreased skin turgor.
- Increased thirst.

A history of oliguria, restlessness, lethargy, sunken eyes, dry mouth, sunken fontanelle and the absence of tears are poor signs of mild to moderate dehydration in children. In general, for:
- <4% bodyweight loss there are no clinical signs
- 4–6% bodyweight loss there are clinical signs present, and the severity of the signs is a guide to the degree of dehydration
- ≥7% bodyweight loss there may be hypotension and acidosis.

In general, fluids to replace the existing deficit are given over the first 24 h. For hypernatraemic or hyponatraemic dehydration, at least 48–72 h should be taken for replacement.

Electrolyte deficit

The type and amount of electrolyte deficit depends on the diagnosis; e.g. in gastroenteritis, the loss of base leads to acidosis; in pyloric stenosis, the loss of acid and chloride leads to hypochloraemic alkalosis.

The rate of infusion of potassium must not exceed 0.4 mmol/kg per h. Concentrations of potassium greater than 40 mmol/L should be used with extreme caution.

Electrocardiographic monitoring should be considered in massive potassium replacement, and infusions of concentrated solutions should be controlled with the use of a pump.

Continuing losses

It is essential to have an accurate recording on a fluid balance chart of the volumes of vomitus or gastric aspirates, drainage from fistulae, diarrhoea, urine output and other fluid losses. These will determine both the volume and type of fluid and electrolyte replacement required (see Table 6.5). It is also important to monitor weight and clinical features during rehydration: weigh every 6 h for the first 24–48 h.

Table 6.5 Composition of some body fluids in children

Fluid	Na+ mmol/L	K+ mmol/L	Cl− mmol/L	HCO_3^- mmol/L	Other
Gastric fluid	20–80	10–20	100–150	0	H+ 30–120
Bile	140–160	3–15	80–120	15–30	
Pancreatic fluid	120–160	5–15	75–135	10–45	Basal state
Jejunal fluid	130–150	5–10	100–130	10–20	
Ileal fluid	50–150	3–15	20–120	30–50	
Diarrhoeal fluid	10–90	10–80	10–110	20–70	
Sweat					
Normal	10–30	3–10	10–35	0	
Cystic fibrosis	50–130	5–25	50–110	0	
Burn exudate	140	5	110	20	Protein 30–50 g/L
Saliva	10–25	20–35	10–30	2–10	Unstimulated

Maintenance requirements

These are given in addition to the replacement of the existing deficit and continuing losses.

ACID–BASE PROBLEMS

The maintenance of pH within narrow limits is a result of two mechanisms:

- Buffer systems – the bicarbonate system is quantitatively the most important in plasma (70% of the total).
- Excretory mechanisms – via the kidneys and lungs.

Acidosis (low pH) and alkalosis (high pH) may be respiratory or non-respiratory (metabolic) in origin. Respiratory disorders result from changes in the excretion of volatile carbon dioxide and, consequently, in the levels of carbonic acid. Metabolic disorders occur with changes in concentrations of non-volatile acids and, consequently, in the concentration of buffer base – mainly bicarbonate.

The four primary disorders are:

- *Metabolic acidosis.* This arises from increased production of non-volatile acid (e.g. ketoacids and lactic acid), failure of the kidney to excrete non-volatile acid or conserve base, or excess loss of buffer base (e.g. gastroenteritis or intestinal fistula).
- *Metabolic alkalosis.* This arises from excess loss of non-volatile acid (e.g. pyloric stenosis), excess intake of buffer (e.g. bicarbonate infusion), or potassium depletion where an extracellular alkalosis occurs as hydrogen ions are lost in the urine (e.g. renal tubular syndromes, pyloric stenosis or diuretic therapy).
- *Respiratory acidosis.* Hypercapnia is the result of alveolar hypoventilation from any cause (e.g. central, neuromuscular or pulmonary).
- *Respiratory alkalosis.* This is caused by hyperventilation.

Indicators of acid–base status
pH
This reflects the actual hydrogen ion concentration and alters in response to both respiratory and metabolic changes.

P_{CO_2} (Partial pressure of carbon dioxide)
In arterial and capillary blood samples, this represents the P_{CO_2} in blood leaving the lungs. Alterations reflect the disturbance in the respiratory component of the acid–base state (and not the metabolic component).

Base excess
This is an estimate of the change in total buffer base that would be present if the P_{CO_2} were normal (40 mmHg). Changes in the base excess reflect a disturbance in the metabolic component of the acid–base status (and not the respiratory component). In metabolic alkalosis, the total buffer base is increased, and thus the base excess is positive. Other calculated measures of the metabolic component are the standard bicarbonate and the total buffer base.

Actual bicarbonate

This is the plasma concentration of bicarbonate; it is influenced by both metabolic and respiratory components.

In practice, isolated metabolic and respiratory disorders are uncommon. Most disorders have a metabolic and a respiratory component. Usually one is the primary disorder, and the other occurs secondarily and tends to correct the change in pH. However, sometimes primary metabolic and respiratory disturbances occur together; e.g. in respiratory distress syndrome, when hypoxia leading to lactic acid accumulation produces metabolic acidosis, and carbon dioxide retention produces a respiratory acidosis (see Tables 6.6 and 6.7).

The interpretation of changes in base excess and Pco_2 as primary or secondary changes must be made clinically.

Table 6.6 Changes in arterial capillary blood (before compensation)

	pH (mmol/L)	Pco₂ (mmHg)	Base excess (mmol/L)	Actual bicarbonate (mmol/L)
	7.36–7.44	36–44	–5 to +3	18–25
Metabolic acidosis	Decrease	Normal	Decrease	Decrease
Metabolic alkalosis	Increase	Normal	Increase	Increase
Respiratory acidosis	Decrease	Increase	Normal	Increase
Respiratory alkalosis	Increase	Decrease	Normal	Decrease

Correction of metabolic acidosis

Metabolic acidosis will often resolve rapidly once the cause has been corrected, and administration of bicarbonate is often not required.

A guide to the amount of bicarbonate required is given by:

mmol of HCO_3 required = basic deficit (mmol/L) × weight (kg) × 0.3

The factor (weight × 0.3) represents the volume of extracellular fluid through which the base deficit (negative base excess) is distributed. In babies less than 5 kg, the factor is weight × 0.5 due to the greater percentage of extracellular fluid. It is usual to give only half the amount of bicarbonate suggested by these formulae, and to repeat the blood gas measurement before giving any more.

Table 6.7 Changes in indicators of acid–base status seen in combined disorders

	pH (mmol/L)	Pco₂ (mmHg)	Base excess (mmol/L)	Actual bicarbonate (mmol/L)
Normal	7.36–7.44	36–44	–5 to +3	18–25
Primary metabolic acidosis + compensatory respiratory alkalosis (e.g. gastroenteritis, diabetic ketosis)	Decrease or normal	Decrease	Decrease	Decrease
Primary metabolic alkalosis + compensatory respiratory acidosis (e.g. pyloric stenosis)	Increase or normal	Increase	Increase	Increase
Combined primary respiratory and metabolic acidosis (e.g. respiratory distress syndrome)	Decrease	Increase	Decrease	Normal

The rate of administration of bicarbonate will be determined by the cause of the metabolic acidosis and the clinical state of the patient; e.g. in cardiac arrest infuse bicarbonate rapidly, in gastroenteritis the correction should usually be undertaken over at least 6 h (and mild to moderate acidosis will resolve with rehydration alone). Rapid correction of metabolic acidosis will cause a fall in extracellular potassium.

The principles of correction of metabolic alkalosis are discussed in the section on pyloric stenosis (see below).

MANAGEMENT OF SOME SPECIAL CONDITIONS

Pyloric stenosis

Hydrogen ion and chloride loss predominate, with consequent hypo-chloraemic alkalosis. Losses of potassium in vomitus and urine can lead to significant hypokalaemia. In severe cases, hypokalaemia will lead to a renal compensatory mechanism, in which an additional hydrogen ion is lost in an attempt to conserve potassium. This leads to paradoxical aciduria.

The duration and severity of vomiting will, to a large extent, determine the degree of fluid and electrolyte imbalance.

Assessment

All patients require biochemical assessment, but not all will require intravenous therapy pre-operatively. Any child who is clinically dehydrated or has significant biochemical derangement requires intravenous therapy.

Intravenous therapy

- In severe dehydration (≥7%), commence with 0.9% saline until adequate circulation has been established and continue with 0.45% saline and 5% dextrose.
- In moderate dehydration (4–6%), commence with 0.45% saline and 5% dextrose.
- Await electrolyte results before commencing therapy if only mildly dehydrated.
- Adequate potassium and chloride replacement is necessary for the correction of the acid–base abnormality. As soon as urine flow is established, potassium chloride is given up to a maximum of 0.4 mmol/kg per h. Usually 20–40 mmol/L is adequate.

Acute oliguria and anuria

The definition of severe oliguria is a urine output of less than 0.5 mL/kg per h.

Initial management

Three clinical situations occur:

- Sudden and complete anuria should arouse suspicion of urinary obstruction, provided the catheter is correctly placed and not blocked.
- Renal hypoperfusion causing oliguria should be suspected in the presence of clinical dehydration or septicaemia leading to hypotension; the urinary sodium is usually less than 20 mmol/L. Blood volume expansion is necessary.
- Renal tissue injury (e.g. acute post-streptococcal glomerulo-nephritis or secondary to hypoperfusion or nephrotoxin). The

urinary sodium is usually more than 40 mmol/L. Frusemide (1–2 mg/kg) should be given i.v. and, if there is no response, treatment for continuing anuria should be instituted.

Continuing anuria

Fluid intake is restricted to the previous 24 h urine output and any abnormal losses; approximately 20% of normal maintenance requirements must also be given to replace insensible water loss.

At least 20% of full calorie requirements are given as carbohydrate to spare tissue protein from catabolism for energy, which accentuates the rise in blood urea. Intravenous 10–20% glucose, or oral Caloreen or Polyjoule are suitable.

Peritoneal dialysis or haemofiltration will be required for hyperkalaemia, severe uraemia (blood urea >50 mmol/L), acidosis, or water overload, leading to hyponatraemia, oedema or hypertension, and should always be considered if anuria persists for more than 24 h.

Hyperkalaemia

The management of hyperkalaemia depends on its cause. Serum potassium is increased by acidosis, and reduced by alkalosis. In acute oliguric renal failure, if urine is not formed after i.v. frusemide (see above), the presence of hyperkalaemia (>7.0 mmol/L) is an indication for dialysis. High values (up to 7.0 mmol/L) not requiring treatment may be found in the neonatal period.

If cardiac arrhythmias are present, rapid but temporary benefit may be achieved by giving:
- Sodium bicarbonate 2 mmol/kg, i.v.
- Short-acting (regular) insulin 0.1 unit/kg given with 2 mL/kg of 50% dextrose, i.v.
- Calcium gluconate 10% 0.5 mL/kg, i.v. given slowly.
- Sodium polystyrene sulphonate (Resonium) 1 g/kg rectal or nasogastric.

Other conditions

See acute infectious diarrhoea (p. 324), haemorrhagic shock (p. 8), burns (p. 224), diabetes mellitus (p. 271) and *Meningococcal septicaemia* (p. 9).

THE NEWBORN

Babies are different from older age groups because they have:

- More body water in all compartments.
- Greater insensible water losses.
- Reduced renal capacity to compensate for abnormalities.
- Less integrated and responsive endocrine controls.

These differences are of practical importance only in very sick babies – those requiring in-patient care in Level 2 or Level 3 nurseries.

This section highlights major practical differences between the sick newborn and older age groups. However, any baby needing intravenous therapy should be in a Level 2 or Level 3 nursery.

Insensible water losses can vary from around 30 mL/kg per 24 h at term to greater than 200 mL/kg per 24 h below 27 weeks gestation.

The newborn kidney is less able to concentrate or dilute urine, less able to retain Na^+ and K^+ or shed excess loads, and less able to excrete H^+ to shed acid loads.

Water requirements

There is often confusion between babies' water and milk requirements. For normal nutrition, babies need 150–200 mL/kg of milk per 24 h. For most babies this is two to three times their water requirements. This difference is only of practical importance in babies suffering illnesses that are made worse by excess water administration; for example acute and chronic lung disease, heart failure or renal impairment.

Table 6.8 Neonatal body water distribution

	<28 weeks	Term
Total body water	85% (of bodyweight)	75%
Extracellular water	55%	45%
Circulating blood volume	90–100 mL/kg	85 mL/kg

Intermediate gestations lie between these figures.

Water requirements depend on:

- Gestational age – the earlier the gestation the greater the skin losses and the poorer the renal concentration.
- Postnatal age – skin losses decrease and renal function improves steadily from day 1.
- Conditions of nursing – dressed babies lose least; naked babies under radiant heaters lose most. Humidified respiratory circuits (e.g. ventilators) reduce respiratory losses.

Water requirements are summarised in Table 6.9.

Table 6.9 Water requirements in newborn babies

	Days 1–2	Days 6–7
Mature 35 weeks +	40–50 mL/kg per day	60
Immature 27 weeks	80–120	60–80

Intermediate gestations lie between these figures. Lower figures are for babies on ventilators.

Before 27 weeks' gestation, requirements are too variable to tabulate: start at 120 mL/kg and modify 6–12 hourly according to the clinical state, serum Na^+ and urine osmolality.

Sodium

Babies are less able to conserve sodium or excrete excess loads. Daily requirements are 2–4 mmol/kg per 24 h; the earlier the gestation, the higher the need.

Hyponatraemia (Na^+ <132 mmol/L)

This may be due to excess water administration, inadequate sodium administration, excess sodium loss or inappropriate ADH secretion. The cause should always be defined; do not just treat blindly.

It is easy to overload sick babies with water in the first days after birth. This is a common cause of hyponatraemia. In general, intravenous rates greater than 60 mL/kg per 24 h in sick mature babies will provide excessive water in the first 48 h.

When the cause is water overload, serum Na^+ correction by water restriction alone is very slow in the newborn. As serum Na^+ <125 mmol/L can result in fits and may be injurious to the CNS, it should be treated with Na^+ administration, even when the primary cause is water overload. The dose required can be calculated as follows:

Dose of Na^+ (mmol) = bodyweight $\times 0.8 \times (140 -$ current serum $Na^+)$

The aim is to correct this condition slowly over 36 h, once the level of 125 mmol is reached. Using this regimen, serum Na^+ should be checked every 6 h: if correction is occurring rapidly, Na^+ administration can be ceased once the serum levels are safe.

Hypernatraemia (Serum Na^+ >154 mmol/L)

This may be due to excess Na^+ administration, inadequate water administration or excess loss of water in relation to sodium. The cause should always be defined.

It is easy to overload sick babies with sodium-containing intravenous fluids; e.g. 1 mL/h of normal saline = 4 mmol Na^+/24 h – the entire Na^+ requirements of a 1000 g baby, and more than half the daily requirements of a 2000 g baby. The use of sodium bicarbonate for correction of acidosis also often leads to sodium overload.

Hypernatraemia may be injurious to the CNS and should be avoided if possible.

Na^+ should be added to intravenous maintenance fluids from the beginning of day 2, taking into account separate sodium administration as sodium bicarbonate or heparinised saline.

Potassium

Potassium requirements are 2–4 mmol/kg per 24 h. Serum K^+ does not reflect body K^+. With high or low levels the cause should be defined.

Except with anuria, K^+ should be added to maintain intravenous fluids from the beginning of day 2.

With diuretic therapy, Na^+ and K^+ losses are much greater in babies than in older age groups.

Glucose

Blood glucose levels are unstable in sick babies. Fasting babies require intravenous solutions containing at least 10% Dextrose. Average glucose requirements are 4–7 mg glucose/kg per min (6–10 g/kg per day), but some sick babies require more, and others less.

Acid–base problems

Metabolic acidosis is the commonest acid–base disturbance in sick babies. The cause should always be defined. Correction with sodium bicarbonate is controversial, but it is reasonable to begin correcting pH <7.10 fairly quickly, i.e. over 30–60 min, and pH 7.10–7.20 slowly, i.e. over 2–4 h.

$$\text{mmol of } HCO_3 \text{ required} = \text{base deficit} \times \text{weight} \times 0.5$$
$$\qquad\qquad\qquad\qquad\qquad (\text{mmol/L}) \qquad (\text{kg})$$

Acid–base status should be re-evaluated once half the dose of bicarbonate has been given, and the dose adjusted if necessary. When given at the rates recommended there is no need to dilute 8.4% sodium bicarbonate before administration. Other measures to control the acidosis (e.g. volume expansion) should be instituted at the same time.

COMMONLY USED INTRAVENOUS SOLUTIONS

Saline bicarbonate

This solution is made up by adding 60 mL of sodium bicarbonate 8.4% to each litre of 0.45% saline and 2.5% dextrose. The solution is stable for only 24 h.

Five per cent normal serum albumin (5% NSA)

This solution contains human albumin 50 g/L, sodium 140 mmol/L, chloride 125 mmol/L and octanoate 8 mmol/L. It has an osmolality of 260 mmol/kg and a pH of 6.7–7.3.

Albumin (20%)

This solution contains albumin 200 g/L, sodium 46–58 mmol/L and octanoate 32 mmol/L. It has an osmolality of 80 mmol/kg and a pH of 7.0.

Additives

- Molar potassium chloride (0.75 g in 10 mL) = 1 mmol/mL of K^+ and Cl^-.
- Twenty per cent sodium chloride = 3.4 mmol/mL of Na^+ and Cl^-.
- Molar sodium bicarbonate (8.4%) = 1 mmol/mL of Na^+ and HCO_3.

Table 6.10 Commonly used intravenous solutions

	Na⁺ (mmol/L)	Cl⁻ (mmol/L)	K⁺ (mmol/L)	Lactate (mmol/L)	Ca²⁺ (mmol/L)	Glucose (g/L)
0.9% NaCl (Isotonic or normal saline)	150	150	–	–	–	–
0.45% NaCl with 5% glucose	75	75	–	–	–	50
0.2% NaCl with 4% glucose	30	30	–	–	–	40
0.2% NaCl with 4% glucose and KCl 20 mmol/L	30	30	20	–	–	40
Hartmann's solution	130	110	5	30	2	–
Hartmann's solution with 5% glucose	130	110	5	30	2	50

- Calcium gluconate 10% = 0.22 mmol/mL of Ca^{2+}, which is 8.9 mg/mL of Ca^{2+}.
- Magnesium chloride for injection (0.48 g anhydrous in 5 mL) = 1 mmol/mL of Mg^{2+}.

FORMULAE AND DEFINITIONS

Conversion factors
- Sodium chloride 1 g contains 17 mmol Na and 17 mmol Cl.
- Potassium chloride 1 g contains 13 mmol K and 13 mmol Cl.
- Sodium bicarbonate 1 g contains 12 mmol Na and 12 mmol HCO_3.

Molarity
Osmolality is the number of osmotically active molecules in a solution per kg of solute (usually mmol/kg of water).

Osmolarity is the number of osmotically active molecules in a solution per litre of solute (usually mmol/L of water).

Useful formulae
- Anion gap = Na – (bicarbonate + Cl); normal <12.
- Number mmol = mEq/valence = mass (mg)/mol. wt.
- Sodium deficit: mL 20% NaCl = wt × 0.2 × (140 – serum Na).
- Water deficit (mL) = 600 × wt (kg) × [1 – (140/Na)] (if body Na normal).
- Non-catabolic anuria: urea rises 3–5 mmol/L per day.
- Bicarbonate dose (mmol) = base excess × wt ÷ 3 (give 1/2 this).
- Osmolality serum = 2Na + glucose + urea (normal 270–295 mmol/L).

CHAPTER 7
INFANT AND CHILD NUTRITION

Julie Bines
Kay Gibbons
Michelle Meehan
Helen Anthony
David James

BREAST-FEEDING

Breast milk alone is adequate nutrition for infants for the first 6 months of life. Breast-feeding is the best means of feeding babies and all efforts should be made to promote, encourage and maintain breast-feeding for as long as possible (see Table 7.1).

Normal variations of breast-feeding
Frequency of feeds

Breast-fed infants usually feed every 2 to 5 h. Young babies feed frequently but demand feeding (i.e. feeding when hungry) will usually have the baby settle into a fairly predictable pattern of feeds. The frequency of the feeds is determined by the baby's appetite and gastric capacity, as well as the amount of mother's milk available. If the baby is feeding very frequently, seems hungry or is not gaining weight as expected, ensure that the baby is being offered both breasts at each feed.

Length of feeds

The duration of the feed is determined by the rate of transfer of milk from the breast to the baby which, in turn, depends on the baby's suck and the mother's 'let down'. This may vary from 5–6 min to 20–30 min. It is the cessation of strong drawing sucks, and the appearance of shorter duration bursts of sucking that indicate the 'end' of the feed – not the time.

If the mother feels the baby is on the breast 'all the time' it is better to look at the point where the pauses between bursts of sucking are longer than the sucking, and take the baby off or swap sides at this time (rather than timing it).

Table 7.1 How to assess good breast-feeding

	Good	Bad
Baby's body position	On side-chest to chest	On back angled away from mother
Mouth	Open wide	Lips close together
Chin	Touching or pressing into the breast	Space between chin and breast
Lips	Flanged out	Tucked in, inverted
Cheeks	Well rounded	Dimpled or sucked in
Nose	Free of or just touching the breast	Buried in breast, baby pulls back
Breast in mouth	Good mouthful, more of bottom part of breast in mouth	Central, little breast tissue in mouth or only nipple in mouth
Jaw movement	Rhythmic deep jaw movement	Jerky or irregular shallow movement
Sounds	Muffled sound of swallowing milk	No swallowing, clicking sounds
Body language of the baby	Peaceful, concentrated	Restless, anxious
Body language of the mother	Comfortable, relaxed	Tense, hunched, awkward
Awareness of feelings during feed	Pain free, may feel a drawing feeling deep in breast or 'let down'	Nipple or breast pain
Nipple, post-feed	Nipple elongated, well shaped	Not elongated, compressed 'stripe' or blanched

Source: Murray S., *Breast Feeding Information and Guidelines for Paediatric Units*, Royal Children's Hospital, Melbourne, 1992.

Appetite spurts

Babies seem to experience appetite spurts at 2 weeks, 6 weeks and 3 months. It is crucial that parents are aware of this or the baby's natural increase in frequency of feeds may be mistaken for diminution of milk supply. This is especially true at 6 weeks when breasts are no longer carrying extra fluid and the supply is settling to the demands of the baby. Unfortunately, many women wean at this time through poor advice. Let the baby feed on demand, even 2 hourly, and this should settle in 48 h.

Appearance of breast milk

Breast milk is naturally thinner in consistency than an artificial formula and may have a bluish tinge – this is normal, healthy and nutritious.

The presence of blood in the milk may cause a red or pinkish brown discoloration. If this is present when the mother first starts expressing colostrum it may be due to duct hyperplasia. This gradually disappears and is of no significance. The most common cause of blood-stained milk (usually first noticed when the baby possets) is trauma to the nipple.

Bowel actions

The motions of breast-fed infants are normally bright yellow and soft to loose. The baby may have a bowel action with every feed (strong gastro–colic reflex) or once every 5–8 days.

Temporary cessation of breast-feeding

If the feeding pattern is interrupted due to illness, a planned fast for a procedure or the mother's absence, the mother will need to express to maintain the milk supply.

- Milk can be expressed by hand or by pump.
- Express as often as the baby would normally feed (i.e. six to eight times a day). Several volumes of expressed milk can be added to the same bottle or storage bag (bags are available from commercial pharmacies), but a new container should be used every 24 h.
- Milk may be kept in the freezer section of the refrigerator for 2 weeks or in the deep freeze for 3 months.
- To thaw frozen milk, place a bag/bottle in a container of cool water and run hot water in until it is standing in hot water. When

the milk is thawed it will be cold; continue to heat in hot water or place in the fridge until required for a feed.
- Thawed milk should be used within 24 h.

How much milk to express?

If the mother wants to express to give a feed by bottle or to substitute a feed as she is weaning, how much will the baby need?

Daily requirements of milk are:
- From 0–6 months: 150 mL/kg per day.
- Over 6 months: 120 mL/kg per day.

Divide this amount by the usual number of feeds to calculate the amount required per feed.

Growth patterns differ between breast-fed and artificially fed infants. Average weights of breast-fed babies are similar to formula-fed until 4–6 months, after which breast-fed babies slow significantly in their weight gains. Length and head circumference remain similar.

There are as yet no standard weight charts for breast-fed infants. It is not appropriate to interpret their naturally slower weight gain, taken in isolation, as abnormal.

Maternal illness

When the mother is unwell, breast-feeding should continue. In the case of maternal infection, antibodies will be passed on in the breast milk to protect the baby.

Maternal drugs

If the mother has to take medication, the cost–benefit ratio should be weighed carefully by the prescriber. The mother should continue to breast-feed unless the use of the drug is absolutely contraindicated during lactation and there is no safe alternative. There are very few drugs that are absolutely contraindicated and almost all have a safe alternative. If the mother is concerned about continuing breast-feeding, even if the drug is safe, suggest that she takes the drug after a feed to minimise the concentration, or to divide the dose if possible.

FORMULA FEEDING

If breast milk is not available, either from the breast or as expressed milk, a commercially prepared iron-fortified formula should be chosen. These are based on cow milk, modified to lower the protein, calcium and electrolytes to levels better suited to the human infant, and contain added amino acids, vitamins and trace minerals (see Table 7.2).

Cow milk-based formulas

- Formulas may be classified as whey dominant or casein-dominant, describing the main protein type in the formula.
- Changes to the formula are made for a variety of reasons. In the normal thriving infant there is little indication to change the formula.

Strengthening formula feeds

Standard formulas provide 270–290 kJ/100mL (65–70 kcal/100 mL or 20 kcal/30 mL). To increase energy to 350 kJ/100 mL (25 kcal/30 mL):

- Use *additional* formula powder (i.e. for formulas where the standard dilution is 1 scoop to 30 mL of water use 1 scoop to 25 mL of water, or for formulas where the standard dilution is 1 scoop to 60 mL of water use 1 scoop to 50 mL of water). This will also increase protein and other nutrient intakes. Care should be taken with infants with renal or liver impairment; or
- Add glucose polymer (polyjoule, polycose) using 2 level teaspoons to the 100 mL formula or 5 mL fat emulsion (calogen, liquigen) to the 100 mL formula. These additions will increase energy value only.

To increase energy to 420 kJ/100 mL (30 kcal/30 mL) use additional formula powder as above with the addition of either glucose polymer or fat emulsion (as above).

Children over 6 months

For infants over 6 months, follow-on formulas can be used. They have a higher protein and renal solute load; however, they are not suitable for infants under 6 months of age.

Table 7.2 Formula composition per 100 mL

Feed	Dilution Scoop:mL	kJ kcal.	Prot. (g)	Fat (g)	CHO (g)	Na (mg)	Zn (mg)	Fe (mg)	Phos. (mg)	K (mg)	Ca (mg)	Protein source Whey:Casein	Fat source	CHO source
Whey dominant														
Nan 1 (13.2%) (Nestlé)	1:30	273, 65	1.5	3.4	7.6	16	0.5	0.8	21	66	42	60:40	milk fat, corn oil	lactose
S26 (12.7%) (Wyeth)	1:60	274, 66	1.5	3.6	7.2	15	0.5	0.8	28	56	42	60:40	oleo, coconut, soy, oleic	lactose
S26 Gold (12.7%) LCP's (Wyeth)	1:60	274, 66	1.5	3.6	7.2	15	0.5	0.8	28	56	42	60:40	oleo, coconut, soy, oleic, omega LCP's	lactose
Enfalac (12.8%) (MJ)	1:30	281, 67	1.5	3.7	7.0	15.4	0.38	0.7	29.8	69.1	45	60:40	coconut, palm, soy, safflower	lactose
Heinz Starter (13.18%)	1:50	283, 67	1.5	3.9	7.1	14	0.42	0.8	32	66	45	60:40	milk fat, palm, coconut, soy	lactose
Karicare I.F. (12.4%) (Nut)	1:50	285, 68	1.5	3.8	7.0	17	0.4	0.7	25	58	48	60:40	corn, palm, coconut, soy	lactose
Karicare First LCP's (Nut)	1:50	285, 68	1.5	3.8	7.0	17	0.4	0.7	25	58	48	60:40	corn, palm, coconut, soy	lactose
Amcal from birth	1:60	279, 66	1.7	3.7	7.1	17	0.4	0.8	26	66	46	60:40	milk fat, palm, coconut, soy	lactose
Casein dominant												Whey:Casein		
Lactogen (13.2%) (Nestlé)	1:30	273, 65	1.7	3.4	7.4	16	0.5	0.8	25	57	42	30:70	milk fat, corn oil	lactose
SMA (12.6%) (Wyeth)	1:60	271, 65	1.5	3.6	7	18	0.5	1.2	36	62	46	20:80	oleo, coconut, soy, oleic	lactose
Enfamil (12.8%) (MJ)	1:30	281, 67	1.5	3.7	6.9	19	0.5	1.2	42	83	54	20:80	palm, soy, coconut, corn	lactose

Continued overleaf

Table 7.2 Formula composition per 100 mL Cont'd

Feed	Dilution Scoop:mL	kJ kcal	Prot. (g)	Fat (g)	CHO (g)	Na (mg)	Zn (mg)	Fe (mg)	Phos. (mg)	K (mg)	Ca (mg)	Protein source	Fat source	CHO source
Karicare – goats (12.5%) (Nut)	1 : 50	287, 68	1.4	3.8	7.3	25	0.5	0.8	34	61	65	23 : 77	goat milk, corn, soy, coconut	lactose
Prem formula														
Prem Enfalac 350 kJ (16.5%) (MJ)	1 : 25	340, 81	2.4	4.1	9	33	0.8	0.2	53	100	95	Whey : Casein 60 : 40	MCT (40%), corn, soy, coconut	dried glucose syrup, lactose
S26 LBW 350 kJ (15.2%) LCP's (Wyeth)	1 : 50	334, 80	1.9	4.2	8.4	34	0.8	0.8	42	83	78	60 : 40	coconut, oleic, palm, soy MCT (12.5%)	lactose, maltodextrin
Prenan 350 kJ (16%) LCP's (Nestlé)	1 : 30	335, 80	2.3	4.2	8.6	34	0.6	1.2	54	96	99	78 : 22	milk fat, veg., LCP's (7.3%), egg phospholipid MCT (30%)	
Soy formula														
Prosobee (12.9%) (Kosher) (MJ)	1 : 30	280, 68	2	3.6	6.6	24.4	0.81	1.2	50.7	81	64.2	soy isolate	palm, oleic, soy, sunflower	dried glucose syrup
Infasoy (13.3%) (Wyeth)	1 : 60	274, 65	1.8	3.6	6.9	2.0	0.5	1.2	42	70	60	soy isolate	oleo, coconut, soy, oleic	CSS sucrose
Karicare Soya I.F. (13%) (Nut)	1 : 30	271, 65	1.8	3.6	6.7	18	0.6	0.8	27	65	54	soy isolate	palm, coconut, corn	CSS
Special formula														
Delact (13.5%) (Nut)	1 : 50	286, 68	1.7	3.7	7.5	21	0.7	0.9	28	62	55	casein dominant	vegetable oil	maltodextrin glucose, galactose, < 0.06% lactose
Digestelact (12.5%) (Nut)	1 : 30	280, 71	3.1	3.9	4.7	54	0.37	0.6	87	110	110	casein dominant	milk fat	glucose, galactose, 0.15% lactose

Continued overleaf

Table 7.2 Formula composition per 100 mL *Cont'd*

Feed	Dilution Scoop:mL	kJ kcal.	Prot. (g)	Fat (g)	CHO (g)	Na (mg)	Zn (mg)	Fe (mg)	Phos. (mg)	K (mg)	Ca (mg)	Protein source	Fat source	CHO source
O-Lac (12.8%) (MJ)	1:30	283, 68	1.5	3.7	6.9	20.3	0.4	1.2	37.2	74.4	55.4	whey dominant	palm, coconut, soy, sunflower	dried glucose syrup
S26 LF (13%) (Wyeth)	1:60	274, 65	1.5	3.6	7.2	15	0.5	0.8	37	56	55	whey dominant	oleo, coconut, soy, oleic	CSS
Pregestimil (13.3%) (MJ)	1:60	279, 69	1.9	3.7	6.9	26	0.63	1.25	41.3	73.3	62.6	hydrolysed casein	MCT (55%) soy, corn, sunflower	dried glucose syrup, dextrose, corn starch
Nutramigen (13.6%) (MJ)	1:30	283, 67	1.9	3.4	7.5	31.8	0.68	1.2	42.6	74.4	63.5	hydrolysed casein	palm, soy, coconut, oleic	dried glucose syrup, corn starch
Alfare (13.6%) (Nestlé)	1:30	272, 65	2.2	3.3	7.0	39.0	0.49	0.8	34.0	82.0	54.0	hydrolysed casein	MCT (43%), butter, corn	maltodextrin, potato starch, trace lactose
Neocate (15%) (SHS)	1:30	292, 70	1.95	3.5	8.1	18	0.75	1.05	34.5	63	48.8	protein hydrosylate synthetic amino acids	safflower, soy, coconut	dried glucose syrup
Portagen (14.4%) (MJ)	1:60	283, 68	2.4	3.3	7.8	37	0.63	1.28	47.4	84.8	63.2	caseinates	MCT (86%), corn	sucrose, dried glucose syrup
3232A (8.6%) + 6.23% CHO (MJ)	86g : 1 L +CHO	283, 68	1.9	2.9	9.1	29.1	0.42	1.27	42.3	74.0	63.4	hydrolysed casein	corn, MCT (85%)	tapioca starch + CHO
Generaid plus (22.1%) (SHS)	22g : 100 mL	420, 100	2.42	4.2	13.6	15.2	0.59	0.9	51.7	103	68.6	73% whey, 27% a.a.; 31% b.c.a.a.	MCT (35%)	
Kindergen P.R.O.D. (20%) (SHS)	20g : 100 mL	411, 98	1.5	5.2	12.0	46	0.84	0.96	18.6	24	20	whey, amino acids	safflower, soy, coconut	dried glucose syrup
Anti-reflux formula														
Enfalac AR (13.5%) (MJ)	1:30	287, 69	1.7	3.6	7.5	23.6	0.67	0.76	43.9	84.4	55.3	whey : casein 20 : 80	soy, coconut, sunflower, palm	lactose, rice starch, maltodextrin
Enfalac AR (MJ)	1:30	283, 67	2.2	3	7.9	32.9	0.68	1.2	61.2	100	77.8	whey : casein 20 : 80	palm, coconut, soy, safflower	lactose, glucose syrup, rice starch
Follow-on (13.5%)	1:60	271, 65	1.5	3.6	7	18	0.5	1.2	36	62	46	whey : casein 20 : 80	oleo, coconut, soy, oleic	lactose, corn syrup solids, corn starch
S26 AR (12.9%) (Wyeth)	1:60	271, 65										whey : casein 20 : 80		
Karicare AR (12.5%) (Nut)	1:50	284, 68	1.8	3	8.4	27	0.55	0.72	50	82	73	whey : casein	vegetable, milk	lactose, carob bean flour

Continued overleaf

Table 7.2 Formula composition per 100 mL *Cont'd*

Feed	Dilution Scoop:mL	kJ kCal.	Prot. (g)	Fat (g)	CHO (g)	Na (mg)	Zn (mg)	Fe (mg)	Phos. (mg)	K (mg)	Ca (mg)	Protein source Whey:Casein	Fat source	CHO source
Follow on														
S26 Progress (13.3%) (Wyeth)	1:60	271, 65	2.2	3.2	7.2	22	0.8	1.2	50	87.5	70	18:82	oleo, coconut, soy, oleic	lactose
Nan 2 (13.6%) (Nestlé)	1:30	274, 65	2.3	3.2	7.3	26	0.5	1.2	50	84	67	30:70	milk fat, corn oil, vegetable	lactose
Enfapro (14.3%) (MJ)	1:30	280, 67	2.5	2.7	8.3	36	0.4	1.2	67.2	110	84	18:82	corn, palm, soy, coconut	lactose, dried glucose syrup
Karicare follow on (12.4%) (Nut)	1:50	280, 67	2.1	3.6	6.6	17	0.4	1	32	58	61	60:40	palm, canola	lactose
Karicare goats follow on (12.4%) (Nut)	1:50	285, 68	2.2	3.7	6.6	27	0.5	0.8	65	110	100		soy, coconut, vegetables, corn, goat	lactose
Heinz follow on (14.5%)	1:50	276, 66	2.2	3.0	8	21	0.4	1.1	52.4	78	78	20:80	coconut, canola, milk, sunflower	lactose
Amcal follow on	1:60	272, 65	2.3	3.4	6.7	33	0.4	0.9	46	105	66	47:53	milk fat, soy, coconut, palm	lactose
Infasoy progress (13.9%) (Wyeth)	1:60	271, 65	2.5	3.2	6.9	23	0.8	1.2	58	100	94	soy isolate	oleo, coconut, soy, oleic	corn syrup solids, sucrose
Karicare Soya (Nut) follow on (14.5%)	1:30	294, 70	2.2	3.6	7.7	23	0.8	0.8	58	101	94	soy isolate	palm, coconut, corn	corn syrup solids

Continued overleaf

Table 7.2 Formula composition per 100 mL *Cont'd*

Feed	Dilution	kJ kcal.	Prot. (g)	Fat (g)	CHO (g)	Na (mg)	Zn (mg)	Fe (mg)	Phos. (mg)	K (mg)	Ca (mg)	Protein source	Fat source	CHO source
Polymeric feeds														
Osmolite (Abbott)	ready to feed	445, 106	3.72	3.76	14.5	64	1.2	0.95	53	102	53	caseinates, soy isolates	MCT (20%) safflower, canola	hydrolysed corn starch
Ensure Powder (23%) (Abbott)	6 : 200 mL	440, 106	3.72	3.72	14.5	84.6	1.2	0.96	53	156.4	53	caseinates, soy isolates	corn	corn syrup, sucrose
Nutrini (Nut) (Abbott)	rtf	420, 100	2.75	4.5	12.2	53,	0.73	0.73	39	104	50	caseinates	veg. oil	maltodextrin
Jevity (Abbott)	ready to feed	445, 1.6	4.44	3.59	15.2	93	1.7	1.37	75.8	157	91	caseinates	safflower, canola, MCT 20%	corn starch, soy polysaccharides
Ensure Plus (Abbott)	ready to feed	630, 150	5.5	5.32	20	105	1.59	1.27	70.5	194	70.5	caseinates, soy isolates	corn oil	corn syrup, sucrose
Resource Plus (Nov)	rtf	630, 152	5.5	4.6	21.0	131,	2.53	1.9	1.6	194,	127	caseinates, soy isolates	sunflower, soybean, corn	corn syrup, sucrose
Elemental feeds														
Vivonex TEN (Nov)	26.8%	420, 100	3.8	0.3	21.0	60,	1.1	0.9	50	95,	50	free amino acids	safflower	hydrolysed corn starch, modified starch
Vivonex Paediatric (Nov)	19%	336, 80	2.4	2.4	12.6	40,	1.2	1.0	80	120,	97	free amino acids	MCT (68%) soybean	maltodextrin, modified starch
Vivonex Paediatric (Nov)	24%	423, 101	3.0	3.0	15.8	50,	1.5	1.25	100	150,	121	free amino acids	MCT (68%) soybean	maltodextrin, modified starch

Source: Royal Children's Hospital Department of Nutrition & Food Services, June 1999.

Note: Information printed in this document was considered accurate at the time of printing. The composition of infant formulas does change and therefore it is recommended that the contents are revised regularly. No responsibility can be made for errors in this chart.

Soy formulas

If a soy-based feed is chosen, a soy infant formula should be chosen. These are nutritionally adequate for infants. Follow-on soy formulas are available.

Antiregurgitation (AR) formulas

Thickened formulas are aimed at reducing regurgitation. Their use should be limited to the stepwise treatment of gastro-oesophageal reflux (see Gastrointestinal Conditions, chapter 23). Not recommended in healthy infants without regurgitation.

Low-lactose formulas

Infant formulas with a low lactose content are recommended only in cases of proven lactose intolerance (see Gastrointestinal Conditions, chapter 23).

NUMBER OF FEEDS

Babies under 6 weeks of age usually feed every 3 h; however, they may take more each time and feed 4 hourly. Babies rarely sleep through the night before 6–8 weeks. When they miss a night feed (usually sleeping 5–6 h straight) they will have five feeds. They will consequently have more milk each feed. Babies who sleep longer in the day (e.g. 5 h between feeds) often need to feed overnight to maintain adequate intake. Parents may need to wake the baby after 4 h in the daytime. There is no need to wake a baby overnight if the intake and weight gain are adequate.

INTRODUCTION OF WHOLE COW MILK

The introduction of cow milk products as part of an expanding diet is appropriate, but the main milk intake should be breast milk or formula until 12 months of age because of the risks of iron deficiency and allergy. Small amounts can be used on cereal, in custard and yoghurt from about 7 to 8 months.

Full cream dairy products should be used for children up to 2 years; skim milk should not be used for children under 5 years.

INTRODUCTION OF SOLIDS

Breast milk or formulas will meet all nutrient needs for the first 4–6 months. From this time solids can be introduced, to increase the intake of nutrients such as iron and as part of the educational process of learning to eat.

Solids can be iron-fortified baby cereal, smooth vegetables or fruits. Foods should be introduced one at a time to allow observation of tolerance. Meat can be introduced at about 6–7 months. Texture should be increased so that by about 8–9 months the infant is managing lumps and varying textures, and is starting to manage finger foods. By about 12 months most family foods can be offered. By 12 months the intake of milk should be reduced to about 600 mL.

Much higher intakes of cow milk will limit the intake of other foods; in infants, continued high intakes of such milk, with its low iron content, are associated with the development of iron deficiency.

Iron deficiency and associated anaemia is the commonest nutrient deficiency in children in Australia. It is associated with the early introduction of cow milk, high intake of cow milk in the second year and low intake of iron-rich foods, such as meat and pulses.

WEANING

There is no set rule for weaning time. Solids should be introduced by 6 months and cup-drinking started as a skill by 7–9 months. There is no need for the baby to be weaned to a bottle – if he or she is old enough he or she can go straight on to a cup.

Sudden cessation of breast-feeding leaves the breasts at risk of developing mastitis. Ideally, weaning is achieved by reducing the feeds by one a week. Start by offering a drink in a cup or bottle instead of a breast feed at midday, and gradually increase these other drinks.

Many mothers retain the early morning feed or the last feed at night for a little longer.

Persistent difficulty in weaning usually requires someone to support the mother, giving the baby a feed and allowing the baby some time away from the mother to help with mutual separation. Both need to be ready to let go. Mother and baby units, especially those with a day-stay program, are helpful here.

TODDLERS WHO WILL NOT EAT

An assessment of the toddler who refuses food includes the following steps:
- Plotting weight and height to assure the parents of the baby's normal growth.
- Demonstrating by the chart that the growth rate normally slows in the second year.
- Linking this to a lessened need for food and subsequent drop in appetite.
- Emphasising developmental progress.

Advise parents that:
- A healthy child will eat when hungry – *quit the fight!*
- Showing independence is an important part of toddler development – choosing and refusing food is an expression of independence.
- Serve small portions – lower your expectations.
- Serve food that you know they like. Cereal is okay for lunch! A lack of variety is not a major worry at this age.
- Try to avoid arguments over food. Remember: 'It's my job to offer food, it's the child's job to eat it!'
- Avoid filling up on milk and juice – large volumes of milk (over 600 mL a day) can make the child feel full. Juice is not necessary in the child's diet.
- Give the child time to enjoy the meal without comment. Remove the food after 1/2 h or if they dawdle or lose interest.
- Learning to eat is fun. Switch to finger food if they refuse to be fed.
- Try not to use food as a punishment or reward. It only increases its potential power.

FOOD NEEDS OF PRESCHOOLERS

The following is a guide to the quantities suitable for the 2–5 year olds. Many parents are surprised at how little children of this age need. However, because total needs are small there is relatively little place for high-fat, high-sugar extras such as savoury snack foods and soft drinks.

Daily
Milk group

Three serves (1 serve = 250 mL of milk, 200 g of yoghurt or 35 g of cheese).

Full cream products are recommended.

Bread and cereal group

Four to five serves (1 serve = 1 slice of bread, 1/2 cup of pasta or 2 cereal wheat biscuits).

Vegetable and fruit group

Four or more serves (1 serve = 1 piece of fruit or 2 tablespoons of vegetables).

Meat or protein group

Two serves (1 serve = 30 g of lean meat, fish or chicken, 1/2 cup of beans, or 1 egg).

OBESITY

Obesity is an increasingly prevalent problem among children in Australia. Up to 20% of Australian children and young people can be defined as overweight.

Childhood obesity increases the risk of adult obesity, and is associated with substantial psychosocial morbidity in childhood and adolescence.

Childhood onset obesity that persists into adulthood accounts for a disproportionate share of severe adult obesity.

A history of childhood obesity is associated with increased mortality and morbidity independent of adult weight.

Parental obesity is the strongest factor for the persistence of obesity in children.

Definition

- Greater than 120% of the expected weight for height, estimated from the growth chart.
- A clinically useful definition that reflects excess body fat and is simple to use is the body mass index (BMI).

  BMI = bodyweight in kg divided by the square of height in metres (kg/m^2).

  — Overweight = BMI greater than the 85th centile for age and sex.
  — Obesity = BMI greater than 95th centile for age and sex.

What causes obesity?

Children become obese because their energy intake exceeds their energy requirement. Our understanding of the factors that influence this energy balance equation is incomplete: genetic, hormonal, metabolic and environmental factors interact to contribute to the development and maintenance of obesity. Genetic factors may account for 25–40% of obesity. The gene pool changes slowly and lifestyle changes appear to be the fundamental genesis of the current increased prevalence of obesity. Lifestyle factors include increased sedentary activities such as television and computer games, less time partaking in physical activities, and increased access to a dietary intake high in fat.

Endocrine causes of obesity are rare and are usually associated with growth retardation, which distinguishes them from the accelerated linear growth accompanying exogenous obesity. Consider:

- Hypothyroidism
- Cushing's disease
- Hypopituitarism.

Syndromic causes of obesity are often recognised by the presence of a significant developmental disability and less frequently by dysmorphic features.

Clues

- Height <50th centile (or < genetic potential).
- Dysmorphic features.
- Developmental disabilities.

Complications

- Psychosocial – depression, teasing, school avoidance and low self-esteem.
- Cardiovascular – hyperlipidaemia, hypertension, increased heart rate and cardiac output, and exercise intolerance.
- Endocrine – glucose intolerance, insulin resistance, non-insulin-dependent diabetes mellitus (NIDDM), accelerated linear growth and bone age, early onset of puberty, polycystic ovary disease, and menstrual dysfunction.
- Orthopaedic – Blount's disease, slipped capital femoral epiphysis and coxa vara.
- Respiratory – obstructive sleep apnoea.
- Gastroenterological – gall-bladder disease and hepatic steatosis.
- Dermatological – intertrigo, furunculosis and acanthosis nigricans.
- Neurological – benign intracranial hypertension.

Management

Assessment

The aim is to identify:

- High-risk individuals
- Underlying syndromes
- Complications.

For high-risk factors check the family history of obesity, heart disease, diabetes, hypertension, dyslipidaemias and other complications of obesity.

A detailed personal, family, developmental and past history complemented by a thorough dietary and activity history, and a detailed physical examination will be sufficient in most cases.

The physical examination should include an assessment of body build, posture, distribution of adiposity, pigmentation, striae, and the pubertal and neurological status.

Blood pressure should be measured, and the height and weight plotted on percentile charts.

Investigations

- Screening for hyperlipidaemia, diabetes and hepatic steatosis should be considered in the child with obesity, and is advisable when complications or a strong family history of adiposity-related morbidities are present.
- When obesity is suspected to be secondary, further investigation is required; e.g. chromosomes, specific DNA tests, thyroid function tests, 24 h urinary-free cortisol, and so on (see also Endocrine Conditions, chapter 20).

Treatment

The goals are to diminish morbidity and morbidity risk, rather than to achieve a normal bodyweight. The weight goal is generally to maintain weight over time as the height increases, or to slow weight gain compared to normal weight gain for age.

The highest success in the achievement of sustained weight loss is found in long-term family-based intervention, including behavioural change. The aim is a shift in energy balance achieved by:

- Lowering the energy intake through targeted changes in the family eating pattern and a reduction in energy density. This includes regular meals and snacks, with an emphasis on cereals, fruit and vegetables, lean protein foods and low-fat dairy products, and a reduction in high-fat items.
- Increasing the energy requirement through an increase in age-appropriate physical activities and a reduction in sedentary activities. Endurance walking (>20 min per session) is useful for older children. Organised sport is useful for social activity, but often provides little sustained activity, especially for the overweight child.

Useful approaches include:

1 Intervention, which can begin at any age, after identifying the problem.
2 Identifying the family's readiness to change (consider deferring treatment or referring for family assessment).

3 Providing families with information about:
   - Medical complications of obesity
   - The concept of energy balance
   - Healthy eating
   - Appropriate physical activities
   - Behavioural strategies.
4 Involving all family members and caregivers.
5 Permanent lifestyle changes as oppposed to short-term diets or exercise programs aimed at rapid weight loss. Medications are not indicated.
6 Monitoring diet and physical activities to help maintain changes.
7 Professional input that encourages support and understanding.

You need to refer a patient to specialist treatment when there is:
- Suspicion of pathological causes
- The presence of complications
- A lack of progress
- Massive obesity
- Parental or patient request.

ENTERAL FEEDING

Enteral nutrition is the provision of nutrients to the alimentary tract through a feeding tube. It can be used to provide the total nutritional needs of a patient (either short or long term), or to provide additional nutrients when voluntary oral intake is inadequate.

Enteral feeding has certain advantages over total parenteral nutrition:
- Less risk of infection
- Less risk of metabolic abnormalities
- The nutrients provided to the alimentary tract enhance intestinal growth and function
- It is cheaper.

Indications

Enteral feeding is used for patients who:
- Cannot feed orally (e.g. neurological damage or prematurity).
- Have increased metabolic requirements for nutrients (e.g. burns or congenital heart disease).

- Fail to achieve their nutritional requirements (e.g. failure to thrive or cystic fibrosis).
- Require unpalatable specialised feeds to treat their medical condition (e.g. metabolic disorders or liver disease).

Contraindication

Enteral feeding is contraindicated in patients with a non-functioning gastrointestinal (GI) tract.

Administration

The most commonly used route is nasogastric, its main benefit being ease of intubation. When long-term feeding is required, a gastrostomy tube may be indicated.

When gastric motility is poor or when gastric residues are persistently high, a nasojejunal tube may be of benefit. However, feeding directly into the jejunum limits the choice of formula and may increase the risk of bacterial overgrowth.

Implementing feeds

When choosing a method consider the feeding route, the length of time the feed is expected to be required and the type of feed to be used (see Table 7.3). The introduction of hyperosmolar feeds should be done gradually.

Table 7.3 Types of feeding regimens

	Advantages	Disadvantages
Bolus feedings	Most closely mimics physiological feeding Increases patient mobility Little equipment is needed Volume given can be precisely measured	Can be time consuming for caregiver May decrease voluntary oral intake
Gravity drip	Little equipment needed	Rate of delivery cannot be closely monitored
Pump-assisted continuous	Feeding most likely to be tolerated Feeding can be delivered while patient sleeps Larger volumes can be tolerated than if given by bolus method	Requires feeding pump

Selection of feed

A full nutritional assessment (current nutritional status, current intake, requirements and the consideration of medical condition/fluid restrictions) should be carried out by a dietitian to establish which feed will be optimal.

In general, infants can be managed using breast milk (if available) or an infant formula, or both. The formula will usually require additional fortification with both energy and other nutrients at around 6 months of age; this is suitable for up to about 2 years of age.

Children over 2 years can be managed adequately using a proprietary product (see Table 7.4).

It is generally inappropriate to put pureed foods down feeding tubes as the amount of fluid required to achieve a suitable consistency dilutes the energy and nutrient content, while increasing the risk of microbial contamination and tube blockage.

Monitoring enteral nutrition

When monitoring patients on enteral feeds, mechanical, metabolic, gastrointestinal, nutritional and growth parameters must be assessed routinely. In the early stages of feeding, the patient's tolerance of the feeding regimen is critical to the success of feeding.

Once the feeding plan has been fully implemented, an assessment of the patient's nutrient requirements is needed regularly to ensure that the adequacy of nutritional support is maintained and to indicate when enteral feeding can be ceased.

From total parenteral nutrition (TPN) to enteral feeding

Initiating enteral feeds in critically ill patients (even in small amounts) helps to preserve gut function and structure, and to minimise the hypermetabolic response to stress. When initiating enteral feeds in patients maintained on TPN, an isotonic, lactose-free formula perfused at a low constant rate is usually best tolerated. The transition from parenteral to enteral nutrition should be gradual with a tapering of TPN and advancing enteral feeds. This helps to prevent hypoglycaemia and fluid overload. TPN should be ceased when enteral feeds provide approximately 75% of nutritional requirements.

Table 7.4 Commonly used enteral feeds

Type	Example	Notes
Polymeric foods 1 kcal/mL (4.2 kJ/mL)	Paediasure Osmolite Ensure Isocal	
	Jevity	Contains fibre
	Pulmocare	High fat, low CHO
High energy polymeric 1.5 kcal/mL (6.3 kJ/mL)	Ensure Plus	Hypertonic
2.0 kcal/mL (8.4 kJ/mL)	Twocal HN	Hypertonic
Specialised formula (elemental)	Vital HN Elemental 028 Paediatric vivonex	Contains short chain peptides; not suitable for infants under 1 year
	Neocate*	Suitable for infants
	Generaid Plus	Used in hepatic disorders
Modular feeds Protein source	Promod, Maxipro HBV	Nutritionally
CHO source	Polyjoule, Polycal Douglas Energy Plus	incomplete; requires vitamin and mineral supplement
Fat source LCT	Calogen	
MCT	Liquigen, MCT Oil*	
Fat and CHO source	Duocal	

All feeds are lactose free.
* Australian Pharmaceutical Benefits Schedule listed.

From enteral to oral feeding

The goals for enteral feeding should be set at the outset. Once the patient is able and willing to eat by mouth the enteral feed can be reduced in proportion to the amount consumed orally. Transition from continuous feeds to overnight feeds may help establish oral intake while ensuring the patient is not nutritionally compromised.

Home enteral feeding

The decision to provide home enteral feeding should take into consideration the patient's medical needs and the social, psychological and financial factors that influence the family's ability to cope with a home feeding program.

Children on home enteral feeding, especially those who have minimal or no voluntary oral intake, require close monitoring of their growth and need their feeding regimens altered appropriately.

Common problems

- Gastrointestinal disturbance is the most common problem (diarrhoea, cramping, nausea and vomiting). These problems can be minimised with the correct formula selection and administration in conjunction with a review of medications and their content. High gastric residues should be treated by reducing the rate of feed given or feeding small volumes continuously, reassessing the concentration of feed and assessing GI function. Directing feed into the jejunum alleviates the problems caused by slow gastric emptying.
- Other problems include overhydration, dehydration, electrolyte imbalance, hyperglycaemia, hypoglycaemia and constipation. These need to be assessed and managed appropriately.
- Malnutrition is associated with major changes in electrolyte balance. Enteral feeding should be initiated with caution in patients with significant and long-standing under-nutrition. Serum phosphate, potassium, magnesium and glucose levels should be assessed regularly (see Refeeding syndrome, p. 133).
- Psychomotor development. Young children who have been fed enterally during infancy or for long periods of time may miss important developmental steps in self-feeding. Non-nutritive sucking or taking small amounts of appropriate food/fluid orally will help establish or maintain eating and feeding skills, or both. A speech pathologist may be of assistance in this area.

FEEDING THE SICK NEWBORN

Feed type

The feed types available are:

- Breast milk, including expressed breast milk (EBM)
- Artificial formulas, including specialised 'low birthweight' formulas
- Specialised feeds for pathological states.

Breast milk

Breast milk feeding should be the primary aim for very sick babies. When babies are too ill to suckle at the breast, most mothers can and wish to establish lactation by expression. EBM can be fed by gavage (nasogastric or orogastric) tube or other artificial means until the baby is well enough to be put to the breast.

In this way breast milk feeding can be achieved in extremely premature babies, and for those with the most major malformations, birth defects and other serious illnesses. The only situations in which breast milk feeding is not possible are:

- When an informed mother chooses not to express.
- Inborn errors of metabolism, which require exclusion formulas.
- Some complex malabsorption syndromes (e.g. short bowel syndrome). However, even some of these can succeed with EBM.

Evidence is accumulating that EBM feeding of sick babies reduces morbidity and mortality, and improves the developmental outcome compared with artificial feeding.

Lactation by expression

Every mother embarking on this course needs ready access to nurses trained in lactation or lactation consultants.

Expression by hand or pump should be started within 24 (preferably 4–8) h of delivery. Episodes should be every 3–4 h, lasting about 30 min with a break for sleep. Hand expression is best until lactation is established. EBM, if used with clean and straightforward techniques, does not have to be sterilised or pasteurised.

General

- EBM for sick babies should be from the baby's mother rather than a bank.
- EBM for sick babies should not be frozen; the freshest EBM available at the time should be used first.

Supplements and fortifiers

'Fortifiers', derived from cow milk, are available to add to EBM to increase its content of protein, energy and other nutrients. The effects of adding such substances to the biological properties of breast milk are unknown and may be deleterious; however, it is common practice.

Babies who may benefit from fortifiers are those with greatly increased nutritional requirements (e.g. very low birthweight babies, (VLBW)), and those requiring fluid restriction (i.e. babies with heart failure or chronic lung disease). For babies with greater nutritional requirements it is not appropriate to add calories only (i.e. glucose polymer or MCT oil); such babies need a range of additional nutrients.

VLBW babies may need folate and iron (in addition to a fortifier); extra sodium; and vitamins C, D and E. The addition of fortifier should be delayed until feeds are fully established (i.e. 150–200 mL/kg per 24 h).

Iron should not be started until 12 weeks of age. VLBW babies who receive multiple blood transfusions may not need supplemental iron.

Phototherapy

Phototherapy for jaundice can impede breast-feeding by placing physical and psychological barriers between mother and baby, and by causing diarrhoea. Breast-feeding should be protected by interrupting the phototherapy frequently. Diarrhoea or sugar in bowel fluid are not reasons to suspend breast-feeding. Although insensible water loss is increased by some phototherapy devices, the increase is only 10–20 mL/kg per 24 h. Thus, as long as usual amounts of breast milk are available by suckling or expression, supplements of water or formula are not necessary.

Artificial formulas

These must be used when breast milk is not available. For those sick babies with greater nutritional requirements or in need of fluid restriction, formulas can be strengthened (by adding extra formula powder) from the standard 280 kJ/100 mL to 350–420 kJ/100 mL (66 kcal/100 mL to 82–100 kcal/100 mL).

Low birthweight (LBW) artificial formulas are designed for very premature (<32 weeks) babies. In general, these contain extra protein, more easily assimilated additional calories and increased calcium, phosphorus, trace elements, and some (but not all) vitamins.

LBW formulas may also be used in sick mature babies who need more nutrients or fluid restriction, instead of the concentrated standard formulas described above.

Specialised feeds

Specialised feeds for pathological states are available for the treatment of complex malabsorption, allergy, inborn errors of metabolism, and liver and renal disease.

Feed volumes, frequency and delivery

For sick babies who cannot be fed to appetite or 'demand'-fed babies, schedules specifying volume, frequency and delivery method are required.

Factors determining schedules include:
- Intestinal motility, gut enzyme and hormonal activity, which are low at birth and take time to switch on. This process is depressed by hypoxia, acidosis, sepsis and drugs, especially narcotics. This limits the feed volumes that sick babies can tolerate.
- A full stomach and bowel, which can press on the diaphragm, impairing breathing.
- Sick babies who reflux or vomit more often and are less able to protect their airways so that milk aspiration is an ever-present risk.
- Aggressive schedules that increase the risk of necrotising enterocolitis

Mature babies need 150 mL milk/kg per 24 h. This is usually reached over 5–7 days, starting at 30–40 mL/kg per 24 h and increasing by 30 mL/kg per 24 h as tolerated. The formula is used at three-quarter strength in the first 24–48 h, but EBM should not be diluted this way. Feed frequency should be 3–4 hourly, although with reflux or abdominal distension, smaller volume and more frequent feeds may help.

By using LBW formulas or concentrated standard formulas, adequate nutrition may be achieved with 120–150 mL/kg per 24 h. LBW formulas should be given diluted (15–20 kcal/30 mL or 210–280 kJ/100 mL) until full daily volumes are achieved. Standard strength (24 kcal/30 mL) should then be introduced.

VLBW babies require 180–200 mL/kg per 24 h of EBM or standard formula, or 150–180 mL/kg per 24 h of fortified EBM or LBW formula, starting at 20–30 mL/kg per 24 h, and increasing by 30 mL/kg per day as tolerated. LBW formula should be used diluted (15–20 kcal/30 mL or 210–280 kJ/mL) until close to maximum daily volumes are reached (usually after 2 weeks); LBW formulas are not designed to be given in full strength to sick or unstable VLBW infants. Initial feed frequency should be 1–2 hourly. Hourly feeds may be necessary in babies less than 1000 g.

Intragastric feeding tubes are necessary for sick babies who cannot suck: use No. 5–6 French for babies less than 2000 g and No. 6–8 French for larger babies. Nasogastric tubes should not be used in babies less than 1250 g; they cause significant airways obstruction (use orogastric).

Continuous intragastric infusion of milk rather than intermittent boluses may help if reflux, gastric distension or apnoea are persistent. Transpyloric duodenal or jejunal feeding provide no advantages and additional risks.

THE NUTRITIONAL MANAGEMENT OF THE UNWELL CHILD

In order to define specific nutritional requirements and the optimal method of delivery, an evaluation of the medical history and nutritional status is required. Dietary manipulation or enteral feeding, or both, should always be considered as the preferred delivery route in any patient with a functioning gastrointestinal tract. Children with severely delayed gastric emptying or who are at risk of aspiration may still be successfully fed enterally through a transpyloric tube.

General indications for parenteral nutrition (PN)

- Recent weight loss of greater than 10% of usual bodyweight and a non-functional GI tract.
- No oral intake for more than 3–5 days in a patient with sub-optimal nutritional status and a non-functional GI tract.
- Anticipated need for PN for a minimum of 3–5 days.

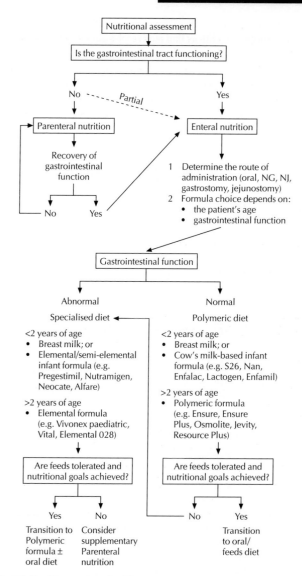

Fig. 7.1 Nutrition support algorithm

Medical/surgical conditions that may require parenteral nutrition

- Patients unable to tolerate enteral feeding because of gastro-intestinal dysfunction; i.e. postoperative neonatal surgery, extensive short bowel syndrome or severe malabsorption.
- Patients with increased metabolic requirements that may not be adequately treated with enteral therapy; i.e. severe burns, cystic fibrosis or renal failure.

DETERMINING NUTRITIONAL STATUS

Medical history

- Type and duration of illness.
- Degree of metabolic stress.
- Treatment (medications or surgery, or both).

Dietary assessment

- Twenty-four hour dietary recall.
- Three-day food record.

Physical examination

- General impression of wellbeing: wasting, oedema, lethargy or muscular strength.
- Specific micronutrient deficiency: pallor, bruising, skin, hair, neurological or ophthalmological.
- Anthropometry:
  - Weight for age
  - Length/height for age
  - Weight for length/height
  - Head circumference
  - Growth velocity
  - Skinfold thickness, mid-arm circumference.
- Laboratory assessment
  - protein status: albumin, total protein, pre-albumin, urea, 24 h urinary nitrogen, carnitine and delayed hypersensitivity testing:
  - Fluid, electrolyte and acid–base status: serum electrolytes and acid–base urinalysis

— Iron status: serum iron, serum ferritin and full blood examination
— Mineral status: calcium, magnesium, phosphorus, alkaline phosphatase, bone age and bone density
— Vitamin status: vitamins A, C, B12, D, E/lipid ratio, folate and INR
— Trace elements: zinc, selenium, copper, chromium and manganese
— Lipid status: serum cholesterol, HDL cholesterol and triglycerides
— Glucose tolerance: serum glucose, HbA1c.

ESTABLISHING A NUTRITION TREATMENT PLAN

Calculating fluid requirement
See chapter 6.

Calculating nutritional requirements
(1) Energy
Estimated energy requirements for the sick child are usually calculated by using either:

- The requirements of a normal well child of the same sex and age.
- An estimate of basal requirements with additional activity.
- Measurement of energy expenditure using indirect calorimetry.

Energy requirements can be expressed as kilocalories (kcal) or as kilojoules/megajoules. The conversion equation is:

$$\frac{mJ \times 1000}{4.2} = kcal$$

Recommended energy requirements for infants
The WHO–FAO–UNU (1985)/NH&MRC (1990) recommendations are generally used to base recommendations of energy intakes for the well and normal child (see Table 7.5a, b and c over page). The recommendations for infants are based on studies in *formula-fed infants*. Recent data suggest that the energy expenditure and energy intake of *breast-fed infants* in the first months of life are significantly less

Table 7.5a Recommended energy requirements for infants

Age (months)	kJ/kg per day (kcal/kg per day)	Age (months)	kJ/kg per day (kcal/kg per day)
0–0.9	520 (124)	6–7	395 (94)
1–2	485 (116)	7–8	395 (94)
2–3	455 (109)	8–9	395 (94)
3–4	430 (103)	9–10	415 (99)
4–5	415 (99)	10–11	420 (100)
5–6	405 (97)	11–12	435 (104)

Source: Recommended Nutrient Intakes Australian Papers, Truswell, A.S. (ed.), Australian Professional publications, 1990, p. 16.

Table 7.5b Recommended energy requirements for children 1–10 years

Age (years)	Males MJ/day	Females MJ/day
1–2	5.0	4.8
2–3	5.9	5.5
3–4	6.5	6.0
4–5	7.1	6.4
5–6	7.6	6.8
6–7	7.9	7.1
7–8	8.3	7.4
8–9	8.7	7.7
9–10	9.0	7.9

Source: Recommended Nutrient Intakes Australian Papers, Truswell, A.S. (ed.), Australian Professional publications, 1990, p. 16.

Table 7.5c Recommended energy requirements for adolescents 10–18 years

Age (years)	Males MJ/day	Females MJ/day
10–11	8.1–9.1	7.3–8.2
11–12	8.7–9.8	7.7–8.7
12–13	9.2–10.3	8.1–9.1
13–14	9.8–11.0	8.4–9.5
14–15	10.5–11.8	8.6–9.8
15–16	11.1–12.5	8.7–9.9
16–17	11.7–13.2	8.8–10.0
17–18	12.0–13.5	8.8–10.0

Source: Recommended Nutrient Intakes Australian Papers, Truswell, A.S. (ed.), Australian Professional publications, 1990, p. 16.

(17 and 27% respectively) than that of formula-fed infants. These differences in energy metabolism are lost after weaning.

Breast-fed infants

- 0–5 months – 100–110 kcal/kg per day
- 6–12 months – 70–80 kcal/kg per day

Preterm infants – parenteral energy recommendation

In acute metabolic stress requirements, 110–120% of basal energy expenditure (~55–65 kcal/kg per day) is required.

If amino acid intake is adequate, an energy intake approaching the resting energy expenditure (i.e. 50–60 kcal/kg per day) should prevent weight loss. To achieve weight gain, more than 60 kcal/kg per day is generally required. Low birthweight infants who receive an energy intake of 80 kcal/kg per day with 3 g/kg per day amino acid intake gain weight at approximately the rate achieved *in utero*. However, this amino acid intake may be difficult to achieve by PN alone if Vamin-N® is used, due to the potential risk of excessive serum concentrations of some amino acids at doses greater than 2 g/kg per day in preterm infants.

(2) Protein

Optimal protein utilisation depends on a balanced energy and protein intake. If energy intake is less than the maintenance energy requirement then protein is shunted through gluconeogenesis to produce glucose. Optimal protein utilisation requires a non-protein energy intake of 60 kcal/kg per day to utilise 2.5 g/kg per day protein (or 0.4 g/kg per day nitrogen), which is a ratio of 150 : 1. This ratio may be altered in metabolic stress.

Amino acid recommendations are usually higher in parenteral nutrition as the patients who require this type of therapy generally have higher protein requirements due to their primary disease or treatment. The following table is a guide to account for these increased requirements.

Table 7.6 Parenteral recommended intake of protein

	Amino acids (g/kg per day)
Preterm infants	1–2 (3*)
0–1 year	2.5
2–13 years	1.5–2.0
13–18 years	1.0–1.5

* The optimal concentration and composition of parenteral amino acids for preterm infants is not known. Preterm infants have incomplete development of metabolic pathways for the metabolism of amino acids, so some amino acids that are not considered essential in adults and children may be essential in preterm infants (cysteine, taurine and glycine).

Increased protein intake is recommended in:
- Protein-losing states; i.e. enteropathy and nephrotic syndrome
- Chronic malnutrition
- Burns
- Renal dialysis
- HIV
- Haemofiltration (~2 g/kg per day).

Reduced protein intake is recommended in patients with:
- Hepatic encephalopathy (0.3 g/kg per day)
- Severe renal dysfunction (not dialysed).

(3) Fat

Fat is a concentrated source of energy and is an integral component of all cell membranes for the transport of fat-soluble vitamins and hormones. Essential fatty acid (EFA) deficiency can occur in neonates within days of initiating fat-free parenteral nutrition. Clinical signs of deficiency include reduced growth rate, poor hair growth, thrombocytopenia, increased susceptibility to infections and impaired wound healing.

EFA deficiency is prevented by intravenous lipid (0.2–1 g/kg per day) or an enteral supplement with corn oil, sunflower oil or safflower oil.

(4) Micronutrients

Special consideration is needed when estimating the micronutrient requirements of sick children (see Table 7.7).

Table 7.7 Diseases that increase micronutrient requirements

Disease	Increased requirement
Burns	Vitamins C, B complex, folate, zinc
HIV/AIDS	Zinc, selenium, iron
Renal failure: dialysis	Vitamins C, B complex, folate (reduce or omit copper, chromium, molybdenum)
Haemofiltration	Vitamins C, B complex, trace elements
Protein energy malnutrition	Zinc, selenium, iron
Refeeding syndrome	Phosphate, magnesium, potassium
Short bowel syndrome, chronic malabsorption states	Vitamins A, B12, D, E, K, folate, zinc, magnesium, selenium
Liver disease	Vitamins A, B12, D, E, K, zinc, iron (reduce or omit manganese, copper)
High fistula output, chronic diarrhoea	Zinc, magnesium, selenium, folate, B complex, B12
Pancreatic insufficiency	Vitamins A, D, E, K
Inflammatory bowel disease	Folate, B12, zinc, iron

ORDERING PARENTERAL NUTRITION

The following basic information is essential:

1   Document the patient's current weight.
2   Assess the venous access available (i.e. central versus peripheral).
3   Establish the fluid volume in mL/kg per day available for parenteral nutrition. In some patients this will equal their daily maintenance fluid requirement, and for others this will be a limited proportion of the total fluid requirement due to the requirements of drug administration or blood products, or both.
4   Establish the nutritional goals.
5   Determine the basic PN solution required. This will be:
    Infants <5 kg – Vamin-N®
    Children >5 kg – Synthamin 17®
6   Determine the standard solution that best meets the patient's requirements (refer to Table 7.8). These have been designed to provide:

Table 7.8 Standard parenteral nutrition solutions

Each litre provides	N1 : 13/100 (<5 kg)	N2 : 20/125 (for <5 kg)	N3 : 33/200 (<5 kg)	P1 : 20/100 (>5 kg)	P2 : 25/200 (>5 kg)	P3 : 30/300 (>5 kg)
Amino acids (g/L)	13	20	33	20	25	30
Glucose (g/L)	100	125	200	100	200	300
Sodium (mmol/L)	20	30	25	30	30	50
Potassium (mmol/L)	20	30	25	30	30	50
Calcium (mmol/L)	12	12	12	6	6	6
Phosphate (mmol/L)	12	12	12	6	6	6
Magnesium (mmol/L)	4	4	4	4	4	4
Multivitamins (mmol/L)	standard	standard	standard	standard	standard	standard
Trace elements	standard	standard	standard	standard	standard	standard
Heparin	nil	nil	nil	1000	1000	1000
Total kilocalories	425	545	876	465	866	1268
Osmolarity (mOsm)	878	1127	1588	914	1520	2206

- Solutions with a 10% glucose concentration. These are suitable for peripheral parenteral nutrition or as day 1 of a centrally administered parenteral nutrition.
- Solutions with a 20% glucose concentration (N3, P2). These should be administered via a central line.
- Solutions with a 30% glucose concentration and maximum amount of amino acid components for the specific use in patients who are severely fluid restricted.

7   If the standard solutions do not meet a patient's specific requirements, options include:
- If fluid requirements are not met, choose the standard PN solution that provides the energy, protein and micronutrient requirements. Additional fluid can be added using a side line of dextrose/saline solution with further electrolyte additions if appropriate. This approach is particularly useful in the first days of parenteral nutrition therapy when there may be frequent changes in total fluid and electrolyte requirements.
- Choose a standard PN solution that provides the total fluid, protein and energy requirements. An increase in electrolyte and micronutrient composition can be made after consultation with Pharmacy.
- Contact the Nutrition Support Service for advice regarding customised parenteral nutrition solutions.

8   Determine lipid emulsion dose in g/kg per day. Lipids should be provided at a minimal dose of 0.5g/kg per day to prevent essential fatty acid deficiency.

9   Calculate total energy (kcal or kJ/kg per day) provided by the prescribed solution.

10   Notify the Nutrition Support Service.

11   Order baseline laboratory investigations (see Table 7.9).

12   Write intravenous infusion orders on the patient's intravenous medication chart or treatment sheet at the bedside.

MONITORING

See Table 7.9.

Table 7.9 Parenteral nutrition monitoring

	Baseline/pre-TPN	Daily	Twice weekly	Weekly	1–3 monthly
Weight	X	X			
Height/length	X				X
Head circumference (<2 years)	X				X
Triceps skin fold thickness	X				X
Mid arm circumference	X				X
Fluid balance	X	X			
Inspect intravenous site	X	X			
Urinalysis	X	X			
Electrolytes	X	X (until stable)		X	
Urea	X	X (until stable)		X	
Creatinine	X	X (until stable)		X	
Acid-base	X	X (until stable)		X	
Glucose	X	X (until stable)	X	X	
Calcium	X	X (until stable)		X	
Phosphate	X	X (until stable)		X	
Magnesium	X		X (until stable)	X	
Triglycerides	X	X (with advancement of fat)	X (until stable)	X	
LFT	X			X	
FBE	X			X	
Zinc/ALP					X
Iron, ferritin					X

B$_{12}$, folate, selenium, manganese, molybdenum, copper, aluminium – 6 monthly or as indicated.

REFEEDING SYNDROME

After a period of prolonged starvation, aggressive nutritional therapy may precipitate a cascade of potentially fatal metabolic complications. These include:

- Hypokalaemia
- Hypophosphataemia
- Hypomagnesaemia
- Glucose intolerance
- Cardiac failure
- Seizures
- Myocardial infarction/arrhythmias

At particular risk are patients with:

- Anorexia nervosa
- Classical marasmus
- Kwashiorkor
- No nutrition for 7–10 days in adolescents (much less in infants and children) with significant metabolic stress
- Acute weight loss of ≥10–20% of usual bodyweight, and possibly metabolic stress, or >20% of usual bodyweight
- Morbid obesity with massive weight loss (i.e. postoperative).

Treatment

- Identify risk and chronicity.
- Identify and treat metabolic stress if present (i.e. infection).
- Establish baseline status: weight, height/length, head circumference, fluid status, electrolytes, urea, creatinine, calcium, phosphate, magnesium, phosphate, magnesium, prior to commencing nutritional rehabilitation.
- Establish modest nutritional goals initially (i.e. basal requirements until stability is assured), then aim to provide for catch-up growth.
- Monitor closely over the first week until a nutritional plan is established with: pulse rate; fluid balance; weight; caloric intake; glucose; electrolytes; urea; creatinine; phosphate; magnesium.
- Administer vitamin and mineral supplement.

CHAPTER 8
ADOLESCENT HEALTH

Susan Sawyer
George Patton

Adolescence is the transitional period of development between relatively dependent childhood and relatively independent adulthood.

Chronological age is not always a good reflection of developmental stage; however, an adolescent is generally considered to be between the age of 10 and 19 years. More recently, the term young person has been used in the context of health policies and young people are arbitrarily defined as those between the age of 10 and 24 years.

A social health perspective

The health profile of young people has changed in recent decades with higher rates of psychosocial disorders such as substance abuse, depression and eating disorders now evident. These health problems have arisen as a result of broad social and economic change in communities. The lifestyles of young people have changed as a result of the longer time elapsing before making key social transitions such as completing education, leaving home, commitment to long-term relationships and having children. In addition, unemployment, poverty and increased drug availability have a special impact on young people who are vulnerable as a consequence of their transitional developmental stage.

Adolescent developmental tasks

Engaging adolescents in a productive therapeutic relationship requires the clinician to have a good understanding of both the social context of young people's lives and the developmental tasks they confront. The key developmental tasks include:

- Autonomy and independence
- Body self-integrity and personal identity
- Peer relationships and recreational goals
- Educational and vocational goals
- Sexuality.

Developmental outcomes as health outcomes

Clinicians must have clear goals of therapy related to the health problems that they are trying to manage in partnership with their patients. Such clear clinical outcomes are necessary in the care of young people; however, they are insufficient. Clinicians must also have a good understanding of the developmental outcomes relevant to the young person and set treatment goals in the context of these developmental goals (see Table 8.1).

The negotiation of treatment goals in a way that takes account of the individual needs of the young person is crucial to engaging him or her in a way that engenders good adherence to treatment regimens.

A CLINICAL APPROACH TO ADOLESCENTS

Consultations with young people are likely to be relatively time-consuming and allowing adequate time is essential to the conduct of a successful consultation. Young people too often perceive that they are not listened to, not given adequate time to put their views across and that their opinions are dismissed. A clinician who listens respectfully and acknowledges a young person's point of view will have made an excellent start in establishing a therapeutic relationship.

Starting the consultation

Greet the young person by name, making eye-to-eye contact and ensuring that they are given your full name. When parents are present, be sure to greet the young person first and then introduce yourself to the parents. The young person is the patient and must be given time alone with the clinician during the consultation at some stage.

Confidentiality

Clinicians should make a clear statement that explains the issue of confidentiality at the beginning of the first contact with every adolescent. Maintenance of confidentiality enhances trust and honesty, which enables more appropriate health care. Although the adolescent may be an integral member of a family, he or she, not the family, is the patient. Young people may require added reassurance before being able to trust clinicians with important information.

- In general, all information gained from an adolescent should be regarded as confidential until this issue has been discussed and clarified.
- Issues of confidentiality for young people under 16 years of age require negotiation. An agreement to break confidentiality or a compromise agreement may be made by negotiation.
- Exceptions to confidentiality occur if there is a current and substantial risk of the adolescent committing suicide, homicide or being subject to physical or sexual abuse.

Developmental screening

Young people are most likely to present for clinical care as a consequence of a minor complaint, such as a viral illness or injury. Irrespective of the primary reason for presentation, the clinician should take the opportunity to undertake a developmental screening that is related to health promotion and disease prevention.

It may be appropriate to schedule a second appointment to enable this developmental screening. One approach to developmental screening is to use the HEADSS framework to take a psychosocial history (*H*ome, *E*ducation and employment, *A*ctivities, *D*rugs, *S*exuality, and *Su*icide risk) (see Table 8.1). HEADSS involves a series of questions that move from less to more sensitive areas in a systematic manner. Taking a

Table 8.1 Adolescent developmental screening: HEADSS*

	Area	Questions
H	Home	Where do you live and who lives there with you?
E	Education and employment	What are you good at in school? What grades do you get?
A	Activities	What do you do for fun? What things do you do with friends?
D	Drugs	Many young people experiment with drugs, alcohol and cigarettes. Have you ever tried them?
S	Sexuality	Most young people become interested in sex at your age. Have you had a sexual relationship with anyone?
S	Suicide risk/ depression screening	See Table 8.2, p. 142

* Goldenring and Cohen, *Contemporary Pediatrics*, July, 1988, pp. 75–80.

psychosocial history provides a mechanism to engage the young person in the medical consultation, provides a mechanism for understanding the balance of health risk and protective factors, identifies opportunities for early intervention, and provides opportunities for positive feedback when things are going well.

Physical examination

A thorough physical examination should be conducted gently and with consideration. Protection of the adolescent's modesty and privacy is vital. It is helpful during the examination to integrate friendly and reassuring dialogue that explains the reason for the particular examination and gives immediate feedback on the findings.

YOUNG PEOPLE WITH CHRONIC ILLNESSES AND DISABILITIES

This is a special group, with many requiring the skills of a multi-disciplinary team. Young people in these categories are frequently the most experienced consumers of the health system in the paediatric environment. Clinicians must be extremely careful to acknowledge and respect the experience and views of such people and their families.

Conflict of priorities

It is not uncommon for a conflict of priorities to occur between the therapeutic goals articulated by the clinician (focused on disease management), and the developmental goals that are frequently the dominant concern of young people. Clinicians need to recognise the potential for this conflict to occur, and be prepared to negotiate a successful resolution through clear and open discussion.

Adherence

Engendering adherence with treatment regimens is a challenge for clinicians irrespective of the age of the patient, but it may be more difficult with adolescents. This is because of the apparent contradiction that exists between the young person's (developmentally appropriate) pursuit of independence and the clinician's desire to give clear instructions on health care. Careful and respectful negotiation is required. Practical tips include:

- Keep language and instructions simple.
- Ensure that the treatment regimen is practical.
- Consider the acceptability of treatment to peers.
- Be consistent and do not 'nag'.
- Keep communication open and avoid the use of threats.
- As appropriate, encourage parents to either be more involved or to 'back off' and not be over-protective.

Multidisciplinary teams and mixed messages

The value of the multidisciplinary team is well established. However, there is a considerable potential for individual health professionals within the team to give conflicting and mixed messages to young people and their families, thereby confounding the achievement of satisfactory disease and developmental outcomes. Excellent communication within the team is crucial to ensure that a mutually agreed to common set of themes and messages is delivered to the young person and their family.

Working across the sectors

The emotional health and wellbeing of young people is influenced by many factors, including families, peers and schools. Consideration needs to be given to both gaining information from and communicating information to those who work with young people, whatever the setting. These include:

- School and educational agencies
- Community-based youth organisations
- Welfare agencies
- Recreational programs
- Peer support groups.

High-risk young people

A small proportion of young people are considered to be at a very high health risk. This includes those who are socially disadvantaged by homelessness, those within the juvenile justice setting and those engaged in multiple health risk behaviours. These young people deserve appropriate health care, but for a range of reasons, often do not receive it. Close consultation and liaison with case-workers is a priority, as is linking high-risk young people to appropriate community-based facilities. This might include youth mental health services, youth substance abuse services, or sexual abuse services.

Transition to adult health care

The concept of transition can be defined as the purposeful and planned movement of adolescents and young adults with chronic physical and medical conditions from child-centred to adult-oriented health-care systems. This is a process that, ideally, has been anticipated by patient, parents and health-care professionals alike, with strategies put in place to increase the likelihood of success. This contrasts with the event of transfer, the physical move from one service or professional to another.

Principles of transition

Experience suggests some key principles that help promote continuing comprehensive care for young people with complex conditions. Anticipation of physical transfer from the time of diagnosis is one way of ensuring that the physical move is truly part of a transition process. A planned, coordinated approach is essential. An adult physician or team that is both interested and capable of providing tertiary care is fundamental. Compilation of a detailed medical and allied health summary is important, as is good communication between paediatric and adult providers. Community providers, such as general practitioners, are an important source of continuity of care.

Adolescent medicine referrals

Specialist adolescent medicine units are a resource for general practitioners and other health professionals for early referral of adolescents with difficult or complex problems.

Common reasons for referral include:
- Health problems that are relatively unique to the adolescent age group, including eating disorders (see p. 142), deliberate self-harm and suicide attempts (see p. 141), school-based problems and behaviour disorders.
- Problems occurring at the interface between adolescent general health and adolescent mental health, such as early depression and psychosomatic disorders.
- Complex interactions between young people, diseases and disease treatments.
- Concerns about physical growth, puberty and sexual behaviour.
- Problems that involve a knowledge of and access to networks and programs dealing with young people.

ADOLESCENT MENTAL HEALTH

The notion that adolescence was a time of inevitable emotional turmoil, with few implications for future mental health, has given way to a view that the teens and early twenties are critical years for the development of major psychiatric disorders that persist into adulthood (see also Child Psychiatry, chapter 12). Major disorders with high rates of first onset in young people include:

- Depression
- Anxiety disorders
- Obsessional neurosis
- Schizophrenia
- Bipolar affective disorders
- Substance abuse
- Personality disorders
- Anorexia and bulimia nervosa.

The recognition and early diagnosis of adolescent mental disorders is a clinical challenge. Many of these disorders will present with less well-developed features than in an adult population. The mounting evidence that psychological and social treatments are most effective at this early stage of illness underlines the necessity for effective early diagnosis and referral for treatment.

Adolescent mental health disorders generally arise in a context of interpersonal and social problems. During assessment and treatment, consideration should be given to recent stresses arising from grief (e.g. death or illness in the family or among friends), conflict (e.g. victimisation by peers or arguments with parents), relationship break-downs and problems with school work. For many young people there are longer standing problems with parents, school and a lack of emotional and interpersonal skills to deal with the developmental tasks of adolescence (e.g. difficulties in initiating social contact, dealing with new sexual feelings and negotiating greater independence within the family).

DEPRESSION, DELIBERATE SELF-HARM AND SUICIDE

Suicide is, after motor vehicle accidents, the most common cause of death in 15–25 year olds in Australia. Factors most commonly associated with completed suicide are a history of deliberate self-harm, major depression, substance abuse and antisocial behaviour (see also Child Psychiatry, chapter 12).

About one in 200 young people present to emergency departments each year for deliberate acts of self-harm, typically in the form of an overdose. An even greater number do not present for medical care. In most instances, deliberate self-harm is not true suicidal behaviour with the intent of causing death: most self-harm is associated with a degree of psychiatric disturbance. Key features of assessment of the potentially suicidal adolescent are shown in Table 8.2. Assessment of the act of self-harm should include:

Table 8.2 Assessment of suicide risk in young people*

Area	Questions
Suicidal ideation: current	
Attitude to death	Is life worthless/hopeless?
Suicidal thinking	Is there a plan? (clarity, lethality)
	Is there access to weapons/drugs?
	Have any steps been taken?
Suicide attempts: previous	
Method	Potential of methods to cause death
Planning	Length of planning period. Preparing for death (e.g. bequests, wills)
Intent	What was hoped would occur? Attitude to previous attempts
Mental health disorder: current	
Substance misuse	How much? How often? Consequences of use?
Depression	Low mood. Poor concentration on studies. Tiredness. Sleep disturbance. Negative feelings. Isolated and withdrawn
Personality disorder	Disturbed past relationships and behaviours. Responses to stress

* Patton and Bowes, *General Practitioner*, 1994; **2**: 18–19.

- Attention to suicidal intent
- Perceived lethality of the act
- Actual harm incurred
- Degree of planning
- Actions taken by the patient after the event.

Assessment should also be made of any associated psychiatric disorders, and the level of social and interpersonal difficulties in a teenager's life.

Depression is the most common major psychiatric disorder of young people with symptoms similar to those found in adults (see p. 189). Typical symptoms include:

- Pervasive boredom
- Extended periods of low mood with feelings of being unwanted
- Fatigue
- Loss of self-confidence and social anxiety
- Social withdrawal from friends
- Impaired concentration and difficulties with school work
- Suicidal ideas.

In most instances a teenager will give a better account of these symptoms than parents or other informants. Assessment should include the consideration of organic causes (e.g. recent steroid therapy or substance abuse). Both psychological (cognitive behavioural and interpersonal psychotherapies) and medication treatments have parts to play in the management of adolescent depression.

EATING DISORDERS

Anorexia nervosa and bulimia nervosa typically arise in the early to mid-teens. The commonest eating disorders to present clinically are subsyndromal forms where the mental state is similar but the full picture has not developed. Such disorders may pass spontaneously but should be treated seriously. Where symptoms persist after 3 months, referral for more specific treatment is warranted.

Adolescent dieting is the usual forerunner of an eating disorder. Although most dieters do not go on to develop an eating disorder, preoccupation with dieting that leads to the avoidance of other activities (e.g. not going out with friends because of feeling fat) deserves attention.

Anorexia nervosa

Anorexia nervosa is characterised by a relentless pursuit of thinness through the use of extreme weight control strategies, amenorrhoea and an intense fear of gaining weight.

Indices of the severity of post-pubertal anorexia nervosa include the current weight, rate of weight loss, methods employed (e.g. abstinence, self-induced vomiting, purging and exercise) and any associated depression.

Consideration should be given to the exclusion of other primary psychiatric disorders (e.g. major depression or obsessional neurosis) and physical disorders (thyrotoxicosis and malabsorption).

Admission is indicated where weight loss is extreme (to <70% standardised bodyweight for age), where physical complications supervene (e.g. hypokalaemia and hypothermia) or where out-patient treatments have failed.

Bulimia nervosa

Bulimia nervosa is characterised by frequent loss of control of eating (bingeing), self-induced vomiting and fear of fatness.

Intercurrent depression and difficulties with impulse control in other areas (e.g. alcohol use, sexual behaviour and deliberate risk-taking) are common. The psychosocial context in which bulimia arises is often similar to that found in depression, but an antecedent history of dieting is usually evident.

Treatment is usually on an out-patient basis and focal psycho-therapies such as cognitive–behavioural therapy (CBT) are effective both in individual and group treatment settings. Antidepressant medications, such as SSRIs, are indicated where more severe depressive symptoms are evident.

CHAPTER 9
COMMON BEHAVIOURAL AND DEVELOPMENTAL PROBLEMS

Rick Jarman
Jill Sewell

Behavioural and developmental problems are best understood in a transactional framework, where symptoms and signs are the result of the interaction between inborn biological attributes of the child and factors within the environment.

INFANT 'COLIC'

Colic is defined as the excessive crying of undetermined cause in young infants. The crying develops during the early weeks of life and may persist until the baby is 3 or 4 months of age. Crying often lasts for several hours, is worse in the late afternoon and evening, and is associated with a drawing up of the knees and passage of flatus as if in pain. However, there is no evidence that colic is associated with abdominal pain, or that it represents anything more than the upper limit of crying seen in all young infants over the early months of life. Wessel's[1] definition of 'paroxysms of irritability, fussing or crying lasting for more than 3 h per day for 3 or more days per week for 3 or more weeks' identifies a group of infants who cry more than 90% of other babies their age.

Colic should be distinguished from:
- Otitis media, raised intracranial pressure, corneal abrasion, intestinal obstruction, urinary tract infection via history, examination, and urine examination.
- Cow milk intolerance (rare without vomiting, abdominal distension, diarrhoea or skin rashes).
- Lactose intolerance (frothy stools and abdominal distension).
- Gastro-oesophageal reflux with oesophagitis (rare without vomiting).

Management

- Reassurance that the infant is not sick or in pain, and that some babies cry more than others in early infancy because of an intrinsic sensitivity or environmental overload, or both.
- Regular supportive contact with parents; monitor for maternal depression.
- Reduce environmental overstimulation: noise, light and excessive handling.
- Adherence to routines.
- Demand feeding, keeping in a semi-upright posture and quiet room, using subdued lighting and comfortable chair.
- Carrying in an infant *snuggly*, using a dummy, giving baby massages, gentle rocking and patting.
- Medication (e.g. phenobarbitone) is rarely indicated.
- Random changes of feed/formula are not advised, nor are trials on antireflux therapy unless reflux is strongly suspected on clinical grounds or confirmed on oesophagoscopy/pH monitoring (see Gastrointestinal Conditions, chapter 23).

SLEEP PROBLEMS

Most new babies do not establish nocturnal sleeping patterns until 3 months of age, or sleep through the night until 6 months. Up to one-third of Australian children continue to wake once or more per night until 3–4 years of age. In the majority of cases these 'abnormal' sleep rhythms are learned behaviours, the child never having learned how to drop off to sleep on his or her own, or to get back to sleep after rousing through the night as part of the normal cycle of sleep without parental help. If parents and children are not unduly distressed by this behaviour there is no reason to intervene. Behavioural techniques are best reserved for dealing with sleep problems in infants over 6 months of age.

Medical causes of sleep disturbance are rare and can be ruled out on history, examination and limited laboratory investigation before a behavioural program is commenced. Think about *otitis media with effusion, upper airway obstruction causing obstructive sleep apnoea, gastro-oesophageal reflux, nocturnal seizures and raised intracranial pressure* as conditions that might cause night time 'arousals'. Psychosocial stresses such as family conflict, maternal depression, parental separation, moving house or other major disruptions to routine can also trigger sleep problems. However, serious psychological problems in children with sleep disturbance are uncommon.

Management

Ask parents to keep a 24 h diary of the child's sleep patterns for several days prior to any intervention.

To settle problems at bedtime

- Note the time and duration of daytime naps and set a temporarily later bedtime.
- Adhere to a strict pre-bedtime routine, so that the child moves through the same sequence in the same order each night.
- Ensure quiet time immediately prior to bedtime.
- Feed the baby/toddler before taking them to the bedroom.
- Farewell other family members and take the child into the bedroom awake.
- Use a night light and a fur toy for toddlers and preschoolers, and place a door gate across the doorway for children old enough to be in a bed.
- Leave the room within a few minutes; prolonged parental presence in the bedroom exacerbates separation difficulties.
- Return the child to his or her room if he or she comes out and use a door gate to block the escape route if this becomes a persistent problem.
- Ignore requests for drinks, snacks, back rubs, and so on after bedtime.
- Use 'extinction' or 'controlled crying' for persistent crying after leaving the bedroom (see below).
- If this is too difficult, sit with the child until he or she falls asleep, and use minimal handling.

For frequent waking through the night

One of three standard behavioural techniques can be used. The primary goal of these techniques is to teach the child to get back to sleep with less and less help from the parents, and any associated props, until he or she can do this on his or her own.

(i) *Extinction* – ignore the child's crying until he or she drops back to sleep.

(ii) *Controlled crying* – respond to the child's crying at progressively lengthening intervals until he or she drops back to sleep. For example, let the child cry for 2 min and then go into the bedroom. Soothe the child and leave the room. Wait 4 min before going back the second time, 6 min before going back the third time, 8 min before going back the fourth time, and so on, until the child cries himself or herself back to sleep.

(iii) *Camping out* – one parent sleeps in the child's room for 2 weeks on a camp stretcher next to the child's bed/cot. When the child wakes the parent touches and soothes by talking softly until he or she drops back to sleep. Over the next 2 weeks the parent progressively moves the camp stretcher further and further away from the child's bed/cot, and tries to soothe the child with less and less input until the child drops back to sleep spontaneously. The parent then moves back to his or her own bed.

A graded approach where props (e.g. parental presence, feeds and dummies) are withdrawn one at a time over several weeks suits many parents better than trying to do this all at once.

Whichever behavioural technique is used, it is important that spontaneous arousals are not reinforced by feeding, or the use of dummies or excessive parental attention through the night.

Sedative medication given nightly for 1–2 weeks (Trimeprazine 2–4 mg/kg per dose (max 25 mg), Chloral hydrate 25–50 mg/kg per dose (max 2 g)) can be used as a supplement to the behavioural techniques listed above, but only in children over 12 months of age.

Parasomnias

Parasomnias such as night terrors, sleep-walking, and sleep-talking are not true night-time arousals because they occur in deep stage 4 sleep. *Night terrors*, the most disturbing of these disorders, are characterised by the child suddenly screaming and thrashing about through the night, and occasionally running around the house in a state of high agitation. The child is usually inconsolable and has no memory of the event afterwards. The parasomnias cluster in two age ranges: 2–3 year olds and 6–9 year olds. They are self-limiting over a period of weeks to months, and usually require no active treatment other than to usher the child back to bed and sit with him or her until the agitated state has settled. Persistent problems may be treated with scheduled waking (waking the child 30 min before an expected arousal) or medication (imipramine 0.5–1.5 mg/kg per dose (max 25–75 mg), or both, or clonazepam 0.02 mg/kg per dose (max 0.5 mg) for 6–8 weeks).

OPPOSITIONAL BEHAVIOUR

Resistant and oppositional behaviour is universal in young children from time to time, and is rarely an indicator of individual or family psychopathology. Surveys indicate that over 75% of parents of 2, 3 and 4 year olds report their children to be stubborn and disobedient on a frequent basis. Most oppositional behaviour in school-age children and adolescents is also developmentally normal, provided it is not associated with violent or antisocial behaviour, or serious school difficulties. Diagnostic interviews with the child and family are necessary to exclude serious pathology that might warrant referral for psychotherapy. Standardised child behaviour checklists completed by parents or teachers, or both, help quantify the severity of the behaviour disturbance objectively, and can be used as an important adjunct to the above.

Management

In most instances, general supportive counselling and behaviour modification is highly effective in working with parents of younger children, as follows:

Praise and reward the child's 'good' behaviour

When children are being difficult they rarely receive much attention for good behaviour. To redress this balance, parents can be encouraged to 'catch the child being good' as often as possible. Verbal praise works best if it is immediate and specific, and if the parents 'praise the behaviour and not the child'.

Special behaviours can be acknowledged with concrete rewards, given after the fact, not offered as a bribe beforehand. Green marks with a texta pen or stamps on the back of the child's hand work well for toddlers. For the over 2 year olds, 'good boy' or 'good girl' sticker charts attached to the refrigerator door are very powerful visual reinforcers of positive behaviour. Lucky dips or points/poker chips that can be cashed in later for an agreed-on set of rewards are effective for older children. Rewards and punishments should be kept separate, lest the difficult child quickly slides into debt!

Prioritise the child's difficult behaviour

Parents need to save their energy for the behaviours that matter most. Punishments lose their effectiveness if overused. Parents should nominate and agree on two or three high-priority behaviours that they will tackle actively in the first instance; everything else by definition becomes a lesser priority behaviour.

Ignore lesser priority difficult behaviours

Many irritating behaviours are exacerbated by the parental attention they attract. Breaking eye contact, staying calm and walking away will lessen these behaviours if all family members are consistent and parents can persist with this for at least several days.

Provide immediate discipline for high-priority difficult behaviour

Consequences work best if they are applied immediately for high-priority behaviours such as non-compliance, oppositionalism and physical aggression. Parents should work towards staying calm, avoiding threats and applying consequences immediately without second chances.

Time out is the preferred disciplinary consequence for children over 18 months of age. *Time out* can be applied in a playpen, a chair in the corner, the bedroom, the back steps, or if away from home, against a fence or in the car. The child should stay in time out for a maximum of 1 min per year of age; if they leave time out without permission they should be returned and the time started again.

Withdrawing privileges is effective for children over 6 years old. Withdrawals work best if they are enacted as soon as possible after the offending behaviour occurs, and if the punishment is over and done with within 24 h. Punishments do not have to cause suffering to be effective.

Refining the way parents handle young children is often all that is necessary to bring many non-compliant behaviours under control. These techniques can be applied sequentially by the doctor over three to four 30 min sessions.

TEMPER TANTRUMS

A normal developmental task of toddlers is to assert their independence and test parental limits. The 'terrible two's' and the resultant tantrums that herald this developmental stage actually start in most children at 15–18 months, and often persist until 3–4 years of age.

Management

Based on the principles listed above, tantrums are best ignored, providing both parents persist with this strategy and follow the guidelines below:

- Stay calm.
- Look away.
- Move away.
- Say nothing.
- Go into another room and busy yourself with something else (lock the door if necessary).
- Persistently ignore this behaviour until the tantrum stops.
- Praise appropriate behaviour as soon as it occurs.

Ignoring a behaviour that has previously attracted attention will result in its escalation over the first few days before the behaviour starts to decline.

BREATH-HOLDING

Breath-holding has a peak incidence in the toddler years, occurring in 5% of all children. Both cyanotic and acyanotic (pallid) events have been described, the former being much more common. Cyanotic spells are inevitably triggered by the child encountering frustration, becoming distressed and crying intensely. The child then holds his or her breath at the end of expiration and becomes centrally cyanosed, often losing consciousness in the process. Occasionally, the loss of consciousness is followed by a generalised seizure. Consciousness is usually regained within 15–30 s. Discrimination from a primary seizure disorder is made on the basis of the breath-holding child becoming cyanosed *before* losing consciousness, with the prodrome as described above.

Acyanotic 'breath-holding' attacks are vasovagal spells (simple faints) that occur in response to fear or pain. Crying is minimal, with the child suddenly becoming apnoeic and losing consciousness. The child is pale and bradycardic during such episodes.

Management

- Reassurance that breath-holding spells are harmless and require no active treatment.
- Avoid reinforcing the tantruming behaviour through excessive parental anxiety or attention (see Temper tantrums above).
- Coma position until the child regains consciousness spontaneously.

HEAD-BANGING

Head-banging is a common distressing behaviour manifest by young children, occurring in 5–15% of normal infants and toddlers. Head-banging typically occurs up to 60–80 times per min and lasts for several minutes to 1 hour or more per episode. The child almost always appears undistressed; in fact, the association between head-banging and other repetitive behaviours in children (e.g. body-rocking and thumb-sucking) has led most experts to view this activity as one of self-soothing. The child almost never sustains significant injury as a result of head-banging, although mild bruising and abrasions are common. In developmentally delayed, autistic or severely emotionally deprived children, head-banging may occur with enough force to warrant the use of helmets or psychotropic medication (e.g. thioridizine), or both. In these cases referral to a behavioural paediatrician is warranted.

Management

- Reassure parents that head-banging is a normal self-limiting behaviour in most children and will not cause brain damage.
- Avoid reinforcing the behaviour through excessive parental attention or punishment, or both.
- Distraction or ignoring such behaviours are the 'treatments' of choice, although spontaneous resolution almost always occurs by the age of 3.

EATING/FEEDING PROBLEMS

See also Infant and Child Nutrition, chapter 7.

Through the second and third year of life the normal growth rate of children decreases dramatically, as does the relative requirement for most nutrients. The average monthly weight gain in children between 6–12 months of age is 500 g, compared to 183 g for children between 12–24 months and 166 g for children between 2–3 years of age. Most parents are concerned about the apparent poor weight gain and food intake of their toddlers, even though they may have been reassured that their child is growing at a normal rate for that particular age. This concern arises at the very time toddlers are asserting their independence and coming to a rapid understanding about the power that not eating has on their relationships to their parents! It is a truism that if a child is physically healthy and active, most meal-time problems are behaviour problems not medical problems.

The correlates of poor eating behaviour in toddlers include:
- Variable meal times
- Grazing between meals
- Excessive juice or milk (or both) intake
- Excessive parental attention to eating.

Management
- Rule out physical causes of poor eating such as reflux oesophagitis, milk allergy, lactose intolerance, pharyngeal incoordination and neurological disorders.
- Monitor the child's growth velocity on standardised charts.
- Help the parents to adopt reasonable expectations about the child's eating behaviour and support them in their anxiety about the child not eating. Help the parents to 'back off'!
- Establish clear meal-time routines and insist that the child sit with the family at meal times.
- Restrict milk or juice (or both) intake.
- Restrict between-meal grazing.
- Encourage independent feeding with finger foods.
- Ignore poor eating behaviour.

- Don't prepare special meals or pander to 'exotic' tastes.
- Praise and reward appropriate eating behaviour.

PHYSICAL AGGRESSION

Physical aggression is a common reaction to frustration in young children and is often modelled on similar behaviour within the family or social environment. The origins of serious aggressive behaviour are multi-faceted and are usually the result of a complex series of interactions between the following:

- Child factors – temperament, genetic endowment, brain injury, low IQ, learning difficulties, chronic illnesses and psychopathology.
- Family factors – parenting incompetence, inadequate monitoring, poor modelling, parental criminality, parental psychopathology, physical/sexual abuse and poverty.
- Social factors – sociocultural norms, media influences, school failure, socioeconomic disadvantage and lack of vocational opportunities.

The doctor should explore these issues with the child and family, and formulate probable contributing factors. At a practical level the doctor can work with parents on fine-tuning the way they handle such behaviours (see Oppositional behaviour). Providing clear and consistent disciplinary limits will help the child to develop better self-control. Also, when smacking is used as a punishment, it models physical violence and sends an ambiguous message to children about the appropriateness of hitting another person. It should therefore be avoided. Time out, the withdrawal of privileges, or both, as described above, are the consequences of choice for aggressive behaviour for children under 10 years of age.

Management

Referral for psychotherapy is indicated if aggression is:

- Repeated
- Severe
- Causes injury
- Is associated with a lack of remorse, other delinquent/antisocial behaviours or family psychopathology.

STEALING

Isolated minor theft is surprisingly common in school-aged Australian children, and while not acceptable, it is usually not an indication of serious pathology. Isolated theft is often associated with one or more of the following characteristics:

- Low self-esteem in a child searching for peer acceptance.
- A reaction to recent family or psychosocial stress.
- A cry for help and attention, with a subconscious desire to be caught.
- Typical school-age risk-taking behaviour.

Stealing may also be associated with the same child, family and social factors seen in children with other conduct/antisocial behaviours (see Physical aggression).

Management

- Insist that the child returns the stolen goods or personally apologises/confronts the person(s) they were stolen from, or both.
- Make the child pay partially for the stolen items through a deduction in pocket money, or by working off the debt.
- Punishment may include the withdrawal of privileges such as grounding, the restriction of TV, and so on.
- Refer the child for psychotherapy if stealing is recurrent, associated with a lack of remorse, or other antisocial/delinquent behaviours.

ATTENTION DEFICIT HYPERACTIVITY DISORDER (ADHD)

ADHD is not a disease. It is merely the most recent label used to describe children who display developmentally inappropriate degrees of inattentiveness, impulsivity and sometimes overactivity relative to what one would expect for their age. Many children with ADHD are not hyperactive at all, some may be under-active. Three subtypes of ADHD have now been described, based on the presence or absence of hyperactivity/impulsivity:

- A predominantly inattentive subtype.
- A predominantly hyperactive/impulsive subtype.
- A combined subtype.

For the diagnosis to be confirmed the clinician must obtain a history that the child has been like this since early in life, that the behaviour has been a problem in more than one situation (at home and at school), and that medical and other psychiatric conditions that may mimic ADHD have been ruled out. Most importantly, the DSM IV criteria (see Table 9.1) need to be fulfilled.

ADHD appears to have a strong biological basis, but its manifestations are modified by family and social factors. Differences have been noted between ADHD and non-ADHD children in brain neurochemistry, autonomic arousal, cerebral blood flow, frontal lobe electrical activation patterns and CNS glucose metabolism. A genetic component to ADHD is now established. At this time, however, it is impossible to reconcile the results of this disparate research under a unifying biological theory. More than one biological contribution may exist in any given child.

Assessment

Assessment of ADHD should include some or all of the following:
- A child and family interview.
- Physical and neurological examination.
- Assessment of visual acuity.
- Referral for audiological assessment, including testing in background noise.
- Serum lead level in children from high-risk groups.
- Observation of the child's behaviour in the office is *not* a reliable guide to the child's behaviour in other settings and should not be used to either confirm or refute the diagnosis of ADHD.
- Standardised child behaviour checklists completed by parents and teachers enable the child's behaviour to be compared with same-age children and is one of the most important tools of diagnosis.
- Referral for formal cognitive testing – 25% of children with ADHD have coexistent learning disabilities.

Management

This involves a combination of the following:

Table 9.1 DSM IV diagnostic criteria for ADHD

A. Either 1 or 2

1. *Inattention*

   At least six of the following nine symptoms have persisted for at least 6 months to a degree that is maladaptive and inconsistent with developmental level

   - Often fails to give close attention to details or makes careless mistakes in school work, work or other activities
   - Often does not seem to listen to what is being said to him or her
   - Often has difficulty sustaining attention in tasks or play activities
   - Often does not follow through on instructions and fails to finish schoolwork chores or duties in the workplace (not due to oppositional behaviour or failure to understand instructions)
   - Often has difficulty organising tasks or activities
   - Often avoids or strongly dislikes tasks (such as schoolwork or homework) that require sustained mental effort
   - Often loses things necessary for tasks or activities (eg. school assignments, pencils, books, tools or toys)
   - Often easily distracted by extraneous stimuli
   - Often forgetful in daily activities

2. *Hyperactivity/Impulsivity*

   At least six of the following nine symptoms of hyperactivity/impulsivity have persisted for at least 6 months to a degree that is maladaptive and inconsistent with developmental level

   Hyperactivity
   - Often fidgets with hands or feet and squirms in seat
   - Leaves seat in classroom or in other situations in which remaining seated is expected
   - Often runs about or climbs excessively in situations where it is inappropriate (in adolescents or adults may be limited to feelings of restlessness)
   - Often has difficulty playing or engaging in leisure activities quietly
   - Is often on the go and acts as if driven by a motor
   - Often talks excessively

   Impulsivity
   - Often blurts out answers to questions before the questions have been completed
   - Often has difficulty waiting in line or awaiting turn in games or group situations
   - Often interrupts or intrudes on others

B. Onset no later than 7 years of age
C. Symptoms must be present in two or more situations (eg. at school, at home and/or at work)
D. The disturbance causes clinically significant distress or impairment in social, academic, or occupational functioning
E. Does not occur exclusively during the course of a pervasive developmental disorder, schizophrenia, or other psychotic disorder, and is not better accounted for by a mood disorder, anxiety disorder, or dissociative disorder, or a personality disorder

Parent training

Parents often benefit from working with a doctor or psychologist to fine-tune the way they handle their child's behaviour at home. Good handling often helps the ADHD child's behaviour settle. Ideas for praising and rewarding good behaviour, ignoring minor irritating behaviour, giving directions, and providing consequences for serious negative behaviour are usually addressed in parent training.

Advice to schools

School is often the area where ADHD children have most difficulty because of the demands placed on the child's concentration and behaviour. The ADHD child will require clear rules and routines, a centre-front seating position, more one-on-one attention, positive reinforcement for focused and attentive behaviour, and frequent stretch breaks.

Counselling

Children and parents sometimes benefit from the opportunity to talk through their feelings of distress with a counsellor, and to resolve issues of conflict that are making their lives unhappy. While counselling will not make ADHD go away, it can help people understand the basis for the conflict at home and to find solutions. Family sessions, individual therapy or anger management/social skills training can be incorporated into a counselling framework depending on the nature of the problem.

Medication

Medication treatment is not a cure for ADHD but can ameliorate its symptoms. Of all the treatments available, medication is the most dramatically effective and may augment the success of other strategies such as parent training. Although stimulants (dexamphetamine 0.2 mg/kg (max 10 mg) orally, daily increasing to a max of 0.6 mg/kg (max 30 mg) 12 hourly and methylphenidate 0.25 mg/kg daily, orally increasing to a max of 2 mg/kg daily are the most widely used and effective medication treatments, antidepressants (tricyclics, SSRIs and reversible MAO inhibitors), alpha-adrenergic agonists (clonidine), and neuroleptics (thioridazine, risperidone) can be used either alone or in combination, depending on the target symptoms that are most troublesome.

Dexamphetamine and methylphenidate are usually given in two divided doses at breakfast and lunchtime, with an occasional after-school dose in older children to help with homework. Weekend and holiday breaks off the medication are occasionally given but are not necessary. About 80% of ADHD children treated with stimulants display dramatic improvements in behaviour, academic performance, cognitive processing and socialisation. Side effects include decreased appetite, insomnia, tearfulness and nausea, most of which are transient.

Prognosis

Despite the short- and medium-term efficacy of treatment, about 80% of ADHD children will have symptoms through adolescence/adulthood, with 30% having ongoing major problems with academic underachievement, early school dropout, antisocial behaviour and delinquency.

TICS AND TOURETTE'S DISORDER

A tic is a sudden, rapid, recurrent, non-rhythmic and stereotyped motor movement or vocalisation, experienced as irresistible but suppressible for a varying length of time. Tics may be motor or vocal, simple or complex. Motor tics include eye blinking, neck jerking, facial grimacing and shoulder shrugging. Vocal tics may involve throat clearing, grunting, sniffing, barking or involuntary repeating of words or phrases out of context. When children display multiple motor tics and one or more vocal tics occurring many times per day over 1 year, the condition is called Tourette's Disorder. Tics of any origin or severity almost always disappear during sleep, and may be exacerbated by anxiety or attention.

The associated features of this disorder include obsessive–compulsive disorder (OCD), ADHD and learning difficulties. Tics may be exacerbated or unmasked by stimulant medication or stress. Tics need to be distinguished from partial epilepsies; particularly, central spike rolandic epilepsy.

Management

Tics are harmless but require treatment if they become socially disabling, or are associated with OCD or ADHD symptoms, or both. Start with antidepressants (tricyclics or SSRIs) if anxiety symptoms are pronounced. Clonidine is particularly useful if there are associated ADHD symptoms.

Pimozide or haloperidol are used if symptoms persist despite the above. Stimulant medication (dexamphetamine or methylphenidate) used to treat associated ADHD should be reduced but not necessarily stopped in children with tics, and only discontinued if tics remain incapacitating.

SPEECH AND LANGUAGE PROBLEMS

Delayed development of speech and language is common. The delay may occur alone or be associated with other conditions such as hearing impairment, general developmental delay, autism or social–emotional deprivation.

Indicators of speech and language difficulties may include parental concern, lack of babbling or vocalisation, unintelligible speech, poor language comprehension, lack of speech and dysfluency (see Table 9.2). Early referral to a speech therapist is important and should be considered as part of the paediatric assessment (see Table 9.3).

LEARNING DIFFICULTIES

Problems with learning affect 10–15% of the school-age population. Learning difficulties may be the result of global impairments in

Table 9.2 Indicators of language delay

Age (years)	Reason for concern
0.5	No response to sound, not cooing, not laughing
1	Not localising sound, no babble, no vocalisation
1.5	No meaningful words except *mum/dad*, not pointing to wanted things
2	Expressive vocabulary less than 20 words
2.5	Expressive vocabulary less than 50 words or no two-word combinations, not understanding simple instructions without gesture, stuttering
3	Not understood within family, not using early syntax (e.g. verb + ing *running*, noun + plural *hats*)
4	Not understood outside family, not using complex sentences (e.g. *and, but, because, if, when, so, before, after*)
5	Speech not reasonably clear, not fluent, not complex, not understood

Table 9.3 Assessment of language delay

What to consider	What to do
Hearing	Audiology referral
	ENT referral
Developmental delay	Paediatric assessment
Social–emotional context	Psychological assessment
Family history of speech/language/ fluency problems	Speech pathology referral
Specific speech/language disorder	Speech pathology referral
Stuttering	Speech pathology referral

cognitive capacity (intellectual disability), hearing or vision problems, chronic illness, medication side effects, severe emotional disturbance, primary attention deficits, low motivation, poor teaching, or specific deficits in the processing of spoken or written language – termed *specific learning disabilities*. Specific learning disabilities are characterised by a discrepancy between the child's overall intelligence and achievement in school that is not accounted for on the basis of conditions listed previously. Failure in school of any origin may cause secondary problems with self-esteem and behaviour.

Assessment

Assessment should include:
- History from the parents *and* teachers of the child's school difficulties. Request previous school reports, psychometric testing results, and details of behaviour at home and at school.
- Standardised child behaviour checklists completed by parents and teachers are an important adjunct to behavioural assessment; they enable the child's behaviour to be compared with other children's the same age.
- Physical and neurological examination to rule out chronic illnesses and underlying gross neurological problems. The traditional neurological examination is usually normal, although minor neurological signs may be present and include subtle abnormalities of tone, reflexes, motor coordination and sensory function.
- Referral to a paediatrician for neuro-developmental assessment. These tests sample aspects of development that are important for learning in school, including gross and fine motor coordination,

visual–spatial orientation, short-term auditory memory, visual sequencing, and language skills. Although neuro-developmental testing will shed further light on the child's strengths and weaknesses that might partially or fully explain their school difficulties, it is no substitute for formal psychological testing.

- Referral to an educational psychologist for formal cognitive testing, including tests of intelligence and academic achievement.

Management

- Individualised and dependent on cause(s).
- Collaborate with teachers and parents, and ensure that everyone (including the child) has a common understanding of the basis of the learning difficulty, and the accommodative strategies that can be used.
- Foster and promote the child's strengths.
- Individualised or small group remedial educational assistance is the cornerstone of intervention for most children. There is no single best approach. The clinician can advocate for extra resources in the classroom to assist the child, or recommend outside tutoring if help at school is not available.
- Behavioural counselling, social skills training, medication for attention deficits, and so on, can be recommended, depending on the associated problems identified.
- Monitor progress and re-evaluate at intervals.

Reference

1 Wessel, M.A., Cobb, J.C., Jacobsen, E.B., *et al.* (1954) Paroxysmal fussing in infancy, sometimes called 'colic', *Pediatrics*, **14**, pp. 421–4.

CHAPTER 10
DEVELOPMENTAL DELAY AND DISABILITY

Catherine Marraffa
Dinah Reddihough

ASSESSMENT OF CHILD DEVELOPMENT

Developmental surveillance is a flexible continuous process of skilled observation as part of providing routine health care. It should occur opportunistically whenever a child comes into contact with a health professional.

Approximately 3–5% of children have developmental delay of at least mild–moderate severity that may remain undiagnosed unless specific assessment is undertaken. In general, problems affecting motor development and speech present early, while problems affecting receptive language, socialisation and cognition present late. The clinician's role is to ascertain whether a child's development is significantly aberrant for his or her age and to determine the underlying reasons for this, realising that most developmental delay does not have a clearly identifiable medical basis.

DETECTION OF DEVELOPMENTAL DELAY

If a parent is concerned about a child's development it is highly likely that the child will have developmental delay after further definitive evaluation. However, a lack of concern from parents is no guarantee that the child's development is normal.

Informal clinical judgement is unreliable as a method for detecting developmental problems.

The milestone checklists (see Table 10.1) serve as an aide to memory by recording what is expected of the average child at each age in several domains of developmental function. Because they record average expectations for each age it is often difficult to distinguish

Table 10.1 Developmental milestones

Age*	Gross motor	Fine motor adaptive	Language	Personal–social
1 m	Lifts head momentarily while prone (0–3 w)	Visual following to mid-line (0–5 w)		Watches face (0–4 w)
2 m	Lifts head momentarily to erect position when sitting	Hands predominantly open	Vocalizes (0–7 w)	Smiles responsively (0–7 w)
3 m	Lifts head to 90° while prone (0–10 w)	Visual following past mid-line (0–10 w)	Laughs (6–10 w)	
4 m	Head steady when held erect (6–17 w)	Plays with hands together (6–15 w)	Goos and gurgles	Excited by approach of food
5 m	No head lag when pulled to sitting (3–6 m) Rolls over	Grasps rattle (10–18 w) Reaches for object with palmar grasp (3–5½ m)	Squeals (6–18 w)	Smiles spontaneously (6 w–5 m)
6 m	Lifts head forward when pulled to sit (19–19 w)	Passes block hand to hand (4½–7½ m)	Turns to voice (3½–8½ m)	Friendly to all comers
8 m	Maintains sitting position without support		Repetition of syllables (e.g. baba, Dada)	Feeds self biscuit (5–8 m) Tries to get toy out of reach (5–9 m)
10 m	Stands holding on (5–10 m)	Index finger approach	'Mum', 'Dad' without meaning (6–10 m)	Shy with strangers Plays peek-a-boo
12 m	Walks holding on to furniture (7½–12½ m)	Crude finger–thumb grasp (7–11 m)	Imitates speech sounds (6–11 m)	Gives up a toy

Continued overleaf

Table 10.1 Developmental milestones Cont'd

Age*	Gross motor	Fine motor adaptive	Language	Personal–social
15 m	Walks alone (11½–15 m)	Neat pincer grasp of pellet (9–15 m)	'Mum', 'Dad' with meaning (9–15 m)	Indicates wants (10½–14½ m)
1½ y	Walks well (11½–18 m)	Builds tower of two blocks (12–20 m)	Three words other than 'Mum', 'Dad' (12–20 m)	Drinks from cup (10–17 m)
2 y	Walks up steps without help (14–22 m)	Scribbles (12–24 m)	Points to one named body part (14–23 m)	Feeds self with spoon (12–24 m)
2½ y	Throws ball (15–32 m)	Builds tower of four blocks (15–26 m)	Combines two words (14–27 m)	Helps in house – simple tasks (15–24 m)
3 y	Pedals tricycle (21 m–3 y)	Imitates vertical line (18 m–3 y) Copies circle (2½–3½ y)	Uses three word sentences	Puts on clothes (2–3 y)
4 y	Balances on one foot (2¾–4½ y)	Copies square	Gives first and last name (2–4 y)	Dresses with supervision (2½–3½ y)
5 y	Hops on one foot (3–5 y)	Draws person in three parts (3–5 y)	Knows some colours (3–5 y) Knows age	Dresses without supervision (2½–5 y)

w, weeks; m, months; y, years.
* Age indicates when at least 90% of a normal group of children will achieve the test. Figures in parentheses represent the range from 25th to 90th centiles for achievement.

the child with true developmental delay from the normal child with below-average milestone attainment.

Formal screening tests such as the *Denver II* and the *Australian Developmental Screening Test* allow the objective discrimination of the child who *probably* has a developmental delay from the child who *probably* does not. Results of screening tests are not definitive; a fail on such a test requires referral of the child for formal developmental assessment.

Formal assessment involves a synthesis of the findings from history, physical and neurological examination, and developmental testing using standardised assessment tools such as the *Bayley Scales of Infant Development* and the *Griffiths Developmental Scales*.

The type of testing undertaken depends on the presence or absence of several risk factors for developmental delay:

Children at a very high risk of developmental problems

This includes those who show signs of developmental regression, abnormal neurological examination, dysmorphism, chromosomal abnormality, hearing or vision problems. In such cases:

- Bypass the developmental screening examination.
- Refer for comprehensive developmental assessment.

Children with a moderate risk of developmental problems

This includes those whose parents suspect developmental delay, history of severe pre- or perinatal insult, very low birthweight (<1500 g), family history of developmental delay, severe socioeconomic or family adversity. In such cases administer a formal screening test. Possible results and strategies include:

- Pass – reassure that development is within normal range and continue to monitor through a local doctor/maternal and child health nurse.
- Questionable – repeat the test 4 weeks later.
- Fail – refer for comprehensive developmental assessment.

Children at a low risk of developmental problems

This includes those with no parental or professional concerns, and with no other risk factors. In such cases, informal monitoring by a local doctor/maternal and child health nurse.

Should there be later parental or professional concerns a formal screening test is recommended. If there are no further concerns continue informal monitoring.

Children with confirmed developmental delay require:
- A referral to an early intervention program for developmental facilitation.
- A baseline investigation of the cause.

DEVELOPMENTAL DELAY AND DISABILITY

Children with developmental delay or disability, or both, have the same basic needs as non-disabled children. They have the potential for further development and the principles of normal development apply.

Specific disabilities in one area may cause secondary disabilities in other areas (e.g. children who have motor disabilities with reduced opportunity for exploration may suffer delayed development of their comprehension abilities).

Transient developmental delay may be associated with:
- Prematurity
- Physical illness
- Prolonged hospitalisation
- Family stress
- Lack of opportunities to learn.

Causes of *persistent developmental delay (developmental disability)* include:
- Language disorders
- Intellectual disability
- Cerebral palsy
- Autism
- Hearing impairment
- Visual impairment
- Degenerative disorders
- Neuromuscular disorders.

Once the suspicion regarding a child's development has been raised, a complete paediatric consultation is required. This should include full details of the family, obstetric, neonatal and developmental histories. Liaison with the family doctor and a maternal and child health nurse to obtain background information is often helpful. A history of loss of previously attained developmental skills is suggestive of regression rather than delay, and requires more comprehensive investigation to exclude neurodegenerative conditions. Observation of how the child looks, listens, moves, explores, plays, communicates and socialises is essential prior to the formal examination. Understandably, parents will be anxious and a sensitive approach is essential at all times.

Developmental assessment provides the family with an understanding of the child's development, and outlines developmental goals and strategies to facilitate development and reduce any handicapping effects of the disability. Assessment and management may include input from physiotherapists, speech pathologists, educationalists, occupational therapists, psychologists and social workers.

Principles of assessment

These include:

- Utilisation of play as a fundamental assessment tool
- Promotion of optimal performance of the child
- Gearing of the assessment towards remediation rather than merely producing a profile
- Involvement of the parents in the assessment process
- Close linking of the assessment service with those offering help and support.

Early intervention

Early intervention includes prevention and early detection of disabilities, as well as health, educational and community services that assist the child, family and community in adapting to the child's disability and developmental needs. Services are based on the principles of normalisation and the least restrictive alternative.

The aims of early intervention are to minimise the handicapping effects of the child's disability on his or her development and education, and to support the family in understanding and providing for their child's individual needs. Services include individual teaching and therapy (physio, speech and occupational therapy), family support and counselling, resourcing and support to child care and preschools, and respite care. Services are usually regionally based and are provided by government and non-government agencies.

Education

There are a range of special educational strategies to optimise learning and development, dependent on the child's abilities and disabilities, with increasing opportunities for integration as resources are moved from special to local schools. A range of special schools is also available.

Family supports

Parents need to be aware of the services that are available to them to assist in the care of their child with a disability. Supports include social security benefits, home help and respite care through foster agencies and community residential units. Consumer organisations can provide parent support, information and advocacy.

INTELLECTUAL DISABILITY

The definition of intellectual disability comprises three elements: (i) a significantly sub-average general intellectual functioning (i.e. two standard deviations below the mean of the intelligence quotient) that exists concurrently with; (ii) deficits in adaptive behaviour; and (iii) manifests during the developmental period.

This definition is used by service providers, as well as academics and legislators. The term *developmental disabilities* is used increasingly to reflect the complexity of development.

Up to 2.5% of children have an intellectual disability: approximately 2% mild and 0.5% moderate, severe or profound.

Causes of intellectual disability
Prenatal

- Chromosomal; e.g. trisomy 21 and Fragile X syndrome.
- Genetic; e.g. tuberose sclerosis and metabolic disorders.
- Syndromes; e.g. Williams and Prader–Willi.
- Infections; e.g. CMV.
- Drugs; e.g. alcohol.
- Major structural anomalies of the brain.

Perinatal

- Trauma.
- Hypoxia.
- Infections.
- Metabolic abnormalities.

Postnatal

- Head injury.
- Meningitis or encephalitis.
- Poisons.

Presentation

- At birth with a known syndrome or malformation.
- At the follow up of high-risk infants.
- Language delay.
- Global developmental delay.
- Learning difficulties.
- Behaviour problems.
- With associated medical complications (e.g. epilepsy).

The timing and type of insult can be determined in approximately 70% of children. The majority are caused by CNS insults during the prenatal period with 15% due to perinatal and 10% postnatal insults. The two most common causes of intellectual disability are trisomy 21 and Fragile X.

Investigations

Aetiological diagnosis is important to establish in order to understand prognosis, provide genetic counselling and to ensure that associated problems are detected.

The following investigations are important:
- Chromosomes, especially Fragile X, Williams, Prader–Willi using DNA probes
- MRI brain
- Creatinine phosphokinase in boys
- Plasma amino acids
- Urinary organic acids
- Thyroid function tests
- Mucopolysaccharide screen

- Investigation for congenital infection: ophthalmological and audiological examination, maternal/infant serology and viral culture (cytomegalovirus).

Despite thorough investigation, the cause is often not identified.

Management

- Regular assessment of vision and hearing.
- Investigation for associated anomalies (e.g. cardiac and thyroid status with trisomy 21).
- Treatment of associated disorders (e.g. epilepsy).
- Referral to and liaison with other practitioners, early intervention, family support and educational services.
- Monitoring of development.
- Support and information for parents.
- Child advocacy.

CEREBRAL PALSY

Cerebral palsy is a persistent but not unchanging disorder of movement and posture due to a defect or lesion of the developing brain. It occurs in about two per 1000 live births.

Aetiology

Cerebral palsy is not a single entity but a term used for a diverse group of disorders, which may relate to events in the prenatal, perinatal or postnatal periods. The cause is unknown in many children. Perinatal asphyxia accounts for less than 10% of cases, and postnatal illnesses or injuries for a further 10%. There is a significant association with prematurity. Infants with birth weights less than 1500 g are especially vulnerable to cerebral palsy, with a childhood prevalence of 60 per 1000 compared with an overall prevalence of two per 1000.

Classification

This is according to:

- The type of motor disorder (e.g. spasticity or athetosis).
- The distribution (e.g. hemiplegia, diplegia and quadriplegia).
- The severity of the motor disorder.

Associated disorders

- Visual problems.
- Hearing deficits.
- Communication disorders.
- Epilepsy.
- Intellectual disability.
- Learning disabilities.
- Perceptual problems.

Some children have only a motor disorder.

Management

Management of the child with cerebral palsy involves:

- An accurate diagnosis with genetic counselling.
- An assessment of the child's capabilities and referral to the appropriate services for the child and family. Liaising with the kindergarten, school and general practitioner is important.
- Management of the commonly associated disabilities and health problems:
  — All children require a *hearing* and *visual assessment.*
  — Careful assessment and management of *epilepsy.*
- Attention to *nutritional problems* – obesity can occur due to an imbalance between intake and physical activity. Conversely, children may be underweight, particularly in the presence of oromotor problems that may result in major feeding difficulties. Dietary advice is important. The presence of severe failure to thrive, major feeding problems or aspiration, or all of these, may be indications for non-oral feeding by a nasogastric or gastrostomy tube.
- Investigation and treatment of *gastro-oesophageal reflux* that commonly occurs in cerebral palsy.
- Advice regarding *constipation.*
- Management of *drooling* with techniques employed by speech pathologists, or by the use of medication or surgery in a small group of children.
- Awareness that *aspiration and lung disease* may be associated with impaired oromotor control. Chronic cough with wheeze or repeated lower respiratory infections may indicate the presence of chronic lung disease. Videofluroscopy is a useful test for the detection of aspiration.

- Psychological and social difficulties, which require careful attention.

Orthopaedic management

The orthopaedic management of cerebral palsy requires a team approach. Dynamic spasticity, which interferes with function in young children, is best managed by conservative methods; e.g. orthotics, inhibitory casts or the use of botulinum toxin A. Surgery is mainly undertaken on the lower limb, but is occasionally helpful in the upper limb. Some children also require surgery for scoliosis. Physiotherapy is an essential part of postoperative management. Gait laboratories are useful in planning the surgical program for ambulant children.

The critical parts of the body to observe are:

- The hip – non-walkers and those only partially ambulant are prone to hip subluxation and eventual dislocation. Early detection is important and hip X-rays should be performed at yearly intervals or more frequently if there is concern. Dislocation, which may cause pain and difficulty with perineal hygiene, is extremely difficult to treat once it occurs, and prevention by early adductor releases is a better strategy. Hip problems may also occur in mobile children; e.g. those with severe hemiplegia. However, this is rare.
- The knee – hamstring surgery may be necessary to improve gait pattern, or the ability to stand for transfers.
- The ankle – there may be a range of problems around the foot and ankle. Conservative treatments are used in young children but surgical correction is frequently required later.

Referrals

Referral to and ongoing liaison with allied health professionals is essential to enable children to achieve their optimal physical potential and independence.

- Physiotherapists give practical advice to parents and carers on positioning, handling and play to minimise the effects of abnormal muscle tone and encourage the development of movement skills. They also give advice regarding mobility aids, the use of orthoses or special seating. They may provide individual or group treatments or refer to appropriate community services.

- Occupational therapists help parents to develop their child's upper limb and self-care skills, and are also involved in suggesting suitable toys, equipment and house adaptations for home care.
- Speech pathologists provide guidance for those with severe eating and drinking difficulties, and communication and augmentative communication systems for children with limited verbal skills.
- Orthotists provide advice, design, fabricate and fit various braces. These braces are used to improve function, support, align, prevent or correct deformities to different parts of the child's body – more commonly the lower limbs. As part of the allied health team, orthotists work closely with orthopaedic surgeons and physiotherapists to optimise the child's potential.
- Other professionals that may be helpful include medical social workers, nurses, psychologists and special education teachers.
- General practitioners play an important role in supporting these children and their families in the community.

SPINA BIFIDA (MYELOMENINGOCELE)

Spina bifida is the commonest severe congenital malformation of the nervous system. The degree of impairment from the spinal cord pathology varies. Most children have some element of lower limb dysfunction, sensory loss, and a neurogenic bladder and bowel. Eighty per cent have progressive hydrocephalus requiring surgery. Many children have specific learning problems.

Prevention

Periconceptional folic acid supplementation (in the month before and in the first 3 months of pregnancy) has been shown to reduce the risk of recurrence in any at-risk family (by about 75%), as well as occurrence in any family. Recommended doses are:

- Low-risk women (no family history of neural tube defects): 0.5 mg daily.
- Women with a previous child with a neural tube defect (or personal, partner or close family history): 4 mg daily (5 mg if 4 mg formulations are not available).

Note: Multivitamin supplements are not recommended because of the potential risks of vitamin overdose to the developing foetus.

Fortification of staple foods with folate has been recommended in many countries. Fewer children are now being born with neural tube defects due to antenatal diagnosis and termination of pregnancy.

Management

Management requires collaboration between health, education and welfare professionals and the child and family. Most children attend regular schools. Families require a great deal of support.

An interdisciplinary team of physicians, a neuropsychologist, physiotherapist, orthotist, occupational therapist, social worker and stomal therapist develops appropriate developmental and rehabilitation programs, in collaboration with the family, general practitioners and community agencies (including local primary care service providers).

Initial management

- Neurosurgical and paediatric assessment of the newborn infant is undertaken to determine if early surgery to close the spinal defect should be recommended. Clinical and ultra-sound observation to detect and monitor the presence of hydrocephalus is important.
- Orthopaedic and urological consultations and investigations are undertaken in the neonatal period to provide baseline information for subsequent management. A small number of infants require early management of talipes or a high-pressure neurogenic bladder.
- The families must be fully informed about the diagnosis, natural history and prognosis, and be reassured that assistance is available.

Specific aspects of management

Children should be monitored regularly by medical and therapy staff.

Mobility

- Whatever the degree of lower limb impairment, independent mobility is the primary goal of the orthopaedic surgeon, physiotherapist and orthotist.

- Almost all children learn to walk during childhood. The degree of assistance required in the form of surgery, bracing, crutches, and so on, varies with the level of the lesion. Those with high lesions often choose in adolescence to use a wheelchair as their primary method of mobility.

Urinary tract

- The primary goals of the urologist and stomal therapist are the establishment of urinary continence (dryness) at a developmentally appropriate age, and the maintenance of satisfactory renal function.
- Clean intermittent catheterisation is now the preferred method of treatment. Not all children become dry, and additional support may be necessary in the form of medication (e.g. an oxybutinin 5 mg dose 8–12 hourly), protective clothing and condom drainage. Bladder augmentation or the insertion of artificial urinary sphincters, or both, may be required.
- Urinary tract infections (UTI) are common and should be treated in the usual way. Younger children and those with an ileal conduit present with constitutional symptoms. Recurrent UTI require investigation.
- Children with urinary continence problems should have a urological assessment regularly: every 6–12 months in infancy and every 1–2 years in childhood.

Neurological functioning

- The neural tube defect is closed early or late, depending on the form of neonatal management undertaken after discussion among the neurosurgeon, paediatrician and family.
- If hydrocephalus becomes established a ventriculoperitoneal shunt is inserted. Problems with the ventriculoperitoneal shunt are common.
- In those infants for whom conservative early treatment is undertaken, a shunting procedure may precede excision of the lesion. Careful observation of the head circumference should be undertaken in all individuals who survive the perinatal period.
- Careful follow up of shunt functioning is required. Children with shunts should have neurosurgical assessment regularly (in infancy every 6–9 months; in childhood and adolescence at least every 1–2 years). See also Neurologic Conditions, chapter 29.

- Tethering of the spinal cord to surrounding structures occurs in most children. In a small number, traction on the cord causes deterioration in neurological functioning. Regular detailed assessment of muscle strength and function is important to recognise early signs of cord tethering and traction problems. Surgical detethering may be required.
- Children often have specific cognitive difficulties and a neuro-psychological assessment is usually carried out prior to school entry and repeated before transition to secondary school.

Miscellaneous medical problems

- Scoliosis, and possibly kyphosis, are common management problems.
- Pressure sores occur in all children with spina bifida at some time, most commonly on the feet or the buttocks.
- Pathological fractures occur infrequently, and usually in those with a high lesion. Common symptoms are local swelling and erythema, with or without deformity, and usually without pain.
- Constipation is a common long-term difficulty but may present as an acute impaction. Dietary advice, laxatives and enemas may be required. For children with severe continence problems, anal plugs can be used following careful assessment by the stomal therapist.
- Epilepsy. Some 15% of children with spina bifida have epilepsy. Treatment is along the usual lines. See also Neurologic con-ditions, chapter 29.
- Latex allergy. Testing is offered to all children. It is not a common problem but has serious implications. See also Allergy and Immunology, chapter 14.

Adolescent issues

- Delayed or precocious puberty can occur.
- Specific adolescent issues including sexuality, relationship dif-ficulties and contraception should be addressed.
- Mental health should be monitored.
- Vocational support is important.
- Transition and transfer to adult services provides a big challenge and needs careful planning and support for the young person.

CHAPTER 11
CHILD ABUSE AND NEGLECT

Anne Smith

DEFINITIONS

Child physical abuse

Child physical abuse is the physical trauma inflicted on a child. Objective evidence of this violence may include bruising, burns and scalds, head injuries, fractures, intra-abdominal and intrathoracic trauma, suffocation, and drowning. The injury may be caused by impact, penetration, heat, a caustic substance, a chemical or a drug. The definition also includes Munchausen's syndrome by proxy.

Child neglect

Child neglect is the failure of caregivers to adequately provide for and safeguard the health, safety and wellbeing of the child.

Child sexual abuse

Child sexual abuse is the involvement of dependent, developmentally immature children and adolescents in sexual activities that they do not fully comprehend and to which they are unable to give consent.

Psychological maltreatment

Psychological maltreatment of children and youths consists of acts of omission and commission that are judged on the basis of a combination of community standards and professional expertise to be psychologically damaging. Such acts are committed by individuals, singly or collectively, who by their characteristics (e.g. age, status, knowledge and organisational form) are in a position of differential power that renders a child vulnerable. Such acts damage, immediately or ultimately, the behavioural, cognitive, affective or physical functioning of the child. Examples of psychological maltreatment include acts of spurning (hostile, rejecting or degrading), terrorising, isolating, exploiting or corrupting, and denying emotional responsiveness.

Signs of neglect and emotional abuse are often non-specific, but suspicion should be raised when infants, preschoolers or school-age children behave in the following ways:

- They are persistently angry, socially avoidant, defiant, disobedient and overactive.
- They are anxiously attached, watchful of their patients, have a limited ability to enjoy things, or are intensely ambivalent to parents.
- They have low self-esteem, are depressed or unresponsive, have developmental and emotional retardation, poor social skills and over-inhibition.

Signs of sexual abuse are also usually non-specific, but may include the above and various behaviour problems (phobias, bad dreams, eating and sleeping disorders, depression, school problems or delinquency). There may be overt manifestations of sexual preoccupation, including precocious and inappropriate sexual activity, promiscuity and aggressive sexual behaviour.

Psychiatric consultation is often useful in conjunction with the involvement of local child protection services.

IDENTIFYING CHILD PHYSICAL ABUSE

Professionals dealing with injured children must become familiar with the manifestations of accidental and inflicted trauma. A thorough and detailed history must be taken of the alleged mechanism of injury. Determine when, where and how the injury occurred. Note who witnessed the injury. Note the child's developmental capabilities.

When an injury appears to be inflicted rather than accidental it is important to obtain details of the child's past medical, social and family history. A parent or legal guardian must give informed consent prior to the child's physical examination.

A thorough physical examination must be performed. Record injuries on a body chart and use diagrams whenever possible. Accurate measurements are essential. Include details of the site, size, colour and shape of all injuries, and skin lesions (including injuries thought to result from accidental trauma).

Look for:

- Skin injuries such as bruises, petechiae, lacerations, abrasions, and puncture wounds. Note injuries that may be inflicted by a human hand (finger marks from a slap or finger-tip bruising from a firm grip) or an instrument.
- Intra-oral injuries such as a torn frenulum, contused gums, dental trauma or petechiae on the soft palate.
- Nasal trauma such as a nasal septal haematoma.
- Ear trauma – remember to inspect behind the pinnae and examine both tympanic membranes.
- Eye trauma – examine for all objective evidence of injury from the lids to the retinae.
- Internal injuries – injuries to internal organs in the thorax and abdomen.
- Genital trauma.

Investigations

- Consider the carrying out of clotting studies and a full-blood examination for children with bruising.
- X-ray sites of clinically suspected fracture.
- Bone scan if the child is less than 3 years and occult or healing fractures are suspected. (*Note*: a bone scan is not a sensitive tool for the detection of skull fractures, therefore perform a skull X-ray as well if skull fracture is considered.)
- A skeletal survey should be performed if a bone scan is not available for the child less than 3 years and occult or healing fracture is suspected.
- Photography is a very important means of documenting injuries. Note the need for a colour wheel and tape measure. Also note that photography augments a detailed written description of injuries.

Interviewing parents

- A non-judgemental, sensitive approach is essential.
- Ask open, non-directive questions.
- Use verbatim quotes whenever possible.

CHILD NEGLECT

Detail information related to the child's health, growth, nutrition, physical and emotional wellbeing.

Examination includes the nature and appropriateness of a child's clothing, cleanliness of the skin and nails, nutritional status, growth percentiles, evidence of infections and infestations, as well as evidence of other medical conditions.

Medical opinion should reflect the doctor's assessment of objective signs of physical neglect, as well as historical evidence of environmental neglect (e.g. if an infant is left unattended in the bath) or medical neglect (medical conditions not treated).

CHILD SEXUAL ABUSE

Aim for one examination by a suitably trained medical practitioner who has access to facilities for paediatric genital examinations and photo documentation. This doctor should have expertise in the preparation of medical reports and presentation of evidence in court. All other medical practitioners are encouraged to seek advice from regional experts.

These guidelines are for the uncommon situation when the examination cannot be deferred and a clinician with expertise in the assessment of child sexual abuse is not available.

History

A full paediatric assessment is required. The evaluation should include:
- The nature of the sexual contact (digital, penile, vaginal, rectal, oral or a foreign object).
- The time and circumstances of the alleged abuse, whether ejaculation occurred and whether a condom was used.
- The identification of the alleged perpetrator(s).
- Genital complaints (pain, discharge or bleeding).

Examination

An examination should be performed as soon as possible after the alleged assault. Note signs of injury on general examination.

- Ask the child to indicate the exact sites on their body where there was contact with the offender.
- The external genitalia should be carefully examined for debris from the crime-scene and signs of injury.
- Girls may be examined in the frog-leg position using labial traction or labial separation techniques. Adequate visualisation of the posterior hymenal rim may be achieved with the girl in the knee–chest position.
- Boys may be examined in the supine position, flexing the boy's knees to visualise the anus.
- An otoscope provides light and magnification when a colposcope is not available. Semen may fluoresce under ultraviolet light (Wood's lamp).
- Speculum examination is not usually required in prepubertal girls or adolescent girls who are not sexually active. Examination under anaesthetic should only be considered if the clinician suspects internal injuries that may require surgical repair.
- Collect the child's clothing (including underwear) for forensic evaluation. Collect forensic specimens. Seek advice if you are uncertain about what specimens to collect. Forensic swabs should be air-dried, labelled and handed to police. Document the transmission of evidence.
- Swabs and slides for microbiological tests should be performed as clinically indicated. Blood for hepatitis B, hepatitis C, screening test for syphilis (VDRL) and HIV should be considered when the history raises concern about the transfer of body fluids. Note the need for repeat serology after 3 months.
- Consider pregnancy prophylaxis if the child is within 72 h of sexual contact. (Use two contraceptive pills containing 50 μg ethinyl oestradiol plus metoclopramide 10 mg stat. Repeat 12 h later.) Arrange for a follow-up pregnancy test and continuing contraception.
- All abused children and their parents should have access to appropriate counselling.

Management

- Multidisciplinary assessment of the child and their family is recommended for all children in whom child abuse is suspected.

- A child with moderate or severe injuries should be admitted to hospital for evaluation.
- Medical staff are expected to attend a case conference as requested by Protective Services or the police.
- Medical reports should be prepared by the senior medical staff responsible for the child's care. The report should use language appropriate for non-medical professionals. The report should be clear, concise and informative, including an opinion as to the possible causes of the injuries.
- Prior to appearing in court, medical staff are advised to consult with senior medical colleagues who are experienced in this field.

MANDATORY REPORTING

In most states of Australia, medical staff are legally required to notify the relevant statutory authorities of children who have inflicted physical injuries or child sexual abuse.

CHAPTER 12
CHILD PSYCHIATRY

Robert Adler
Ernest Luk
Catherine Marraffa

About 10–15% of the child and adolescent population have adjustment/ behaviour disorders. The majority of them are helped by their families, relatives, friends, school, primary health-care workers, general practitioners and paediatricians. Only a small proportion are seen by mental health services.

A successful use of mental health services requires preparation for the referral process.

PREPARATION FOR REFERRAL

The social stigma of attending a mental health service still exists. It is important for parents to understand that:
- They are not to blame for their child's problem
- It is not a sign of failure and it is positive that they seek help
- It is not unusual for children to have such problems
- It may take some time to find the best way to help their child.

It should be explained directly to the child that referral is not a punishment, but a means to overcome difficulties. A number of discussions may be needed.

It is best to know the setting and the clinical approach of the person to whom you are referring the child. Phoning the professional is often useful.

INTERVIEWING FOR PSYCHIATRIC PROBLEMS IN CHILDHOOD

As well as interviewing the parent(s) and child together, for a more complete picture try to see each separately, if possible. Determine why the family has presented at this particular time. Note that children, the less intelligent or educated, and those with language and cultural disadvantages, are more likely to be misunderstood and to misunderstand questions, to be afraid or hostile, and to use somatic complaints to communicate distress.

Use simple language, and try to understand the predicament of the child and the family. One's own response to the child and the family is a vital aspect of the assessment.

Assess the details of the problem behaviour: history, frequency, context and the responses of family members. Assess the meaning of the problem behaviour to the family and the ways in which they have attempted to solve the problem, including professional advice previously sought.

Inquire about situations such as pregnancy, delivery, the nursing relationship, early development, preschool and school life (educational progress and peer relations), interests, family structure, recent stresses, the marital relationship, family support and the extended social network, inter-generational difficulties, illnesses, and separations.

Observe the following:
- Affect: range, variability and form (e.g. flat or anxious).
- Play: confidence, competence, coordination, activity and creativity.
- Thinking: content (including suicidal thoughts), concentration, organisation, orientation, form of thoughts, dreams, wishes, etc.
- Personality: behaviour style, adaptability/rigidity, openness/defensiveness, and the ability to engage in a relationship.

Often it is very helpful to obtain information from the school. Seek parents' consent before doing so.

FAMILY CRISIS

Children's self-perception, emotional life, understanding of people, and relationships and behaviours are intimately connected with the views and the behaviour of their families. Parental responsibilities and obligations include: nurturance, care and protection of children; the establishment of limits and rules; the provision of security and emotional space to play and develop; and the appropriate education, stimulation and involvement.

Where parental competence is undermined by illness, poverty, ignorance, stress, lack of support and other factors, children may show evidence of behaviour disturbance. Overactivity, aggression, self-stimulation, destructive behaviour, stealing, running away and suicidal behaviour may all be evidence of family difficulty. While these behaviours bring the predicament of the child to the attention of others, they are also often perceived by parents as 'bad' and in turn punished or rejected. A cycle of unsatisfactory interactions develops: the parents feel bad and angry, and the child feels bad and angry.

It is very useful to differentiate families who have been functioning well, but present in crisis because of recent stresses, from those who have had difficulties for a long period of time; e.g. more than 6 months. The latter often require longer term treatment.

At various points in the crisis-filled lives of some families, children may be presented at emergency departments with adjustment problems. They may carry labels such as 'hyperactive', 'suicidal', 'possessed', 'bad' or 'out of control'. At such times it is helpful to focus on the difficulties of the caretakers, as well as on those of the child, and to clarify the interactional cycles or habits that characterise their lives.

One should balance the disadvantages of offering crisis admission with the benefits of being able to establish appropriate responsibilities and community support systems once the problem becomes clearer.

Action
- Refer to crisis social work/psychiatry for assessment.
- Liaise with and refer to the appropriate community agencies.
- Liaise with a general practitioner.

ATTEMPTED SUICIDE

This most often presents as a drug overdose in children beyond 9 years of age, but it may take more violent forms such as wrist laceration or attempted hanging.

Most suicide attempts are an expression of long-standing difficulties between parent(s) and the child. Care, cooperation and communication are unsatisfactory.

Up to 50% are more serious expressions of suicidal intent, often in association with a depressed mood and other depressive symptoms.

It is always dangerous to dismiss a self-injurious act as attention seeking. The most worrying profile is the male adolescent with a history of attempted suicide, access to firearms and who shows symptoms of depression.

Action
- Do not delay any necessary medical attention.
- Interview the child alone, parent(s) alone and the family together. Evaluate the underlying difficulties, strengths and the likely responses of the family to this crisis.
- Consult the local Mental Health Service to determine whether urgent psychiatric assessment, admission or referral for out-patient assessment is required.
- Involve the general practitioner in the management plan.

ANXIETY DISORDERS

These disorders present with high levels of autonomic arousal and subjective fear or panic. They may occur in attacks or as a persistent state, and may lead to avoidance behaviour.

Childhood anxiety may be related to over-worrying, separation from their carer, excessive shyness in social situations, and following stress or trauma. Anxiety problems in children often present as somatic complaints such as headache, abdominal pain and nausea. Diagnosis is based on the absence of an organic cause, a history of other anxiety symptoms and examination (see also Recurrent abdominal pain, Gastrointestinal Conditions, chapter 23 and Chronic and recurrent headache, Neurologic Conditions, chapter 29).

Action

- Define the origin of the fear. The explanation and planned follow up with the family doctor is usually sufficient.
- Discuss the more difficult cases with the child psychiatric service for emergency psychiatric assessment or an urgent out-patient appointment.

Conversion reactions

Such reactions may be associated with paralysis, blindness, deafness, pains or other sensory changes that have no organic basis.

They usually occur in association with recent stresses, family difficulties with emotional communication and difficulties in providing emotional support.

Action

- Admission may be required for full medical and psychiatric assessment.
- Otherwise, consider elective consultation with the local Mental Health Service, a referral to medical out-patients or a follow up with a general practitioner.

School refusal

The child is presented with the complaint of panic and distress that is related to school. The symptom is often a somatic problem or complaint of abdominal pain. This should be distinguished from truancy, where the child avoids school without the accompanying anxiety symptoms and often without the parents' knowledge.

Action

- A full physical examination should precede psychiatric referral.
- An urgent return to school is a high priority.

Aggressive behaviour

Anxious children may present with problems of aggressive behaviour, which is often confined to the home situation in children with a history of dependency. The parent–child relationship may become very confrontational and the child is seen as 'out of control'.

Action

- Helping the carers to understand the underlying basis of the aggression goes a long way towards reducing their anxiety.
- Further work to change the parent–child relationship is needed.
- Severe cases should be referred for emergency psychiatric assessment or an urgent out-patient appointment.

Obsessive–compulsive behaviour

This presents with checking, rituals, compulsive behaviour or intrusive thoughts. Obsessive–compulsive disorder is relatively uncommon. Obsessive–compulsive behaviour is more common, and is often associated with anxiety or depression, and pervasive developmental disorder.

Action

- Provide support and any necessary explanations to the child and family.
- Refer for assessment and management by a psychiatrist.
- Children will respond well to cognitive behavioural therapy alone or in combination with medication.

GRIEVING

Grieving may occur in response to the loss of support (if parents are unavailable or are themselves grieving), as well as following more obvious losses. Protest at the loss with overactivity and rage may be followed by sadness, depression and withdrawal.

Action

- Parents need explanations, and the children need to be supported by adults who can understand their response to the loss.
- Help the family to gain appropriate access to support and counselling.

DEPRESSION

Depression occurs in childhood but it is often missed. Depressive phenomena are often modified because of age and the developmental stage. Children may present with a low mood, poor sleeping patterns, a lack of meal enjoyment, low self-esteem, and negative thoughts that include the contemplation of suicide, poor concentration and irritability.

Depressed adolescents are at an increased risk of suicide. Co-morbidities are common. These include oppositional defiant/conduct disorder, anxiety disorders and attention deficit hyperactivity disorder (ADHD).

Action

- It is very important to recognise depression in children and adolescents. If untreated they run a much higher risk of depression in adulthood.
- Psychiatric referral for an early out-patient appointment is often needed.
- The general practitioner plays an important role in management.

DISRUPTIVE BEHAVIOUR DISORDERS

The separation of ADHD and conduct problems is essential. Many families with a child suffering from ADHD may appear to be coping poorly. This is often secondary to the ADHD and, once the diagnosis is made and appropriate treatment provided, family functioning improves (see Attention deficit hyperactivity disorder, Common Behavioural and Developmental Problems, chapter 9).

Chronic conduct problems (that endure more than 6 months) in childhood seriously affect social adjustment in adult life. They require long-term and multiple forms of treatment.

Action

- The management of ADHD should be left to experienced paediatricians or psychiatrists.
- Chronic conduct problems should be referred to the local Mental Health Service.

AUTISTIC SPECTRUM DISORDER

Definition

Autism comprises three core features that are present by at least 3 years of age:

- Qualitative impairment in social interaction
- Qualitative impairment in communication
- Restricted, repetitive and stereotyped patterns of activities, behaviour and interests.

Prevalence

- 9–10/10 000 children[1].
- 3 males : 1 female.

The main diagnostic systems ICD-10 and DSM-IV place autism in the category of pervasive developmental disorders. Autistic spectrum disorder is considered useful clinically and includes Asperger's syndrome. There is intellectual disability in 75% and 20% will develop epilepsy by adulthood. There is also the risk of comorbid psychiatric disorders; e.g. Tourette's, ADHD and affective disorders.

Aetiology

It is unknown. However, research suggests a genetic predisposition, and abnormalities of the left cerebral hemisphere, temporal lobe, limbic system and cerebellum have been described. There is an association with:

- Genetic and metabolic disorders; e.g. Fragile X syndrome
- Tuberous sclerosis
- Epilepsy

- Congenital rubella
- Perinatal brain trauma.

Careful medical assessment to exclude these conditions is important.

Diagnosis

This is best made by a multidisciplinary team with a paediatrician/ child psychiatrist, speech pathologist and psychologist. The diagnosis of Asperger's syndrome is particularly difficult. Controversy exists about whether or not differentiation between Asperger's syndrome and high-functioning autism is needed.

However, Asperger's syndrome is used to describe individuals with:

- Normal intelligence
- No delay in language development
- Impaired social and communication skills, and a narrow range of obsessional interests.

Management

Early intervention is vital and includes a well-structured and pre-dictable environment with:

- Behavioural modification
- Special education
- Speech and language augmentative communication
- Sensorimotor programs.

Drugs are used to treat the comorbid psychopathology. Support and information for families through parent organisations is available. Home help and respite is important.

PSYCHOSIS

Psychosis is a general term for states in which the mental function is grossly impaired, so that reality testing and insight are lacking, and delusions, hallucinations, incoherence, thought disorder or dis-organised behaviour, or both, may be apparent.

In the case of 'organic' psychosis there may also be a clouding of consciousness, confusion and disorientation, as well as perceptual disturbances. Short-term memory impairment is common in organic brain syndromes.

Anticholinergics, anticonvulsants, antidepressants, antimalarials and benzodiazepines have been associated with psychotic reactions in young people, as have substances of abuse (amphetamines, cocaine, opiates and hallucinogens). Organic brain syndromes may follow even minor head injury.

Adolescents may occasionally present in an acutely psychotic state with no prior history of drug ingestion or head injury. In this case the possibility of a 'functional' psychosis, schizophrenia or manic-depressive disorder should be considered. The latter often presents with an elated mood, grandiose ideas, increased energy and reduced sleep requirements.

Action
- The doctor should make a clinical evaluation and psychiatric referral.
- Most of these children will require admission for full psychiatric and medical examination.
- Do not sedate the child before a complete assessment unless it is essential.

BASIC TREATMENT PRINCIPLES IN PSYCHIATRIC PROBLEMS

Explanation
- Treatment should involve the collaboration of the parents, child and the professional.
- The parents should be informed of the diagnosis, the formulation of the problem, the treatment plan and the steps it takes to achieve the treatment goals.
- The child should also be informed, using age-appropriate language.
- With the parents' consent, the school and family doctor should be contacted to share relevant information and to help the child whenever appropriate.

Supportive psychological work/basic behaviour modification
- Some families will improve following explanations, advice and through referral to the appropriate reading materials.

- Behaviour modification based on observation, recording and learning principles can also be used.
- Consultation or advice from psychologists or psychiatrists should be sought, as described above.

Use of psychotropic drugs

- Psychotropic drugs should be used with care. They are only part of the whole package of treatment. However, in some cases they can be extremely important.
- Before prescribing them, it is advisable to consult with an experienced paediatrician or child psychiatrist. The common indications are psychosis, some cases of ADHD, tic disorder and severe behaviour problems in children with brain damage or mental retardation.
- Anxiety problems are rarely treated with drugs except when related to severe pain. This happens in some cases of severe separation anxiety, in severe acute stress and before a surgical operation.
- Psychological treatment is the first line of treatment for depression. Medication should be considered for melancholia, psychotic depression and refractory depression.

Monitoring and referral

- The monitoring of progress is essential. Initially, families should be seen weekly or bi-weekly.
- The more severe, chronic or refractory cases should be referred.

Reference

1   Tonge, B.J. (1996) Autism: time for a national approach to early assessment and management, *MJA*, **165**, pp. 242–5.

CHAPTER 13
THE DEATH OF A CHILD AND SUDDEN INFANT DEATH SYNDROME

Peter McDougall
John Rogers
Hubert van Doorn
Margaret Loughnan

The death of a child causes an intense grieving process in surviving family members that may last for years. For the family's future well-being it is very important that the health-care team ensures that the processes surrounding death are carried out in a sensitive and caring manner. The purpose of this chapter is to provide some practical guidelines.

BEFORE DEATH

Often the death of a child can be anticipated. This particularly occurs in preterm infant hospital patients with multiple problems or term infants with major congenital abnormalities, overwhelming sepsis or metabolic disease. Death usually occurs in older children following a chronic illness or trauma. The majority of these children spend time in hospital and become involved with many members of staff, as well as their family doctor and community nurse.

The interview in a hospital setting
Personnel
The consistency of the health-care team in a child's final illness is essential. Medical interviews in hospital with families should be led by a senior doctor together with a junior doctor, nurse, social worker or member of the clergy. The presence of more than two of these people at an interview may be difficult for the family. Other health-care team members, especially the family doctor, community nurse and others outside the hospital, must be closely informed.

Comfort

Choose a physically comfortable location where interruptions can be avoided. The open ward or corridor are not the places for interviews.

Information should be clear and simple

- Begin by asking the family to give their understanding of the situation.
- The prognosis is usually best given first.
- Give an explanation of the disease process.
- Avoid the use of unexplained medical jargon.
- Avoid information overload unless requested. There is time to deal with complex medical issues at later interviews.
- Avoid ambiguous phrases such as 'we might lose the battle' or 'he's passed away'. The words death, die or dying should be used.

Respect silences

When bad news is delivered it is best to remain silent until the parent responds. This sometimes takes minutes and can be very uncomfortable. These are important moments; they should not be interrupted.

Responsibilities of the accompanying members of the health-care team

At a medical interview, the accompanying members of the health-care team need to be sensitive to the parents' needs and to watch for misunderstandings. If they do not understand the medical message, it is unlikely that the parents will. At an appropriate time, the accompanying team member may ask the doctor to clarify some of the explanations given, but it is important not to interrupt a train of conversation or the silences that occur.

The senior doctor will, when appropriate, inform the family that all possible reasonable measures were taken to preserve their child's life. It is not necessary to repeat this message.

Adequate relief of pain and distress of the child

This needs to be attended to and the parents assured of its importance.

Interpreters

The availability of trained interpreters for people with a language other than English is essential. Do not use other family members or friends as interpreters.

Preparations for death

Time and space

The health-care team must not overwhelm families. Parents need to spend time alone together and with their child, either in the hospital ward, a quiet room, at home, or at a children's hospice.

Arrangements

These may need to be made for baptism, religious advice, photographs, videos and other memories of the child.

Permission

Many families have specific needs and sometimes they are unsure whether these are permissible. If these issues can be anticipated and discussed, the family's wishes may be facilitated.

The child

The preparation for death is largely dependent on the age and particular illness of the child. The older child with a chronic illness is often aware of impending death, and the health-care team needs to be sensitive to the family's and child's wishes in the delivery of information.

The place of death

Decisions need to be made about where the child will die. This largely depends on the family, but it may be at home, in a hospice or the hospital. When appropriate the child may be included in this planning.

SUDDEN UNEXPECTED DEATH

The sudden death of a child from a wide variety of causes may occur in the community, the emergency department, or the ward of a hospital. Sudden infant death syndrome (SIDS; see below) is particularly traumatic because it is the unexpected and unexplained death of a previously well infant. Although most of the preceding guidelines are applicable, there are some additional considerations regarding sudden death.

Resuscitation

This is frequently attempted either at home or in hospital. Some parents may wish to be present and they should not be excluded, but an experienced health professional needs to be available to provide them with support.

When it becomes clear that further resuscitative attempts are futile, it is the responsibility of the senior hospital doctor, general practitioner or senior ambulance officer to inform the family. An experienced health professional needs to:

- Establish a relationship of trust.
- Listen to the family's account of the events.
- Allow the family to express their emotions.
- Provide a non-judgemental understanding for any pre-existing difficult family relationships.
- Provide access to telephones for the notification of relatives.
- Facilitate the attendance of siblings and other important family members at the hospital.

In the case of a death in the community, the general practitioner generally assumes the above responsibilities.

The family response

The immediate responses to sudden death vary from emotional withdrawal to outbursts of profound grief. Unexpected reactions commonly occur; e.g. anger towards health-care providers who have done their best. Any response is appropriate, provided it does not threaten other people.

Brain death

Occasionally it becomes clear that a child who is dependent on mechanical ventilation is brain dead. In such a situation:

- The senior doctor needs to explain the meaning of brain death. Avoid the use of confusing words. The unambiguous message that death has occurred, together with the distinction between brain death and coma, needs to be clearly explained.
- It can be helpful to say that, although the child's body is still alive, the brain is dead and therefore the person is dead.
- It frequently helps parents to understand that their child has died by encouraging them to witness some or all of the brain death tests.
- The request for organ donation generally requires a separate interview, made in a positive manner, without coercion, and

with the clear acknowledgement of the family's vulnerability. Issues related to organ donation need to be discussed in order to receive an informed consent.

AFTER DEATH

The moment of death

Although usually anticipated, the moment of death is an important event and needs medical confirmation.

Mementos

Offer the family mementos such as photographs, locks of hair, hand and footprints together with personal belongings. Remember that:

- Black and white photographs of the dead child produce better looking pictures.
- If parents do not initially want mementos, these need to be stored as some families request them at a later date.

Viewing the body

This can be valuable for family members. It may eliminate the disbelief that death really occurred or, in the case of stillbirth, that the child was profoundly abnormal.

- A private area should be provided where the family can spend uninterrupted time with their child.
- Families should be offered the opportunity to wash and dress their child as a last act of love and care.

Autopsy

Discussion is best done before an anticipated death. Explanations need to include the following:

- The autopsy procedure.
- The provision of information about the risk of recurrence to the couple and their other offspring.
- More information about the nature of the problem.
- That a doctor will perform the autopsy like an operation, with care and respect.
- The process does not interfere with funeral arrangements.
- The full results will not be available for some weeks after death.

Coroner's cases

Following a sudden unexpected death, referral to the coroner is a statutory requirement. The coroner then decides whether or not an autopsy is to be performed. Parents can request (on a special form) that the coroner does not direct that an autopsy be performed. In many cases where the cause of death is not in doubt (e.g. severe head injury), the coroner will respect the wish of the family.

Funeral options

These need to be discussed and the family assisted to make their own arrangements with a funeral director and religious personnel as appropriate. Encouragement is given to the family to involve siblings in this important ritual.

Sedation

Unless a parent has a well-defined psychiatric illness, sedation should be avoided for the acute stages of grief as it interferes with and suppresses the normal mourning process.

Breast-feeding

Advice needs to be given to the breast-feeding mother regarding suppression of lactation.

The surviving siblings

Children react in their own way to their sibling's death. They may blame themselves and will fear their own death. This fear is often unspoken. Parents often need help and support to understand the responses of their surviving children who need repeated reassurance.

The availability of the health-care team

The availability of the health-care team to the family after death needs to be assured and follow-up procedures arranged. In particular, notify the health professionals who have been and who will continue to be involved with the family following the child's death, including the referring doctor or institution, the family's general practitioner, and the maternal and child health nurse. It is usually important to both families and team members that farewells be made.

Other families

The death of a child often affects the parents of other children in the hospital ward or local community. The acknowledgement of a child's death with these families is very important.

FOLLOW UP

Medical interview

Whether an autopsy is performed or not, it is essential that an appointment be made for the parents to see the child's treating doctor. Some parents are reluctant to attend, but most see the interview as a 'final farewell'. The discussion should include the autopsy results, the child's period of illness, future child bearing and issues related to bereavement.

If the child has died in hospital the child's doctor should see the family for one or more follow-up visits, although he or she may not be the best person to conduct ongoing bereavement counselling. It is necessary for that doctor to ensure that an appropriate subsequent follow up is arranged, often through the family doctor.

Ongoing support

Information needs to be provided to families about the support groups that are available both at the hospital and in the community. If someone is struggling more than expected, formal referral for psychotherapy should be considered. Medication is not a solution for grief.

SUDDEN INFANT DEATH SYNDROME (SIDS)

Sudden infant death syndrome is the sudden death of any infant or young child that is unexplained by history and in which a thorough post-mortem evaluation fails to demonstrate an adequate cause of death.

Epidemiology

Until 1990 about 550 babies a year died of SIDS in Australia, approximately 140 of these in Victoria, which correlated with the national and international average of two SIDS cases per 1000 live births.

Following the 'Reducing the Risks' campaign initiated in 1990 the rate in Victoria has steadily fallen to 0.47 per 1000 live births in 1997. A drop in incidence has also been observed in Europe and New Zealand where similar campaigns have been promoted.

SIDS accounts for 28% of deaths that occur between the ages of 1 month and 1 year. It most commonly occurs in babies under 6 months of age, and rarely in those over the age of 12 months. Although the incidence of SIDS is slightly higher in subsequent siblings of a SIDS infant, when matched for birth order with controls, there is no significant difference in occurrence.

'Reducing the risks' campaign

The 'Reducing the risks' campaign advises that:

- Infants should be put on their back to sleep, not on their side or face down.
- Cigarette smoking during pregnancy should be avoided and a smoke-free home should be maintained.
- The infant's head should remain uncovered during sleep.

Further information on the campaign can be obtained from the appropriate SIDS organisations.

APPARENT LIFE-THREATENING EPISODE (ALTE)

ALTE is defined as an episode that is frightening to the observer and that is characterised by some combination of apnoea, colour change, marked change of muscle tone, choking or gagging. The terms 'near miss SIDS' or 'aborted cot death' should not be used as it implies a close association between ALTE and SIDS.

- Less than 7% of infants who die from SIDS have a preceding history of ALTE.
- No cause is found in over 50% of cases presenting under the age of 6 months.

Associations that have been found with ALTE are:

- Gastro-oesophageal reflux – a small number of infants with this common condition experience coughing and choking episodes, and occasionally apnoea. These episodes occur most frequently when the infant is awake and are often recurrent. Most resolve within a month of onset but some persist for up to a year.

- Respiratory syncytial virus – can cause apnoea, particularly in preterm infants. Other viruses and pertussis can also be associated
- Upper airway obstruction – due to mid-nasal narrowing or adenoidal hypertrophy. It is usually suspected by a history of snoring and sleep disorder.
- Epilepsy – usually suggested by a good history. Investigations of ALTE by electroencephalogram (EEG) are usually fruitless.
- Cardiac arrythmia – this is an uncommon cause.

Most infants with ALTE need minimal resuscitation. However, some need cardiopulmonary resuscitation and these infants have at least a 10% chance of further episodes.

A cause will usually be found in infants presenting with ALTE over the age of 6 months. If no cause is found in this age group and the episodes are recurrent, Munchausen by proxy should be considered as a possibility. Formal sleep polysomnography should be performed before this diagnosis is considered.

All infants presenting with ALTE should be admitted to hospital for monitoring, investigation and counselling of the parents. However minor the episode may appear to health-care professionals, the parents usually believe that their infant's life was endangered by the episode.

HOME APNOEA MONITORING

No study has been able to demonstrate that widespread home apnoea monitoring programs reduce the incidence of SIDS.

Although we do not recommend widespread home apnoea monitoring there is a community awareness of its existence and, despite some medical advice to the contrary, a small demand for its use. The following are our recommendations for consideration of home apnoea monitoring:

- Subsequent siblings of SIDS victims – many of these parents conduct a 24 h watch on their infants and for these people home monitoring is of benefit.

- ALTE – particularly if mouth-to-mouth resuscitation has been used.
- If the SIDS victim has a twin.
- For extremely premature infants – most of these families have a high exposure to monitors and the reality of death in the intensive care nursery.

Counselling and instruction of cardiopulmonary resuscitation, together with a complete medical and service back-up, are essential to a home monitoring program.

CHAPTER 14

ALLERGY AND IMMUNOLOGY

Mimi Tang
Andrew Kemp

ALLERGIC DISEASES

Allergic disease is a common problem in our community. It affects up to 20% of children. The allergic conditions include asthma, eczema, allergic rhinitis, and allergies to food, insects or drugs. Children who have allergic diseases are often atopic; i.e. they produce IgE antibodies to common allergens such as house dust mite, animal dander, pollens and foods. The presence of IgE antibodies to these allergens does not necessarily cause disease; however, exposure to an allergen to which a patient is sensitised may exacerbate or even precipitate symptoms (e.g. inhalant, food, insect or drug allergy).

Allergy tests: What are they, who should have them and what do they tell us?

Skin-prick test and radioallergosorbent tests (RAST)

Skin-prick and RAST tests detect specific IgE antibodies against allergens. Skin testing is the preferred test – it is highly sensitive, inexpensive, simple and rapid. RAST has reduced sensitivity, is expensive and slow – it is best used to assess sensitivity to a single allergen (e.g. cats). More extensive testing should be performed by skin testing. RAST is a useful alternative to skin testing if there is dermatographism or widespread skin disease, history of anaphylaxis, or the inability to discontinue antihistamines. Skin and RAST tests are available for numerous relevant and irrelevant (e.g. chocolate) allergens. An appropriate panel of test allergens must be selected, based on knowledge of the allergens relevant to the diseases, population and geographical area being studied. Testing should be individualised for each clinical situation.

Skin tests may be affected by medications. Antihistamines should be withheld for 2–4 days, and skin tests delayed for 6 h after oral or parenteral adrenaline. Inhaled beta 2 agonists, oral theophylline and corticosteroids do not interfere with skin-prick tests. Age is not a contraindication to skin testing. Skin testing can be performed from early infancy. Dermatographism may complicate the interpretation of skin tests.

Interpretation

When ordering these tests the question that is being asked is: 'Are there IgE antibodies present?'. These tests will not necessarily answer the question: 'Is this antigen causing the patient's symptoms?'. A positive skin-prick or RAST test only identifies the presence of specific IgE against an allergen. *A positive test does not prove that an allergic illness exists, nor does it necessarily predict that the patient will develop symptoms on exposure to that substance.* For example, only 50% of individuals with a positive skin test to a food allergen will develop symptoms when exposed to that food. Skin test results must be correlated with history and examination findings.

Indications for skin testing

A detailed allergic evaluation is indicated in any patient with asthma or rhinitis who requires maintenance anti-inflammatory therapy to control symptoms. Skin testing is also indicated in patients with moderate or severe eczema despite appropriate medical therapy. Skin testing can identify major allergic factors that may exacerbate or contribute to symptoms and can guide the application of appropriate environmental modification.

Skin testing is also indicated in evaluation of suspected IgE-mediated food reactions. A negative skin test almost eliminates the possibility that a food will induce an IgE-mediated immediate reaction. A positive skin test must be correlated with the history. When there is a clear history of reaction to a specific food, a positive skin test can confirm food allergy. However, if the history is uncertain, a positive test only indicates the possibility of food allergy, and food challenge may be required to confirm the presence or absence of allergy.

In vivo challenges

In vivo challenges are primarily used for diagnosis of food allergy. The clinical relevance of a positive skin test should generally be confirmed by a challenge unless the history clearly implicates a food or there is a history of anaphylaxis. Less than half of the patients with a positive skin test to a food will react to the food during a challenge. Diagnosis of delayed non-IgE-mediated reaction to foods requires a formal food challenge as there are no skin or blood tests for this type of food reaction. *In vivo* challenges are also used for the evaluation of antibiotic reactions.

ALLERGIC RHINITIS

Allergic rhinitis refers to nasal symptoms of paroxysmal sneezing, itching, congestion and rhinorrhoea caused by sensitivity to environmental allergens. Symptoms may be present throughout the year (perennial rhinitis), related to a particular season (seasonal rhinitis/hay fever) or related to a specific allergen (e.g. cats or horses). Diagnosis requires the demonstration of an allergic basis for symptoms. Other causes of rhinitis should be considered: non-allergic rhinitis with or without eosinophilia, infective rhinitis, vasomotor rhinitis, hormonal rhinitis or rhinitis medicamentosa (rhinitis induced by excessive use of topical decongestants). Allergic rhinitis has a major impact on the quality of life and school performance. Appropriate recognition and treatment is important.

Perennial allergic rhinitis can occur at any age. In preschool and primary school children, perennial rhinitis is more common than seasonal rhinitis. House dust mite is the major allergen involved but concurrent sensitivity to pollens is also common. Sneezing and congestion are prominent. Symptoms are greatest on waking in the morning. There may be significant nasal obstruction and snoring at night. It is important to consider the possibility of perennial allergic rhinitis in any atopic child – this diagnosis is frequently missed.

Seasonal rhinitis is more frequent in teenagers and young adults. Sneezing, itching and rhinorrhoea are prominent. Sensitivity to pollens is the major finding. Symptoms occur in the relevant pollen season. In general, trees pollinate in early spring, grasses in the late spring and summer, and weeds in the autumn, although there is some overlap. Rye grass is the commonest provoking antigen in Australia, but multiple sensitivities to tree, grass and weed pollens are also seen. Nasal symptoms are frequently associated with ocular symptoms of itchy, red and watery eyes. The diagnosis is suggested by the seasonal nature.

Examination

Airflow through the nostrils should be assessed and an examination made of the nasal airway and mucosa. Pale oedematous mucosa and swollen turbinates indicate ongoing rhinitis. In seasonal rhinitis, examination may be normal outside the relevant pollen season.

Management

Topical corticosteroid nasal sprays (beclomethasone or budesonide) are the treatment of choice for perennial and seasonal allergic rhinitis, as well as perennial non-allergic rhinitis. Topical sodium cromoglycate is generally not effective. Topical anti-inflammatory treatment must be taken regularly for benefit. Improvement may not be apparent for 3–4 weeks and an initial course of treatment should last for 2–3 months. Continuous topical corticosteroid therapy for perennial rhinitis has not been shown to cause suppression of the hypothalamic–pituitary– adrenal axis. In seasonal rhinitis, treatment is commenced 1 month prior to the relevant pollen season and continued over the symptomatic period.

Appropriate allergen avoidance measures should be recommended where possible for all patients placed on topical anti-inflammatory therapy. Major allergic factors contributing to symptoms can be identified by history and skin testing.

Antihistamines are not helpful in relieving nasal obstruction and are not indicated as first-line treatment for rhinitis. They may be used in seasonal rhinitis for control of break through sneezing, itching or rhinorrhoea while on topical corticosteroid therapy or prophylactically prior to allergen exposure in allergen-specific rhinoconjunctivitis (e.g. cats or horses). Second-generation non-sedating antihistamines (loratadine and cetirizine) are well tolerated. Terfenadine and astemizole should be avoided as they may cause cardiac arrhythmia when taken with other medications.

FOOD ALLERGY

Milk, egg, wheat, soy, peanut, tree nuts, fish and shellfish are responsible for 90% of food allergies in children and adults. Food allergy is commonest in infancy. Most food allergies resolve by 5 years of age. The exceptions are peanut, tree nut and shellfish allergies that usually persist.

Allergic reactions to food fall into two broad groups:

IgE-mediated food reactions

These are common and occur within 1–2 h of food ingestion. They typically occur in young infants and frequently resolve by the age of 3–5 years. The common foods that provoke reactions are milk, eggs and peanuts. The common symptoms are erythema, where food touches the skin; urticaria, which may be facial or generalised; angioedema, which is usually facial; and vomiting immediately after the ingestion of the food. More severe reactions (anaphylaxis) involve the respiratory tract with stridor, wheezing, or hoarse voice; and/or cardiovascular system with hypotension and collapse.

Management

Patients with a suspected food allergy should be referred for specialist allergy advice. Practitioners should advise patients to avoid the suspected food until further evaluation. Parents should not challenge or force children to eat a suspected food in the home environment – severe reactions and even death have occurred.

Suspected IgE-mediated immediate food reactions are investigated with skin testing. A negative skin test almost eliminates the possibility of an immediate IgE-mediated reaction to that food. A positive skin test may confirm food hypersensitivity if there is a convincing history. However, if the history is uncertain, further evaluation by formal challenge is required. In an infant with a suspected reaction to one food, skin testing should also be performed with the other common food allergens as reactions are often multiple.

Non-IgE-mediated food reactions

These are generally delayed reactions occurring within 24–48 h of food ingestion, although some infants may have immediate non-IgE-mediated food reactions that occur within 1–2 h of food ingestion. Non-IgE-mediated food reactions are much less common and will often need specialist consultation to confirm. Typically, gastrointestinal symptoms are prominent with vomiting, diarrhoea and abdominal cramps. Occasionally there may be malabsorption, weight loss or failure to thrive. In severe cases there may be cardiovascular collapse. A worsening of eczema may also occur. Cow milk and soy proteins are the most common foods implicated. Diagnosis requires elimination of the suspected food followed by formal food challenge. Skin testing is not helpful.

MEASLES IMMUNISATION AND EGG ALLERGY

See also Immunisation, chapter 5.

Egg allergy is *not* a contraindication to measles, mumps and rubella (MMR) immunisation. Suspected egg-allergic children should be referred to an allergy immunology specialist for further investigation and management.

ATOPIC DERMATITIS (ECZEMA)

See also Dermatologic Conditions, chapter 18.

Atopic dermatitis has a major impact on the lives of patients and their families. Allergic factors may play an important role in the exacerbation of eczema and this possibility should always be considered in moderate or severe disease. Avoiding the relevant allergic factors can improve symptom control. However, allergic factors are not the sole cause of disease and allergen avoidance is only one component of overall management. An important triggering factor is *Staphylococcus aureus* infection and colonisation. Treatment of acute staphylococcal infection and reduction of staphylococcal loads on the skin can provide significant improvement of eczema control. Staphylococcal infection or colonisation, or both, must be controlled before the benefits of other allergen-avoidance measures can be assessed.

House dust mite sensitivity is an important exacerbating factor in atopic dermatitis. Dust mite allergen is ubiquitous in the home environment, particularly in the bedroom where a child spends up to 10 h each day. In cases of sensitivity to house dust mite allergen, instituting the appropriate avoidance measures may be beneficial.

Immediate food hypersensitivity reactions can act as exacerbating factors, particularly in young children with severe atopic dermatitis and generalised erythema. Investigation is as outlined in the section on food allergy above. In a small number of the more severe cases, delayed reactions to foods may also exacerbate dermatitis. There are no skin or blood tests that can reliably identify whether a delayed reaction to a food is occurring. The implementation of a restricted diet and a systematic reintroduction of suspected foods is used to assess this. These dietary manipulations are often complex and difficult to interpret. Specialist advice is required in the administration of the diet and in the interpretation of results. Appropriate case selection is important. Dietary restrictions should not be instituted in children with mild atopic dermatitis that can be readily controlled with the appropriate topical medication.

ASTHMA

See also Respiratory Conditions, chapter 32.

Allergic factors may contribute to the symptoms of asthma, particularly in cases of chronic persistent asthma. Investigation for allergens to which a patient is sensitised should be pursued in any patient requiring more than low-dose maintenance anti-inflammatory corticosteroid therapy, particularly those with interval symptoms.

The avoidance of relevant allergic factors represents a simple, inexpensive and non-pharmacological approach to anti-inflammatory therapy. However, allergen avoidance only represents one component of the overall management of asthma and patients should understand that allergic factors are not the sole cause of asthma. The major allergens implicated are the indoor inhalants (house dust mite, cat and dog dander). Pollens may also contribute to seasonal exacerbations of asthma, especially if the patient also suffers from seasonal allergic rhinitis.

Allergic rhinitis can exacerbate asthma and untreated persistent rhinitis may be one of the reasons for a failed response to standard anti-asthma therapy. The possibility of allergic rhinitis should be considered in all patients with asthma – it is common and treatable.

Foods generally do not induce asthma symptoms apart from immediate hypersensitivity reactions when respiratory symptoms are associated with cutaneous eruptions. In some patients with chronic asthma, the preservative metabisulphite can provoke acute exacerbations of asthma. Confirmation of this requires specialist consultation.

URTICARIA AND ANGIO-OEDEMA

Urticarial rashes are raised areas of erythema and oedema, which move over several hours. They are usually itchy. Angio-oedema is the swelling of deeper tissues and often involves areas of low tension, such as the eyelids, lips and scrotum. Angio-oedema is not necessarily itchy. When faced with the problem of urticaria the lesions should be classified as acute (<6 weeks duration) or chronic (>6 weeks duration).

Acute urticarias often only last a few days. In the vast majority of cases, no precipitating factor is identified. The most important step is to take a careful history to look for possible exposure to drugs (especially antibiotics and aspirin) or foods that may have induced an immediate hypersensitivity reaction. If a precipitating factor cannot be identified on history, skin tests and RAST tests will generally not provide additional information. Some cases follow viral or streptococcal infections.

Chronic urticarias can persist or occur intermittently for months. The possibility of a physical urticaria (e.g. heat, cold or cholinergic) should be considered. In protracted cases, it is important to consider the possibility of an underlying connective tissue or autoimmune disorder that may rarely present as chronic urticaria. In these cases, there are usually other suggestive features such as arthritis, or vasculitis. Chronic urticaria is rarely caused by specific allergic factors and therefore investigation with skin testing and RAST testing is not helpful.

Treatment of both acute and chronic urticarias is symptomatic with second-generation antihistamines. Cetirizine (0.2 mg/kg (max 10 mg) p.o. 12 hourly) is particularly effective. Manipulation of the diet is generally not helpful and is not indicated in children. A small number of subjects may respond to a preservative and colouring-free diet; however, this should only be considered if symptoms are particularly troublesome. The institution of such a diet and the interpretation of the result require specialist advice.

ANTIBIOTIC SENSITIVITY

Reported sensitivity to antibiotics in children is common. However, many patients are incorrectly labelled as 'antibiotic sensitive' and careful history is required to identify those patients who are likely to have experienced true antibiotic reactions. Reactions may be IgE mediated or non-IgE mediated. The most common presentation is a cutaneous eruption, either urticarial or maculopapular. More severe reactions are anaphylaxis with angio-oedema and bronchospasm or laryngeal oedema, exfoliative dermatitis, Stevens-Johnson syndrome, or serum sickness with arthralgia. Multiple antibiotic sensitivity where a child is reported to react to a significant number of antibiotics is not uncommon.

Reactions to penicillin and amoxicillin are generally due to a sensitivity to the major or minor determinants of penicillin. Reactions to amoxycillin and cephalosporins may also be induced by sensitivity to the individual side chains. Reactions to other antibiotics (e.g. sulphonamides) are less well characterised.

Management

There are no completely adequate *in vitro* or *in vivo* tests to diagnose drug allergy. The detection of IgE antibodies by RAST or skin testing may be helpful in the evaluation of penicillin or amoxicillin reactions. A negative skin test indicates that a patient is unlikely to react on re-exposure and any reaction is likely to be mild. A positive skin test is less helpful as the presence of IgE antibodies does not necessarily indicate a reaction after re-exposure. Skin-testing regimens have been established for the penicillin metabolites; however, this is not widely performed in Australia as the test reagents are not readily available. Skin testing for other antibiotics is less helpful. In most cases an oral challenge initiated under observation and then continued on an out-patient basis is required to confirm sensitivity.

An assessment should be made of the severity of the reaction. Each case must be judged on its merits. If there has been significant anaphylaxis with respiratory problems or hypotension, or both, the patient should not be challenged with the drug again except in exceptional circumstances and after an appropriate evaluation. Other contraindications to challenge include severe mucocutaneous reactions such as Stevens-Johnson syndrome or exfoliative dermatitis and serum sickness. In these instances, an alternative class of antibiotic should be selected. In deciding whether to proceed with a challenge, a judgement should also be made regarding the importance of the antibiotic in question. In the vast majority of cases with the question of multiple antibiotic sensitivity, a challenge is performed with a single antibiotic selected as being appropriate for future use and the challenge is completed without reaction.

LATEX SENSITIVITY

Latex products contain two types of compounds that can cause reactions: chemical additives that cause dermatitis and natural proteins that induce immediate hypersensitivity reactions. The majority of reactions to latex in the hospital setting involve disposable gloves; however, other items including catheters, dressings and bandages, intravenous tubing, stethoscopes, and airways may contain latex. Common latex products used in the community include balloons, baby bottle teats and dummies, elastic bands, and condoms. Reactions to latex products may be irritant or immune mediated.

Irritant dermatitis

Irritant dermatitis is the most common problem encountered with the use of latex gloves. This is a non-allergic skin rash characterised by erythema, dryness, scaling and cracking. It is caused by sweating and irritation from the glove or its powder, or by irritation as a result of frequent washing with soap and detergents.

Immediate hypersensitivity to latex

Type I hypersensitivity reactions to latex are the most serious reactions; they are potentially life threatening. They are caused by IgE antibodies to latex proteins. Reactions may occur after contact with latex (e.g. gloves and catheters) or the inhalation of airborne powder particles containing allergenic latex proteins. Sensitisation may occur following direct exposure of mucosal surfaces to latex (e.g. catheterisation). The severity of the reaction may vary widely, ranging from isolated allergic rhinoconjunctivitis, urticaria or asthma to anaphylaxis and death. Certain populations are at high risk for developing latex allergy: children with spina bifida or other urogenital anomalies, and individuals undergoing multiple surgical procedures, particularly if they are atopic. Skin-prick testing and RAST testing is useful in confirming suspected hypersensitivity. Skin testing is more reliable than RAST; however, well-standardised skin-test extracts are not widely available. There is no cure for latex allergy. The best approach is to avoid exposure. There may be cross-reactivity between latex and certain foods, in particular avocado and banana. If latex-allergic individuals experience discomfort in the mouth or throat while eating these foods, such foods should be avoided.

Contact dermatitis

This is a delayed Type IV hypersensitivity to chemical additives used in processing latex. Reactions are limited to the site of contact. Use of rubber gloves results in eczematous lesions on the dorsum of the hands. The skin may become dry, crusted and thickened. Oral reactions caused by dental appliances or balloons, and genital reactions caused by condoms have been described. The use of cotton-lining gloves inside latex gloves or a change to gloves that do not contain the chemicals contained in latex gloves usually reduces the problem. Patients with irritant and contact dermatitis are at an increased risk of developing immediate hypersensitivity to latex, and exposure to latex should be minimised.

IMMUNOTHERAPY

There are relatively few indications for immunotherapy in paediatric practice. Immunotherapy with purified bee venom is indicated for life-threatening anaphylactic reactions to bee stings in children. Referral should be made to a paediatric allergist/immunologist for allergy testing and further management. Severe local reactions are not an indication for immunotherapy and do not require further investigation with skin-prick testing. Immunotherapy may be an option in severe seasonal allergic rhinitis if the symptoms are not controlled with maximal topical anti-inflammatory medication and antihistamines, particularly if a limited number of allergens can be identified. Extreme caution is required in administering immunotherapy to unstable asthmatic patients as deaths have resulted.

GUIDELINES FOR THE INVESTIGATION AND TREATMENT OF IMMUNODEFICIENCY

When to suspect immunodeficiency

It is important to remember that normal, immunocompetent children average five to 10 viral upper respiratory tract infections per year in the first few years of life (even more if the child attends child care or has older siblings). Therefore, recurrent viral infections in a well, thriving child do not suggest immunodeficiency. Immune deficiency should be suspected when there is a history of severe, recurrent, or unusual infections. Recurrent or chronic bacterial infections (e.g. persistently discharging ears or purulent respiratory secretions) or more than one severe pyogenic infection may indicate antibody deficiency. Severe or disseminated viral infections, persistent mucocutaneous candidiasis, chronic infectious diarrhoea and/or failure to thrive in infants suggest a severe T-cell deficiency. These children should be investigated for Severe Combined Immune Deficiency (SCID). The presence of auto-immune cytopenias, together with recurrent sinopulmonary infections, raises the possibility of less severe forms of Combined Immune Deficiency. Recurrent pyogenic infections affecting lymph nodes, skin, lung and bones suggest a neutrophil defect. Recurrent meningococcal disease suggests a late component complement deficiency. Early component complement deficiencies may present with clinical features that are similar to antibody defects or with autoimmune disease.

Which tests to order

Basic immunodeficiency screen

A full blood count and immunoglobulin levels (IgG, IgA and IgM) will identify the vast majority of treatable primary immunodeficiencies (e.g. Agammaglobulinaemia, Common Variable Immune Deficiency, selective IgA deficiency and Severe Combined Immunodeficiency). If these tests are normal and the clinical suspicion of immune deficiency persists, referral to an immunology specialist for further evaluation is indicated.

Specific antibody responses and IgG subclasses

These are only considered when there is evidence of persistent or recurrent suppurative upper or lower respiratory tract infection, or both, and hypo-gammaglobulinaemia has been excluded. When considering these studies, one should ask: 'If an antibody defect is found, does this clinical condition warrant regular gammaglobulin therapy?' Specific antibody responses should generally be performed in conjunction with IgG subclasses. Reduced absolute levels of IgG subclasses do not necessarily indicate the presence of abnormal antibody production. The most important question is whether appropriate antibodies can be made to specific protein and polysaccharide antigens. Abnormal IgG subclass levels may be a clue to an evolving antibody deficiency. However, isolated abnormalities of IgG subclasses with normal specific antibody responses rarely result in clinical problems. In general, regular gammaglobulin therapy is only indicated for severe recurrent infections when a specific antibody defect has been identified.

T-lymphocyte numbers and function

These tests are used predominantly in the first 6 months of life to help in the diagnosis of severe combined immunodeficiency and Di George syndrome (absent thymus, hypocalcaemia and cardiovascular anomalies). The use of delayed hypersensitivity skin tests and a chest X-ray to look for absent thymic shadow may be helpful when suspecting a T-lymphocyte defect.

Neutrophil function tests

Specific defects of neutrophil function (e.g. Chronic Granulomatous Disease and Leucocyte Adhesion Deficiency 1) are very rare. They are almost always associated with gingivitis and careful examination of the mouth is important when considering abnormalities of neutrophil function. Markedly elevated circulating neutrophil counts and delayed separation of the umbilical cord suggest the possibility of an adhesion molecule deficiency.

Complement studies

Deficiencies of complement are rare. The best screening test for congenital deficiency is a CH50 that measures the function of the classical complement pathway.

HIV tests

HIV testing should be considered in the setting of recurrent, severe or unusual infections, particularly if there is hyperglobulinaemia.

Specialised immune function testing is best undertaken in consultation with a clinical immunologist.

Immunodeficiency treatment

Immunisation

See also Immunisation, chapter 5.

As a general rule all live virus vaccines should be avoided unless advised by a specialist. In certain circumstances measles immunisation may be given to patients with a T-cell defect (e.g. Di George syndrome or paediatric HIV infection) as the risks of wild-type measles infection are considerable while adverse reactions to the vaccine are largely theoretical. In cases of antibody deficiency, T-cell deficiency and combined immunodeficiency, immunisation with killed vaccines will not promote a significant antibody response. If the patient is on immunoglobulin replacement therapy, passively acquired antibody will prevent virus infections such as measles and chickenpox. Patients of any age with asplenia should be immunised with Hib, pneumococcal and meningococcal vaccines.

Immunoglobulin therapy

Immunoglobulin therapy (400–600 mg/kg i.v. monthly) is given when a significant deficiency of antibody production is demonstrated in a patient with clinically significant infections that usually affect the sinopulmonary tracts. In hypogammaglobulinaemia, immunoglobulin therapy is generally life long. In patients with combined immunodeficiency, immunoglobulin treatment may be discontinued once normal B-cell function can be demonstrated following bone marrow transplantation. In patients with IgG subclass deficiency immunoglobulin therapy is only indicated if a significant functional antibody deficit is demonstrated and the patient has significant symptoms. In this instance, a trial of immunoglobulin therapy may be used for a restricted period of time to determine if there is clinical benefit. This should only be instituted in conjunction with a clinical immunologist. The finding of a low immunoglobulin subclass level alone is not a sufficient indication for immunoglobulin therapy. Immunoglobulin therapy is not indicated for selective IgA deficiency.

Antibiotics

As immunoglobulin therapy does not provide significant levels of IgA antibody (the mucosal surface antibody), aggressive treatment of respiratory infections in patients with antibody deficiency is important to prevent bronchiectasis and permanent damage to the lungs. In severe cases, prophylactic rotating antibiotics are used to prevent recurrent severe sinopulmonary infections. Antibiotic prophylaxis with cotrimoxazole 2.5/12.5 mg/kg (max 80/400) p.o. twice a day 3 days per week is indicated in patients with T-cell or combined immune deficiency to prevent infection with pneumocystis.

Use of blood products

If it is suspected or known that the patient has a significant T-cell deficiency, blood products that contain cells (e.g. whole blood, packed red cells or platelets) should be irradiated to prevent graft versus host disease. In infants with severe combined immunodeficiency, attempts should be made to provide cytomegalovirus (CMV) antibody-negative blood as CMV infection can be a significant problem in such patients. If this is not possible the blood product should be filtered to remove contaminating white blood cells as it is delivered to the patient. If possible, Epstein–Barr virus (EBV) antibody-negative blood should also be given as EBV can induce lymphoproliferative states in severely immunodeficient subjects.

Bone marrow transplantation

Bone marrow transplantation is the definitive treatment for severe combined immunodeficiency. The cure rate can be of the order of 80% if the transplant is from a matched sibling or a parent. Survival is slightly less, of the order of 50%, if the transplant is only partially matched and from an unrelated donor.

CHAPTER 15

BURNS

Julian Keogh
Russell Taylor

TREATMENT AIMS

- To prevent and treat burn shock.
- To prevent infection.
- To obtain early skin cover.
- To prevent hypertrophic scar formation.
- To restore function and correct cosmetic defects.

ASSESSMENT

Age

The younger the child, the more likely shock will occur for a given extent of burn.

Estimating the surface area burned

The usual adult formula (rule of nines) is not applicable to children, because the proportions contributed by the head and limbs vary at different ages. The burned areas should be plotted accurately on the body chart, and the area calculated with the aid of the Lund–Browder chart (see Fig. 15.1). The extent of the burn is only rarely under-estimated, but overestimation is common and frequently leads to excessive fluid administration.

Assessment of the depth of burn

In most burns, there are varying grades of injury (see Table 15.1).

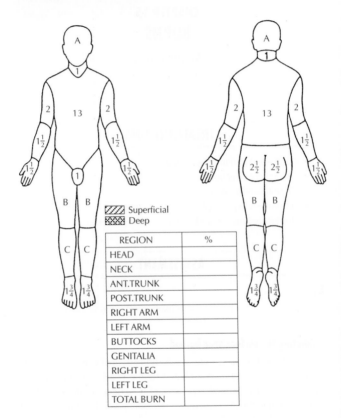

REGION	%
HEAD	
NECK	
ANT.TRUNK	
POST.TRUNK	
RIGHT ARM	
LEFT ARM	
BUTTOCKS	
GENITALIA	
RIGHT LEG	
LEFT LEG	
TOTAL BURN	

▨ Superficial
▩ Deep

Relative percentage of areas affected by growth

Age (years)	0	1	5	10	15	Adult
A $-\frac{1}{2}$ of head	$9\frac{1}{2}$	$8\frac{1}{2}$	$6\frac{1}{2}$	$5\frac{1}{2}$	$4\frac{1}{2}$	$3\frac{1}{2}$
B $-\frac{1}{2}$ of one thigh	$2\frac{3}{4}$	$3\frac{1}{4}$	4	$4\frac{1}{4}$	$4\frac{1}{2}$	$4\frac{3}{4}$
C $-\frac{1}{2}$ of one leg	$2\frac{1}{2}$	$2\frac{1}{2}$	$2\frac{3}{4}$	3	$3\frac{1}{4}$	$3\frac{1}{2}$

Fig. 15.1 Lund–Browder chart

Table 15.1 Assessment of burn depth

Depth	Cause	Surface/colour	Pain sensation	Treatment
Superficial (partial loss of skin)	Sun, flash; minor scald	Dry, minor blisters, erythema	Painful	Expose
	Scald	Moist, reddened with broken blisters	Painful	Non-adherent dressing
Deep superficial	Scald, minor flame contact	Moist white slough, red mottled	Painless	Graft otherwise scarring
Deep (complete loss of skin)	Flame, severe scald or contact	Dry, charred whitish	Painless	Graft

FIRST AID

Instantly remove clothing or smother the flame and apply cold water.

In a minor burn, continue the cold water application in a bowl or by compressing for up to 30 min. In a major burn, bathe for 20 min while awaiting transport to the hospital. Cover to guard against hypothermia or cold injury. Never use ice or ice slush.

Major burns are covered in a special foam transport dressing if available) or plastic cling wrap, with a blanket for warmth. These patients should be given intravenous fluid, oxygen and morphine, if necessary, before admission to the hospital.

Check the tetanus immunisation status and boost with tetanus toxoid +/– tetanus immunoglobulin as appropriate (see Procedures, chapter 3).

MINOR BURNS

Superficial burns of less than 5% of the body surface are suitable for out-patient treatment, unless they occur on the face, neck, hands, feet or perineum. Infants under the age of 12 months are at risk and are more likely to require admission.

Initial management
- Blisters should be left intact.
- Gently cleanse and remove loose skin.
- Dress with tulle gras and an absorbent dressing (polyurethane; e.g. Opsite, Tegaderm; or a combination of polyurethane and absorbent backing; e.g. Melolin).
- Immobilise with a crepe bandage, plaster slab or sling, if indicated.

Subsequent management
- Leave the initial dressing for 5–8 days. If the dressing is soaked by exudate, redress as necessary without disturbing the adherent tulle.

- Consider grafting to the residual areas if the healing process is not complete by the end of the second week. Graft deep second-degree burns by 5–10 days.
- Pain, fever and soiled or offensive dressings indicate that the dressing should be changed earlier than anticipated.

MAJOR BURNS

Superficial burns to greater than 5% of the body surface area, and deep burns, require admission to hospital. *For any child with burns to greater than 10% of the body surface area, transfer to a specialist paediatric burns centre should be considered.* Older children with more extensive superficial burns, such as sunburn, may be managed as out-patients (see Fig. 15.1).

General

- A brief history should document the time, causative agent and circumstances of the burn, the therapy already given and the child's general health.
- Carefully estimate and chart the extent and depth of the burn.
- Weigh the patient if possible – otherwise estimate weight.
- Insert an intravenous line in patients with burns greater than 10%. If a central venous line is needed, a specialist burn centre should be involved. Plan intravenous therapy (see below) and commence treatment with Hartmann's solution.
- Draw blood for baseline laboratory studies, including haemoglobin and haematocrit, serum electrolytes and, in severe burns, blood grouping and cross-matching.
- Insert a silastic urethral catheter for hourly urine volume in all patients with burns greater than 15%.
- Analgesia or sedation should be administered as necessary (see Pain Management in Children, chapter 4).
- Prevent infection. Care should be taken in ward management to guard against cross-infection. Antibiotics are not prescribed routinely.
- Observations of general condition, pulse, respiration rate, temperature, BP and fluid balance (including hourly urine output estimations) are necessary.

- With severe burns to the face, consider early endotracheal intubation. As the face swells, airways obstruction may occur, making intubation very difficult.
- Observe for effects of smoke inhalation that lead to acute respiratory distress syndrome (ARDS) where ventilation perfusion defects result in hypoxaemia, alveolar collapse, shunting and decreased lung compliance.
- Carboxyhaemoglobin (COHb) concentration should be measured in all burn/smoke inhalation patients. Symptoms of hypoxaemia will be manifested at levels greater than 30% COHb. Treatment is simple oxygen therapy as CO binding to Hb is reversible.

Fluid resuscitation

See Fig. 15.2.

Fluid volume

Use 3 mL/kg bodyweight per 1% burn surface area (BSA) for the first 24 h. In less severe burns 2 mL/kg bodyweight per 1% BSA may be sufficient.

Type of fluid

Use 5% normal serum albumin solution (NSAS) and Hartmann's solution. Fifty per cent of each type of solution is used concurrently.

Fluid maintenance
Type of fluid

Use 0.45% saline in 5% dextrose to provide extra sodium.

Rate of infusion (first 24 h)

- First 8 h: one-half resuscitation fluid plus one-third maintenance fluid.
- Second 8 h: one-quarter resuscitation fluid plus one-third maintenance fluid.
- Third 8 h: one-quarter resuscitation fluid plus one-third maintenance fluid.

The 24 h period commences from the time of burning, not from the time of admission. Adjustments are made according to the hourly urine output, which is the best guide to the adequacy of fluid replacement. Expected flow is 0.75 mL/kg per h in children; in the infant and toddler, a urine output of up to 1.0 mL/kg per h is required. Specific gravity of

BURNS SURFACE AREA (BSA).......%
TIME OF BURN.......24 h CLOCK
WEIGHT IN KG.......

TIME IV COMMENCED......24 h CLOCK
DATE.......

	1st 24 h (volume)	1st 8 h (volume)	2nd 8 h (volume)	3rd 8 h (volume)
A BURN RESUSCITATION				
* 3 × kg × % = ...mL				
TYPE OF INFUSION				
** 1 5% Normal Serum Albumin Solution (NSAS)	_____ mL	$\frac{1}{2}$ of 24 h vol. _____ mL	$\frac{1}{4}$ of 24 h vol. _____ mL	$\frac{1}{4}$ of 24 h vol. _____ mL
*** 2 **Remainder as Hartmann's Solution**	_____ mL	_____ mL	_____ mL	_____ mL
50% of each type solution is used concurrently				
B MAINTENANCE FLUID				
See oral fluids information below				
0.45% saline in 5% dextrose (estimated volume on bodyweight in kg)	_____ mL	$\frac{1}{3}$ of 24 h vol. _____ mL	$\frac{1}{3}$ of 24 h vol. _____ mL	$\frac{1}{3}$ of 24 h vol. _____ mL
TOTAL A & B				
BURN RESUSCITATION + MAINTENANCE FLUID				

URINARY OUTPUT EXPECTED 0.75 mL/kg per h = _____ mL

ORAL FLUIDS: Most children with burn injury tolerate oral fluids. Initially all children may be offered small amounts of milk and, if tolerated, the quantity is increased at hourly intervals. Usually after a few hours the patient is receiving most maintenance fluid by mouth, except for those patients with very severe burns.

IF ORAL FLUIDS ARE NOT TOLERATED SEE (B) ABOVE.

NOTES: * In less severe burns 2 mL × kg × 1% in the first 24 h may be sufficient.
** Normal Serum Albumin Solution (NSAS) is interspersed and not given as one bolus.
*** If no Hartmann's available use normal saline.

2nd 24 h: After the initial 24 h of fluid replacement, the type of fluid replacement will depend on urinary output, serum electrolytes and haemoglobin. The volume of burn resuscitation fluid is approximately $\frac{1}{2}$ that given for the first 24 h.

Fig. 15.2 Resuscitation of a burnt child during the first 24 h

the urine is recorded, as is the osmolality of urine and serum if renal function is poor.

Repeated haemoglobin, haematocrit and electrolyte estimations are made. Restlessness may indicate inadequate fluid replacement.

Rate of infusion (second 24 h and onwards)

Replacement fluid: approximately one-half of the volume for the first 24 h; maintenance fluid as before. Total volume is given at an even rate over 24 h, and the volume and type of fluid given are adjusted according to urine flow and electrolyte estimations, and decreased as the shock diminishes over the succeeding days. Diuresis occurs 2–3 days post-burn.

Oral fluids

Most children will tolerate small amounts of milk (30–60 mL/h) after 4–8 h. If this is tolerated, increase the quantity to 4 hourly. In minor burns, oral fluids may be commenced earlier. If gastric dilatation associated with vomiting occurs, a nasogastric tube should be inserted.

After 48 h, the majority of fluid intake is usually oral. Children who refuse to drink, or who have burns to the face and mouth may require tube feeding.

Blood

Whole blood is not required initially except in severe, deep burns, and then usually only 24 h post-burn, when the haemoglobin concentration is falling.

Local wound care

Minimal debridement of loose skin is performed initially and management continues by exposed or closed methods.

Escharotomies should be considered if the peripheral circulation to a limb is jeopardised, but before commencing this procedure contact with a paediatric burns unit is desirable.

Respiratory difficulties require particular attention; intensive care or escharotomy to the trunk may be required.

Exposure

- Indications: for burns on the face, perineum, or one surface of the trunk.
- Treatment: allow eschar to form if superficial, or apply topical silver sulphadiazine cream. A daily bath is given with warm water and mild soap, followed by the application of antibiotic cream.

Closed

- Indications: for small children and burns on extremities. Except for burns to the face or perineum, nearly all children are ultimately nursed with closed dressings.
- Treatment: an antiseptic tulle gras and gauze for superficial burns, or topical silver sulphadiazine cream and Melolin for deep burns. Fingers and toes are separated with non-adherent tulle and wrapped together (not separately). Before the dressing, a daily bath is given with warm water and mild soap.

Antibiotics

These are usually only given for proven infection and on the basis of sensitivity tests. On admission, swabs should be taken of the burn area, nose, throat and rectum, and the burn area should be re-swabbed twice weekly. In major burns, multiple 3 mL punch biopsy specimens are the most reliable method of detecting infection. If septicaemia is suspected clinically, blood culture should be performed and antibiotics such as gentamicin 7.5 mg/kg (max 240 mg) i.v. daily and flucloxacillin 50 mg/kg (max 2 g) i.v. 4–6 hourly are commenced.

Nutrition

All children with burns should receive a high-calorie diet containing adequate protein, and vitamin and iron supplements. In severe burns there is a marked increase in metabolic rate, and gastric tube feeding with a complete fluid diet (e.g. Isocal or Osmolite) should be instituted early and adjusted to maintain or increase bodyweight. The involvement of a dietitian is recommended.

Room temperature

It is desirable that this is in the range of 22–26°C. If a child is partly exposed and nursed in a cool environment, metabolic requirements will increase.

Special therapy

Physiotherapy and occupational therapy should be commenced early, and continue throughout the course of burn care. Splints and pressure dressings are necessary to control hypertrophic scar formation. The play therapist also has an important role.

Social rehabilitation is important, as many burned children come from disadvantaged homes. *Maltreated children constitute approximately 6% of admissions to the burns unit.* Psychological and psychiatric consultation is often required, and the hospital teacher should liaise with the child's schoolteachers.

Follow up

Healed burns and grafts are kept soft with emollient. Pressure therapy and splintage supervision is continued by a physiotherapist and occupational therapist. Parents and children need continuing support, and further operations are sometimes necessary to correct contractures and relieve cosmetic defects.

CHAPTER 16
CARDIOVASCULAR CONDITIONS
James Wilkinson

WHEN TO INVESTIGATE A MURMUR

- Approximately 70% of infants and 50% of normal school children have soft heart murmurs. While the distinction between 'innocent' and 'organic' murmurs may not be urgent in an asymptomatic child, it is extremely important that the appropriate 'label' be applied as soon as is practicable. No child should continue through childhood without his or her 'murmur' having been clearly designated as innocent (in which case the heart is normal and *no* special precautions, including endocarditis prophylaxis are needed) or otherwise.

- In an asymptomatic child such murmurs most often have the characteristics of a *vibratory murmur* (Still's murmur), a *venous hum*, a *pulmonary flow murmur*, or a *carotid bruit*. Such murmurs are fairly easily identifiable on the basis of their characteristic timing, pitch and behaviour with changes in posture. However, some practice is required to become confident in identifying these common innocent murmurs. The pulmonary flow murmur in particular, if heard after infancy, because of its close similarity to the murmur associated with an atrial septal defect (ASD), should always be investigated further.

- Where doubt exists about the nature of a murmur it is appropriate to arrange an ECG and chest X-ray. If the X-ray or ECG are in any way suspicious, or if the patient has any symptoms that suggest a possible structural cardiac problem, a consultation with a paediatric cardiologist with a view to a possible echocardiogram should be arranged. It should be understood, however, that echocardiography, although it will exclude a range of significant heart defects, cannot 'diagnose' an innocent murmur and may not always exclude an organic basis for the murmur. This still depends on clinical judgement.

- In the first 3 months of life the distinction between organic and innocent murmurs can be particularly difficult. If in doubt the auscultation should be repeated at 3 to 6 months of age, by which time it is usually easier to achieve a firm diagnosis either way.

A simple scheme for analysing murmurs and deciding which justify referral to a specialist is illustrated in Fig. 16.1, p. 232.

HEART FAILURE

Recognition

- The main symptoms in infants are dyspnoea on feeding or at rest, poor feeding and failure to thrive.
- Physical signs include tachycardia, tachypnoea, intercostal and subcostal recession, Harrison's sulci and hepatomegaly.
- Cardiomegaly is almost always present on the chest X-ray and, if not seen, other causes for the symptoms need to be explored.
- A child who is previously well and who presents with recent symptoms and manifestations of cardiac failure requires urgent echocardiography to exclude pericardial effusion or tamponade, or both.

Management

Diuretics

Frusemide: 1 mg/kg (max 20–40 mg) once or twice daily. This should be accompanied by a potassium sparing diuretic (e.g. spironolactone) or potassium supplements.

Digoxin

Rapid digitalisation is not usually necessary (except for patients with supraventricular tachycardia (SVT)). The maintenance dose is 10 µg/kg per day (usually given as 5 µg/kg (max 250 µg) orally, 12 hourly). If rapid digitalisation is considered necessary, give a loading dose of 15 µg/kg stat, then 5 µg/kg after 6 h, and 5 µg/kg (max 200 µg i.v.; 250 µg oral) 12 hourly (give half these doses in preterm infants). Serum digoxin levels are useful in assessing the adequacy of digitalisation. A level of 1.0–2.5 nmol/L is likely to be in the therapeutic range. Infants tolerate somewhat higher levels (up to 3.5 nmol/L).

Vasodilators

These may be helpful. Currently, the favoured agents are usually ACE inhibitors, such as captopril 0.1–1 mg/kg (max 50 mg) orally, 8 hourly. Their introduction usually needs to be done with the patient in hospital so that blood pressure may be monitored. Long-acting agents (enalapril 0.2–1.0 mg/kg (max 40 mg) orally, daily or lisinopril 0.1 mg/kg (max 5 mg) orally, daily) are being used increasingly as the dose frequency is lower and the likelihood of 'post-dose' hypotension is less.

Other measures

- *Oxygen* should be administered if hypoxia is thought to be related to pulmonary congestion or respiratory infection.
- *Sodium bicarbonate* may be used if a correction of severe acidosis is required.
- *Inotropic drugs* (e.g. dopamine or dobutamine) may be infused if severe cardiac failure is accompanied by poor peripheral perfusion. (Dosage – initially 5 μg/kg per min by i.v. infusion. Dobutamine may be given into a peripheral line, dopamine into a central line.)
- *Prostaglandin E_1* infusion (0.01 μg/kg per min = 10 ng/kg per min) should be considered in neonates presenting with manifestations of cardiac failure if it is probable on clinical grounds that they have a ductus-dependent defect, in which part or all of the systemic circulation is compromised as a result of a cardiac defect (e.g. hypoplastic left heart syndrome, critical aortic stenosis, aortic interruption or coarctation syndrome).
- *Positive pressure ventilation* should be considered if the infant is progressing to cardiorespiratory failure.
- *Antibiotics* should be given if a superimposed infection is present or suspected, especially in the sick neonate.

NEONATAL CYANOSIS

Rapidly progressive cyanosis in the early newborn period may be related to the presence of a ductus-dependent cyanotic defect (e.g. pulmonary atresia), or to transposition of the great arteries.

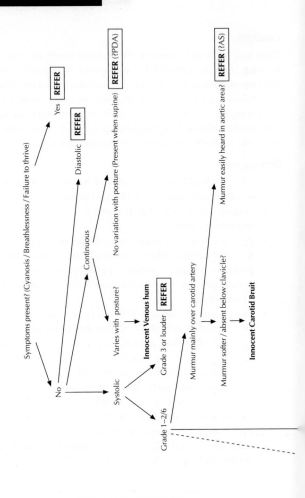

Symptoms present? (Cyanosis / Breathlessness / Failure to thrive)
Yes → **REFER**

No →

Diastolic → **REFER**

Continuous →

No variation with posture (Present when supine) → **REFER (?PDA)**

Varies with posture? → **Innocent Venous hum**

Systolic →

Grade 3 or louder → **REFER**

Grade 1–2/6 →

Murmur mainly over carotid artery →

Murmur easily heard in aortic area? → **REFER (?AS)**

Murmur softer / absent below clavicle? → **Innocent Carotid Bruit**

Symptoms

Timing

Amplitude

Location

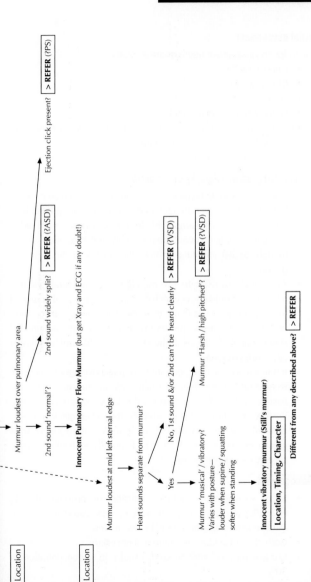

Fig. 16.1 Decision tree for analysis of murmurs and when to refer on for further investigation

Initial assessment

The following assessment methods are available:
- Chest X-ray
- Blood gases
- ECG
- Echocardiogram (if available) or
- Hyperoxic test (in order to decide about the desirability of an urgent transfer for echocardiography)
- A blood group and cross-match.

Hyperoxic test (if echocardiography is not available)

- Arterial Po_2 should be measured before and after the administration of 100% oxygen by face mask, head box or endotracheal tube for 10 min. The sample should be taken from the right radial artery if possible (to avoid the possibility of desaturation related to right to left shunting through the ductus in the newborn period).
- An arterial Po_2 rising to 150 mmHg makes structural cyanotic heart disease unlikely, in which case cyanosis is probably related to lung disease. Most major cyanotic defects (e.g. transposition or pulmonary atresia) presenting in the newborn period will show arterial Po_2 levels in the range of 50–70 mmHg or lower after 100% oxygen.
- If this test is done using non-invasive pulse oximetry to measure oxygen saturations, there is usually little improvement from the baseline values, if the cyanosis is due to cyanotic heart disease. Resting saturation levels of 50–80% (or sometimes lower) will generally rise by 5–10% with oxygen. An improvement by a greater degree (e.g. to 90–100%) is usually indicative of non-cardiac causes of cyanosis.

Management

- Initial management includes infusion of prostaglandin E_1 (10 ng/kg per min). Prostaglandin E_1 may cause apnoea, so intubation for transport should be considered.
- Correction of acidosis is required, if necessary.
- Oxygen may be administered, usually in a concentration of 30%.
- Diagnosis can usually be achieved by echocardiography.

CYANOTIC (HYPOXIC) ATTACKS

- Severe cyanotic attacks are a characteristic feature of Fallot's tetralogy, but may occasionally occur with other cyanotic lesions.
- Episodes may be spontaneous, but are often precipitated by exertion, feeding or crying. They often occur first thing in the morning, and intercurrent infection and dehydration may play a part.
- Attacks are manifested by increasing cyanosis or pallor, or both, shortness of breath, and distress out of proportion to the precipitating situation. Loss of consciousness may occur in severe attacks.

Management

- *First Aid.* Try to stop the child from crying. The child should be picked up, cradled and soothed, and nursed in the knee chest position over the mother's shoulder. Morphine 0.2 mg/kg i.m. may be helpful in severe cases.
- *Oxygen.* The administration of oxygen is of limited benefit, but it may be given provided it does not provoke further distress in the child.
- *Bicarbonate.* Severe acidosis may develop and require correction, but in milder cases that resolve spontaneously the acidosis will correct itself.
- In extreme cases the infant may require intravenous fluid replacement, correction of acidosis, intubation and positive pressure ventilation.
- Beta-blocking drugs (propranolol 0.2–0.5 mg/kg per dose orally, 6–12 hourly). These may be used prophylactically to prevent spells in a child who has started to have attacks. This should only be used as a temporary measure while further investigation and surgery are planned.

SUPRAVENTRICULAR TACHYCARDIA (SVT)

Clinical features
- Pallor, dyspnoea and cardiac failure are the usual manifestations of an episode of SVT in infancy.
- The pulse is very rapid (the rate is usually between 180 and 300 b.p.m.), of small volume and regular.

Diagnosis
- The ECG shows a regular narrow complex tachycardia.
- If P waves can be seen these should be present with each complex. (In many cases, P waves are not readily seen as they are hidden in the T waves.)

Management
Early consultation is advised.
- *'Vagal' manoeuvres.* Place a polythene bag that contains cold water with ice cubes over the upper face (forehead, eyes and nose) for 15–20 s. This will quite frequently lead to a reversion of the tachycardia. If this, or other 'vagal' manoeuvres are unsuccessful, adenosine should be considered.
- *Adenosine.* This is highly effective in terminating SVT. The initial dose is 0.1 mg/kg, diluted in normal saline and given i.v. by rapid bolus injection, with continuous ECG monitoring. It is essential that the bolus reaches the central circulation rapidly; hence, the use of a hand vein may be ineffective. The effect wears off within 1 min and further doses may be given at 2 min intervals, increasing the dose by 0.05 mg/kg for each dose up to a maximum dose of 0.3 mg/kg (max 18 mg). The main side effects in older children are flushing, agitation and a sensation of tightness in the chest, but these are brief and transient.
- *Digoxin.* If adenosine is not available and if the infant's condition is stable and cardiac failure is absent, the next line of treatment is digitalisation (see p. 230). The initial dose of digoxin should be given i.v. The tachycardia will usually not revert for several hours with digoxin alone.
- *Verapamil.* This may be given to children over the age of 1 year, but should be avoided for infants. The initial dose should be

0.1 mg/kg given slowly i.v. (over 10 min), under continuous ECG monitoring. This may be repeated after 15–20 min if there is no response. Intravenous calcium should be available if hypotension occurs. *Verapamil is contraindicated if the complexes are broad or the rhythm is irregular, or both.*

- *DC cardioversion.* If the infant is severely symptomatic, or has evidence of congestive failure, or if drug therapy has failed to revert the tachycardia, DC cardioversion should be considered (1 J/kg shock – synchronised). *Verapamil and DC cardioversion are potentially dangerous, and should ideally only be given by (or under the supervision of) a paediatric cardiologist or intensivist.*

INFECTIVE ENDOCARDITIS

Patients at *high* risk

Those who have:
- Cyanotic heart defects
- Previous endocarditis.

Those who are postoperative and who have:
- Prosthetic valves
- Conduits
- 'Shunts'.

Patients at risk

- All children with structural congenital heart defects (except isolated ASD secundum).
- All children with *operated* heart defects (except repaired ASD secundum and PDA).
- All children with acquired valve disease.
- Children with endocardial pacemakers.
- Patients with intravascular lines/shunts, and so on.

Those in the first two categories are subject to advice from the patient's cardiologist.

Patients not at risk

- Children with murmurs if confirmed 'innocent'.
- Children with non-structural problems (e.g. arrhythmia).
- Children with history of Kawasaki disease.

Presentation

Infective endocarditis is usually caused by organisms of relatively low virulence. The onset of symptoms can be insidious, and often suggestive of an intercurrent viral illness. Fever, anorexia, general malaise and weight loss may persist over many weeks.

The classic physical signs of endocarditis (e.g. splenomegaly, splinter haemorrhages, petechiae and clubbing) may be absent in children with endocarditis.

Diagnosis

Any patient in the above risk groups who presents with such symptoms (especially if they persist for more than 7–10 days without other explanations) should be investigated for possible endocarditis with multiple blood cultures, full blood count, erythrocyte sedimentation rate or CRP, and urinalysis.

Echocardiography is an important investigation and will frequently demonstrate vegetations, *although a negative echo does not exclude endocarditis.*

Endocarditis prophylaxis

See Antimicrobial guidelines.

RHEUMATIC CARDITIS

Rheumatic carditis is associated with acute rheumatic fever and is now very rare in the developed world.

Clinical manifestations

Rheumatic fever follows an infection (usually tonsillitis) caused by a group A, β haemolytic streptococcus (*Streptococcus pyogenes*).

Major criteria

- Migratory polyarthritis mainly affecting large joints.
- Evidence of carditis with one or more of the following:
  - Tachycardia at rest; e.g. while asleep. (This feature alone is insufficient to diagnose carditis as it may occur with other febrile illnesses.)
  - Cardiac enlargement, if presumed to be of recent origin.
  - The development of new murmurs, including an apical systolic murmur of mitral incompetence or diastolic murmurs at the apex (Carey–Coombs murmur), or both, or at the left sternal edge (aortic regurgitation).
  - Pericardial friction rub.
  - The onset of cardiac failure.
- A transient, demarcated skin rash on the trunk (erythema marginatum).
- The development of nodules over bony prominences ('subcutaneous nodules').
- Choreiform limb movements – Sydenham's chorea, often appearing some weeks later than the other features.

Minor criteria

- Fever.
- Arthralgia.
- Previous history of rheumatic fever.
- Raised erythrocyte sedimentation rate or CRP.
- Prolonged PR interval on electrocardiograph (ECG).

All patients with suspected rheumatic fever should be tested for evidence of streptococcal antibodies (ASO titre, anti-DNAse titre). The diagnosis cannot usually be regarded as established unless evidence of recent streptococcal infection is demonstrable (positive throat culture or positive antibody titres). However, if such evidence is found, the presence of one major and two minor criteria, or two or more major criteria is indicative of the presence of rheumatic fever (Jones' criteria).

Management

- Rest in bed.
- *Aspirin* in full therapeutic doses (80–100 mg/kg per day in three to four doses to maintain serum salicylate levels of around 2 mmol/L).
- *Steroids* may be administered in the presence of severe carditis (e.g. prednisolone 1–2 mg/kg per day). These will usually reduce the duration of the acute episode, but probably do not affect the development of chronic valve disease.
- During the initial illness streptococcal infection should be eliminated by the appropriate penicillin therapy. Subsequently, long-term penicillin prophylaxis should be instituted to prevent recurrence and further cardiac damage.

CHAPTER 17
DENTAL CONDITIONS

James Lucas

TOOTHACHE AND INFECTION

Patients presenting with toothache or dental abscess and who have severe pain, elevated temperature, obvious facial swelling and/or associated lymph node involvement will require treatment with antibiotics such as phenoxymethylpenicillin (drug of first choice) 15 mg/kg (max 500 mg) orally, 6 hourly, or they may need admission for i.v. benzylpenicillin 50 mg/kg (max 3 g) 6 hourly. Consultation with a dentist should be made immediately for these patients as treatment requires extraction, surgical drainage, or both.

Children who suffer intermittent toothache only after eating may be given analgesia and referred to a dentist (unless they are medically compromised; e.g. haematology or cardiology patients). This does not apply to the severe spontaneous pain at night that is indicative of pulpitis, periodontitis or early abscess.

LOCAL BLEEDING FROM THE MOUTH

In such cases:
- Always wear gloves.
- If possible, irrigate the patient's mouth with cold water or saline, or remove with gauze or tweezers any loose, broken down or excess clots.
- Identify the source of bleeding, such as a soft tissue laceration or a tooth socket (bone).
- A bleeding tooth socket is usually due to the extraction of a tooth with untreated infection (more rarely a haematological disorder).

Soft tissue laceration

All soft tissue lacerations should be assessed for:
- Any displacement from the bony base (i.e. degloving injury).
- Any requirement for repositioning and suturing.

Bleeding tooth socket

- If the child has been bleeding for an extended period of time, the haemodynamic status of the patient must be assessed, particularly if treatment requires general anaesthesia for the control of the haemorrhage.
- Compress the alveolus between the finger and thumb firmly. Topical Thrombin may be placed on the pack.
- If the child is cooperative, place a gauze pad over the socket. Have the child bite on it for 20 min and change when it is soaked. If the child is not cooperative, a parent should hold the gauze in place. Never pack anything into the socket.
- Sedation is frequently necessary. This should be given immediately if indicated.
- Antibiotics should be given if infection is present, as indicated by a history of preceding pain or abscess formation. Phenoxymethylpenicillin 15 mg/kg (max 1 g) orally, 6 hourly is the drug of first choice.
- A dentist should be contacted for further management or if the bleeding continues – the tooth socket may require suturing and debridement.

TRAUMA TO TEETH AND JAWS

Treatment should be commenced as early as possible if complications such as disturbed jaw growth, malformation or malposition of permanent teeth, tooth loss or pulp death with abscess formation are to be prevented.

Suspected fractures of the mandible and maxilla

- Tetanus prophylaxis (see wound management, Procedures, chapter 3) and antibiotics should always be given for a compound fracture that opens into the mouth or skin. Phenoxymethylpenicillin 15 mg/kg (max 1 g) orally, 6 hourly is the drug of choice initially.

- A dentist or maxillofacial surgeon, or both, should be involved in the management of these children from the time of presentation.

Dento-alveolar injuries

- Tooth fracture can occur to the primary or permanent dentition. This may involve the crown or root of the tooth with or without an associated alveolar bone fracture.
- Assessment is required to establish the extent of the fracture and possible pulp involvement. It is important to determine what has happened to the tooth fragments.
- If tooth fragments cannot be found then a chest X-ray may be indicated to make sure that the fragments have not been inhaled.
- Assess tetanus prophylaxis (see Procedures, chapter 3) and the need for antibiotics.
- Dental consultation is necessary for all injuries to the teeth, soft tissue and alveolar bone.

TOOTH DISPLACEMENT

This may be palatal or labial, an intrusion or a total dislodgement, or an extrusion with a fracture of the labial or lingual alveolar bone, or both. Before the dental consultation assess the following:

- The degree of fracture or the amount of displacement, or both.
- Occlusion (whether the bite is distorted).
- Mucosal lacerations.

If possible, order orthopantomograph (OPG).

Displaced primary teeth

- If a primary tooth is avulsed (knocked out) do not reimplant it.
- The dentist should be made aware of the degree of displacement, tooth fracture and soft tissue or mucosal laceration, and called to assess other injuries of the primary teeth.
- The appropriate treatment will be either extraction or stabilisation of soft tissues.

Displaced or avulsed permanent incisor teeth

- Ideally, the tooth should be reimplanted in the socket immediately. Handle the tooth gently by the crown only, not by the root surface.

Table 17.1 Eruption times of normal dentition

Primary or deciduous teeth (total 20)

	Central incisors	Lateral incisors	Cuspids	First molars	Second molars
Age (months)	6–12	8–10	16–20	12–16	20–30

There is wide variation in eruption times, particularly of the deciduous teeth. At 1 year an infant has six to eight teeth, at 18 months 12 teeth, and at 2½–3 years 20 teeth. *Should there be no teeth erupted by 12 months, dental consultation should be sought.*

Permanent teeth (total 32)

	Central incisors	Lateral incisors	Cuspids	First bicuspid	Second bicuspid	First molars	Second molars	Third molars
Age (years)	6–9	7–10	10–12	10–12	11–12	6–7	11–13	17–21

The first permanent teeth to erupt are the lower first molars and central incisors.

- If it is not possible to reimplant, keep the tooth stored in milk, saliva or plastic wrap until dental treatment can be arranged. It is important that the tooth is replaced within 30 min as there is a high chance of success.
- Order appropriate radiographs: OPG, lateral cephalogram and chest X-ray if the tooth is missing (to make sure it has not been inhaled).
- Once the tooth has been reimplanted, a temporary splint may be constructed from aluminium foil moulded around the tooth.
- Splinting and stabilisation of the teeth will be required, as well as the treatment of associated soft tissue lacerations. Appropriate dental follow up should be arranged.

OTHER DENTAL PROBLEMS

The following problems may present as emergencies, but are generally not so:

- A lost filling (unless associated with significant pain).
- A broken denture or orthodontic plate.
- A loose band or wire of a fixed orthodontic appliance. Tuck the wire out of the way with a haemostat. The sharp end can be covered with chewing gum or blue tac.
- A loose artificial crown.
- A superficially chipped tooth.
- A minor laceration not requiring suturing. Give mouth rinses with warm saline and chlorhexidine gluconate 0.2% (Chlorhex, Savacol).

These patients may be advised to ring their own dentist for an appointment at the earliest opportunity.

RULES FOR DENTAL PREVENTION

- Commence oral hygiene with the eruption of the first tooth (see Table 17.1).
- Do not allow children to sleep with bottles at night.
- Minimise exposure to sugars and other refined carbohydrates.
- Begin dental visits as well baby consultations at 12 months.

CHAPTER 18
DERMATOLOGIC CONDITIONS

Rod Phillips
George Varigos
John Su

INTRODUCTION

The keys to accurate diagnosis and hence to appropriate management of skin disorders in children are a carefully taken history and astute observation of rashes, particularly focusing on their appearance, site and pattern of development. Most children you see will have one of the conditions listed in this section. During the examination ask yourself a few key questions (see also Fig. 18.1).

- Are there any vesicles; i.e. fluid-filled lesions? Finding these narrows greatly the range of possible diagnoses. Small circular erosions may be the only signs of an underlying vesicular process.
- Is the rash raised (papular) or flat (macular)?
- Is the rash red? Redness is from haemoglobin. Most red rashes blanch; i.e. the redness disappears with pressure. If not, the haemoglobin is outside the blood vessels – purpura.
- Is the rash scaly? If so, the epidermis may be broken (eczematous) to give weeping, crusting or bleeding, or it may be intact (papulosquamous).

VESICULOBULLOUS RASHES

Vesicles are usually caused by infections (HSV, varicella zoster virus (VZV), enterovirus, tinea, scabies or impetigo) or contact dermatitis. Also, consider drug reactions and erythema multiforme. Larger blisters may be from Stevens–Johnson syndrome, arthropod bites, contact dermatitis, burns or trauma.

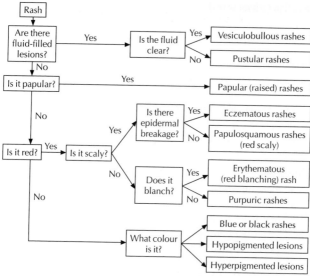

Vesiculobullous rashes
- Impetigo (school sores)
- Eczema herpeticum
- Erythema multiforme
- Single blisters

Pustular rashes
- Acne

Papular (raised) rashes
- Scabies
- Urticaria/serum sickness
- Papular urticaria
- Keratosis pilaris
- Papular acrodermatitis
- Molluscum
- Warts

Eczematous rashes
- Atopic eczema

Red scaly rashes (papulosquamous)
- Seborrhoeic dermatitis
- Psoriasis
- Tinea corporis
- Pityriasis rosea

Red blanching rashes (erythematous)
- Fever and exanthem
- Erythema infectiosum

- Roseola infantum
- Kawasaki's disease

Purpuric rashes
- Enteroviral infection
- Septicaemia
- Leukaemia
- Henoch–Schoenlein purpura
- Child abuse
- Idiopathic thrombocytopenic purpura (ITP)
- Trauma and vasomotor straining

Blue or black rashes
- Vascular malformations
- Haemangiomas

Hypopigmented lesions
- Tinea versicolor
- Pityriasis alba
- Vitiligo
- Post-inflammatory hypo- and hyperpigmentation

Hyperpigmented lesions
- Congenital pigmented naevi
- Acquired pigmented naevi

Fig. 18.1 Classification of skin disorders in children

Impetigo (school sores)

Cause

Staphylococcus aureus or *Streptococcus pyogenes*, or both.

Clinical features

Impetigo presents as areas of ooze and honey-coloured crusts on the face, trunk or limbs. Occasionally, the primary lesions are bullous. Lesions are rounded and well demarcated and may be single, grouped or widespread. Their onset and spread may be rapid or occur over days. In more chronic cases, there may be central healing with peripheral spread to give annular lesions.

Management

- Bathe off crusts.
- Apply topical mupirocin 2% ointment 8 hourly if localised, or oral flucloxacillin 15 mg/kg (max 500 mg) orally, 6 hourly if severe or extensive.
- Isolate the child from other children or from sick adults unless all lesions are covered or treated.
- Look for and treat any underlying condition such as scabies (a common cause of widespread impetigo) or eczema.

Staphylococcal scalded skin syndrome

Clinical features

- Usually seen in younger children.
- Mediated by an epidermolytic toxin released from an often insignificant staphylococcal focus (e.g. eyes, nose or skin).
- Fever and tender erythematous skin are early features.
- Exudation and crusting develops, especially around the mouth.
- Wrinkling, flaccid bullae and exfoliation of the skin are seen – Nikolsky sign ('normal' skin separates if rubbed).
- Blisters are very superficial and heal without scarring.

Management

- Flucloxacillin 50 mg/kg (max 2 g) i.v. 6 hourly if there is evidence of sepsis or systemic involvement.
- Drain any foci of pus if present.
- Monitor temperature, fluids and electrolytes if large areas are involved.
- Handle skin carefully and use an emollient ointment.

Erythema multiforme
Clinical features

This is a specific hypersensitivity syndrome that occurs at any age. Usually symmetric lesions appear most commonly on hands and feet, and often the face. They can be found anywhere.

Typical target lesions have an inner zone of epidermal injury (purpura, necrosis or vesicle), an outer zone of erythema and sometimes a middle zone of pale oedema. They are not migratory. The involvement of mucous membranes is common and can be extensive. Most cases are caused by herpes, some by other infections, uncommonly drugs.

Management
- Fluid maintenance.
- Apply emollient ointment to the lips, if needed.
- If the condition is recurrent, it is highly likely to be related to HSV. Prophylactic aciclovir should be considered if recurrences are frequent, severe and affecting the quality of life.

Stevens–Johnson syndrome/toxic epidermal necrolysis
Clinical features
- Stevens–Johnson syndrome and toxic epidermal necrolysis are believed by many to be variants of the one condition.
- They are characterised by widespread blisters on an erythematous or purpuric macular background, often with extensive mucous membrane haemorrhagic crusting.
- There may be tender erythematous areas with a positive Nikolsky sign ('normal' skin separates if rubbed).
- Conjunctivitis, corneal ulceration and blindness can occur.
- Anogenital lesions can lead to urinary retention.
- Fever, myalgia, arthralgia and other organ involvement can occur.
- Drugs are the most common cause, occasionally Mycoplasma.

Management
- Cease any drug that may be the cause.
- Fluid maintenance.
- Apply emollient ointment to the skin, lips and anogenital areas – this may be required many times a day.

- A regular eye examination with a specialist review for topical steroid drops if any eye involvement is noted.
- Corticosteroids may lessen the severity of the condition.

Note: Stevens–Johnson syndrome is not severe erythema multiforme. They are distinct conditions with different aetiologies. This distinction is important because permanent sequelae are rarely seen in severe EM and concurrent drug use is unlikely to be the cause. Skin lesion morphology is the best discriminating factor; mucous membrane involvement does not discriminate between these two conditions.

Eczema herpeticum
Clinical features

Herpes simplex virus infection in children with eczema is common, but many cases are misdiagnosed as either an exacerbation of the eczema or bacterial infection. Grouped vesicles may be prominent, but more often vesicles are rudimentary or absent and the infection presents as a group of shallow 2–4 mm ulcers on an inflamed base. The infected area may not be painful or itchy and does not respond to standard eczema therapy. If untreated, resolution usually occurs in 1–4 weeks, but dissemination may occur. Recurrences may occur at different sites.

Management

- Collect epithelial cells from the base and roof of the vesicles for herpes immunofluorescence and culture.
- Local disease in an otherwise well child requires regular observation but does not need antiviral therapy.
- A child with fever or multiple sites of cutaneous herpes infection may need admission to hospital and treatment with i.v. aciclovir 5 mg/kg per dose (2–12 weeks), 250 mg/m^2 per dose (12 weeks–12 years), 5 mg/kg per dose (adult) 8 hourly i.v. over 1 h.
- Eye involvement should be managed with topical or systemic aciclovir, or both, and urgent review by an ophthalmologist.
- The underlying eczema can be treated with moisturiser or wet dressings.

Single blisters

For a child who presents with a single blister as an isolated finding, consider an insect bite, cigarette burn, friction or spider bite. The latter can grow over days to become a non-tender blister with a diameter of many centimetres.

PUSTULAR RASHES

Consider acne, folliculitis, scabies and perioral dermatitis.

Acne

Clinical features

Acne mainly affects the forehead and face but other sebaceous gland areas (neck, shoulders and upper trunk) can be involved. Early lesions include blackheads, whiteheads and papules. In more severe cases there may be pustules or inflammatory cysts that can lead to permanent scarring.

Management

Acne is treatable. No person with acne should just be told it is an inevitable part of adolescence. Effective acne therapies are now available and should be used to control the disease.

For mild disease, use topical benzoyl peroxide 2.5–5%. Other topical agents include antibiotics (clindamycin, erythromycin or tetracycline), isotretinoin (not in pregnancy) or azelaic acid. These can be used singly or in combination and an improvement may be noted in 2–8 weeks. All of these topical agents have side effects with which practitioners must be familiar.

Treatment of moderate acne often involves the addition of oral antibiotic therapy (e.g. tetracycline 500 mg twice daily, erythromycin 500 mg twice daily, doxycycline 50–200 mg per day) for 4 to 12 months. Oral hormone therapy can help female patients.

Referral to a specialist for oral isotretinoin therapy is needed if there is scarring or cystic acne, a lack of response to antibiotics or significant depression.

Consider underlying endocrine disorders if acne begins before puberty.

PAPULAR (RAISED) RASHES

If the child is itchy, consider scabies, urticaria, serum sickness, papular urticaria or molluscum. If not, consider urticaria, molluscum, warts, melanocytic naevi, keratosis pilaris and papular acrodermatitis. For soft red, purple or blue swellings consider haemangiomas or vascular malformations. For raised red circles or rings, consider urticaria.

Scabies
Clinical features
An intensely itchy papular eruption develops 2–6 weeks after first exposure to the *Sarcoptes scabiei* mite or 1–4 days after subsequent reinfestation. The characteristic lesion is the burrow several millimetres in length. Burrows are best seen on the hands, especially between the fingers, and on the feet. Early burrows may be vesicular. Papules can occur anywhere including the palms, soles and genitalia. Excoriations and secondary impetigo may be present. There is currently a worldwide pandemic of this contagious disease affecting both adults and children.

Management
- Treatment is expensive and upsetting. If you are not confident of the diagnosis, confirm by scraping to find a mite or refer before treating.
- Use permethrin 5% cream. An alternative for pregnant or neonatal cases is sulphur 2% in yellow soft paraffin. We do not recommend lindane 1% (contraindicated in infants or women who are pregnant or breast-feeding) or benzyl benzoate 25% (too irritant for children and ineffective if diluted).
- At the same time, treat all family members and any other people who have close skin contact with the affected individuals.
- Apply to dry skin (not after a bath) from the neck down to all skin surfaces. For infants, apply to the scalp as well (not face). Use mittens if necessary to prevent finger-sucking.
- Leave the cream on for at least 8 h.
- Wash the cream off. Wash clothing, pyjamas and bed linen at this time.
- The itch takes a week or two to settle and can be treated with calamine lotion or an antihistamine, or both.

- Reinfestation is common. The family should notify all social contacts (e.g. creche, school or close friends) to ensure that all those infected receive treatment.

Urticaria/serum sickness

See also Allergy and Immunology, chapter 14.

Clinical features

Urticaria is characterised by the rapid appearance and disappearance of multiple raised red weals on any part of the body. Individual lesions are often itchy and clear within 1 day. There may be central clearing to give ring lesions. (These are not the so-called target lesions of erythema multiforme that persist for several days.) The child is usually well but may have associated fever and arthralgias (serum sickness). Urticarial episodes usually resolve over weeks or months, and rarely last longer than 6 months. In most cases of short duration, the cause cannot be determined.

Management

- Investigation is usually not required.
- Ask about drugs. Serum sickness commonly follows cefaclor use.
- Treat the itch with oral antihistamine (e.g. chlorpheniramine 0.1 mg/kg (max 4 mg) p.o. 6–8 hourly) or, in severe cases, a few days of oral prednisolone (1 mg/kg per day (max 50 mg)). Bed rest for joint involvement.
- For recurrent or chronic urticaria that persists for weeks look for trigger factors. Consider mast cell degranulating drugs, foods, animals, parasitic infections, heat, cold and physical pressure. Consider investigating with a throat swab (for streptococcal carriage), full blood examination (for eosinophilia and anaemia), antinuclear antibodies, urine culture for bacteriuria, nocturnal check for threadworms and a possible challenge with any suspected agent. Adding cimetidine (10–15 mg/kg (max 200 mg) p.o. 6 hourly) to the antihistamine may help.
- Urticaria may be the first sign of anaphylaxis. If there is associated angio-oedema (prominent subcutaneous swelling) or wheeze, continued observation and appropriate treatment is required (see Medical Emergencies, chapter 1).
- If individual lesions last longer than 2 days or are tender or purpuric, consider investigation for cutaneous vasculitis.

Papular urticaria
Clinical features

This is a clinical hypersensitivity to insect bites. New bites appear as groups of small red papules, usually in warmer weather. Older bites appear as 1–5 mm papules, sometimes with surface scale or crust, or with surrounding urticaria. Vesicles or pustules may form. Individual lesions may resolve in a week or last for months and may repeatedly flare up after fresh bites elsewhere. Itch is often intense and secondary ulceration or infection is common.

Management

- Prevent bites (e.g. adequate clothing, modifying behaviour that leads to exposure, occasional repellent, and the treatment of pets and house for fleas if necessary).
- Treat the itch with an agent such as aluminium sulphate 20% (Stingose), Liquor Picis Carb, 2% in calamine lotion, moderate potency steroid ointment or antihistamines (promethazine (0.2–0.5 mg/kg (max 25 mg) p.o. 6–8 hourly), diphenhydramine (1–2 mg/kg (max 100 mg) p.o. 6–8 hourly). Protective dressings (e.g. Duoderm) can speed the healing of lesions.
- Treat secondary infection with topical mupirocin ointment 2% or oral antibiotics.

Keratosis pilaris
Clinical features

This is an asymptomatic rough, somewhat spiky papular rash on the upper outer arms, thighs, cheeks, or all three areas, with variable erythema. It is common at all ages.

Management

Reassure the patient that this is rarely a problem. Soap avoidance and moisturisers can improve the feel. Steroids don't help.

Papular acrodermatitis
Clinical features

This is characterised by the acute onset of monomorphic red or skin-coloured papules mainly on the arms, legs and face.

It is usually asymptomatic and can be caused by coxsackie virus, echovirus, mycoplasma, EBV, adenovirus and others.

Management

Reassure and advise that clearing can take a few weeks.

Molluscum

Clinical features

Uncomplicated molluscum lesions are easily recognised as firm, pearly, dome-shaped papules with a central umbilication. However, presentation to a doctor is often prompted by the development of eczema in surrounding skin. In such cases, recognition can be difficult as these changes can obliterate the primary lesions. A carefully taken history of the initial lesions is usually diagnostic.

Management

- Education. Molluscum is caused by a virus and is very common. A child may develop a few or a great many lesions and individual lesions may last for months. Complete resolution will not happen until an immune response develops, which may take from 3 months to 3 years.
- Children with molluscum should not be restricted in their activities.
- The treatment depends on the age of the child, the location of the lesions and any secondary changes. Things to note include:
  - Treatment of the surrounding eczema may be all that is required.
  - Uncomplicated lesions not causing problems and not spreading can be left alone.
  - Isolated or troublesome lesions (e.g. on the face) can be physically treated. One method is gentle cryotherapy.
  - Occasionally, children warrant curettage under topical anaesthesia. This is well tolerated and usually curative. Alternatively, the stimulation of an immune response can be attempted with aluminium acetate solution (Burow's solution 1 : 30) for large areas, or benzoyl peroxide 5% daily to small areas and covered with the adhesive part of a dressing.
  - Inflamed lesions rarely warrant antibiotic treatment.

Warts

Many serotypes of the papilloma virus can cause warts. Different serotypes have a predilection for different areas of the skin. The resolution of all warts of the same serotype occurs when immunity develops, but this may take years. No treatment is necessary unless the warts are causing a problem to the child (e.g. social embarrassment, or pain from a plantar wart). Avoid painful procedures unless chosen by older children.

- *Ordinary warts.* If tolerated by the child, paring every 2–3 days with a razor blade or nail file will remove the surface horn. Apply a proprietary keratolytic agent that contains salicylic or lactic acid, or both, each day or two as directed.
- *Plantar warts.* These can be painful and can appear flat. Pare as for ordinary warts. Apply a proprietary keratolytic agent that contains salicylic or lactic acid, or both, each day or two. Alternatively, apply the affected area of sole for 30 min each night to a small pad of cotton wool soaked in 3% formalin and placed in a saucer on the floor. Cryotherapy and surgery are often ineffective and can lead to painful keloid scarring.
- *Plane (flat) warts.* These are smooth, flat or slightly elevated, skin-coloured or pigmented lesions. They may occur in lines or coalesce to form plaque-like lesions. If treatment is needed for plane warts on the hands, apply a formalin solution as for ordinary warts. Lesions on the face are often subtle and may not need treatment. Treatment may cause complications such as pigmentary changes and requires considerable caution.
- *Anogenital warts.* These are soft fleshy warts that occur at the mucocutaneous junctions, especially around the anus. They may be isolated flesh-coloured nodules or may coalesce into large cauliflower-like masses. Management options include awaiting resolution, topical podophyllin, curettage and diathermy and carbon dioxide laser. *Note:* genital warts in children should lead you to consider sexual abuse, but transmission is usually by normal intimate parent–child contact. The presence of genital warts in a young child is not an indication for mandatory reporting to government protective services.

ECZEMATOUS RASHES

Consider atopic eczema, allergic contact dermatitis, irritant contact dermatitis, photosensitivity eruptions, molluscum, tinea corporis and scabies.

Atopic eczema

See also Allergy and Immunology, chapter 14.

Clinical features

Eczema usually begins in infancy. It most commonly involves the face, and sometimes the trunk and limbs as well. In older children, the rash may be widespread but is often localised to flexures. Erythema, weeping, excoriation and rarely vesicles may be seen in acute lesions. Chronic lesions may show scale and lichenification. In some children, the lesions are more clearly defined, thickened discoid areas that may intermittently be itchy. There is usually a cyclical pattern of improvement and exacerbation. Weeping and yellow crusted areas that do not respond to therapy may indicate secondary bacterial or herpetic infection.

Management

- *Education.* Parents need to know that treatments are effective in controlling the disease, that they will not cure eczema and that exacerbations are common. Allergic factors are not the cause, but both environmental and food allergens may contribute to the exacerbation of symptoms in some patients. Allergen avoidance in these children may benefit some.
- *Avoid irritants.* The following may worsen eczema: soaps, bubble baths, prickly clothing, seams and labels on clothing, car seat covers, sand, carpets, overheating or contact with pets. Smooth cotton clothing is preferred.
- *Keep the skin moist.* Use a moisturiser such as sorbolene with 10% glycerine, aqueous cream or paraffin ointment (50 : 50 white soft paraffin/liquid paraffin) as often as several times a day if necessary.
- *Treat inflammation.* In mild or moderate cases, steroid creams can be used intermittently with good effect. Hydrocortisone 1%

is usually adequate. If not, moderate potency (e.g. beta-methasone valerate 0.02%) or potent (e.g. mometasone 0.1% or methylprednisolone 0.1%) ointment can be used for exacerbations in areas other than the face or nappy area. Prolonged use of moderate potency steroids to the skin of young children can cause atrophy and adrenal suppression. Oral steroids are rarely indicated in eczema. For chronic eczema on the limbs, zinc and tar combinations are alternatives to steroids.

- *Control itch.* Advise parents to avoid saying 'Stop itching' all the time and to distract the child instead. Avoid overheating at all times, particularly at night. Wet bandaging may be helpful, and sedation may be required. Antihistamines are often unhelpful but if the itch is not controlled by other measures try hydroxyzine 0.5–2.0 mg/kg (max 100 mg) 8 hourly, trimeprazine tartrate 0.05–0.5 mg/kg (max 25 mg) 6 hourly or promethazine hydrochloride 0.2–0.5 mg/kg (max 25 mg) 8 hourly. Terfenadine (Teldane) and astemizole (Hismanal) should not be used because of occasional fatal interactions if erythromycin is also taken.

- *Treat infection.* Take cultures and treat with simple wet dressings and oral antibiotics (e.g. erythromycin, cephalexin or flucloxacillin). Consider if herpes simplex is present (see p. 250). For a recurrent bacterial infection use antiseptic wash or bath oil (e.g. triclosan) and mupirocin 2% ointment nasally 8 hourly to treat staphylococcal carriage if present.

- *Diet.* A normal diet is usually indicated. If a child has immediate urticarial reactions to a particular food, that food should be avoided. In difficult cases, consider a more formal allergy assessment.

RED SCALY RASHES (PAPULOSQUAMOUS)

Consider seborrhoeic dermatitis (infants), psoriasis, tinea corporis, pityriasis rosea, pityriasis versicolor and atopic eczema. Ichthyosis vulgaris is a common cause of generalised scale without itch or redness.

Seborrhoeic dermatitis
Clinical features

- This condition presents in the first months of life, possibly partly due to the activity of commensal yeasts.
- Red or yellow/brown scaly areas will commonly affect the scalp, forehead and napkin area. The folds behind the ears and around the neck, axillae, groin and gluteal clefts are also commonly affected.
- Resolution by the age of 1 year is usual.

Management

- Imidazole creams, with hydrocortisone 1% cream or with a mixture of salicylic acid (1%) and sulphur (1%) ointment, b.d.
- Anti-yeast shampoos (e.g. selenium sulphide – Selsun) can be helpful. Use carefully to avoid irritation or toxicity.

Psoriasis
Clinical features

Psoriasis can occur at any age. Lesions begin as small red papules that develop into circular, sharply demarcated erythematous patches with prominent silvery scale. Common presentations include plaques on extensor surfaces, generalised guttate (small) lesions, red scaly scalp lesions or moist red anogenital rashes. Itch can be a problem. Nail changes are often seen in childhood.

Management

- The treatment depends on the site and extent of disease and the age of the child. Adolescents are less tolerant of the smell of tar creams.
- Treat isolated skin plaques with either topical steroids (e.g. intermittent mometasone with clinical monitoring) or tar-based creams (e.g. liquor picis carbonis LPC 3%/salicylic acid 2% in sorbolene cream). Generally avoid tars on the face, flexures and genitalia.
- Thick scalp plaques can be softened overnight with a similar tar cream and removed with a tar shampoo.
- Use hydrocortisone 1% ointment on the face and anogenital region. Topical steroids are not used for large areas in childhood

psoriasis because of the possible development of rebound pustular disease.

- Topical calcipotriol can be used in children older than 12 years.
- Widespread psoriasis may need treatment with one or more of dithranol, etretinate, methotrexate, cyclosporine or ultraviolet therapy, all of which are effective.

Tinea corporis
Clinical features

The typical lesion is a slow-growing erythematous ring with a clear or scaly centre. However, tinea corporis can present in a wide variety of ways, particularly if previously treated with steroid ointments. It can be pustular or vesicular, or spread to many sites within days. Tinea should be considered in any red scaly rash where the diagnosis is unclear.

Management

- If in doubt about the diagnosis, confirm by scraping the scale for microscopy and culture.
- Lesions are treated with terbinafine cream (b.d. for 1 week), an imidazole cream (e.g. clotrimazole, miconazole or econazole b.d.–q.i.d. for 4 weeks) or oral griseofulvin for widespread lesions.

Pityriasis rosea
Clinical features

The condition is common between the ages of 1–6 years.

Initially, a pink scaly patch appears, followed a few days later by many pink/red scaly oval macules mainly on the trunk. It is usually asymptomatic.

Management

Reassure the patient. The condition can persist for weeks.

RED BLANCHING RASHES (ERYTHEMATOUS)

Macular erythematous lesions are most commonly caused by viral infections (e.g. coxsackie, echovirus (ECHO), Epstein–Barr virus (EBV), adenovirus, parainfluenza, influenza, parvovirus B19, human herpesvirus 6 (HHV6), rubella and measles) or drug reactions. Consider also septicaemia, Kawasaki disease and mycoplasma infection. Spider naevi can be seen in children as isolated findings.

Fever and exanthem

The onset of fever and exanthem is usually due to a viral illness, often enterovirus. Some infections have specific clinical features that aid diagnosis; e.g. measles and erythema infectiosum. However, in most instances a diagnosis cannot be made with certainty. To manage such a child, consider the *STOP* strategy:

- *S*ick? Is the child lethargic, cold peripherally or young? Consider meningococcal disease, other bacterial sepsis, Kawasaki disease. Investigate and treat.
- *T*aking drugs? Consider ceasing medication.
- *O*ther people at risk? If relatives are immunosuppressed or pregnant, consider serology, stool viral culture, and advising the at-risk person to consult their doctor.
- *P*apular? Consider papular acrodermatitis.

If the answer to all the above is 'no', reassurance and review is probably appropriate.

Erythema infectiosum, Roseola infantum and Kawasaki disease

See Infectious Diseases, chapter 26.

Cellulitis
Clinical features

- An infection of cutaneous and subcutaneous tissue, characterised by erythema, warmth, oedema and tenderness.
- Predisposing factors include a break in the skin (e.g. insect bite, trauma) or a pre-existing skin lesion.
- May be associated with regional lymphadenopathy, fever, chills and malaise.
- Usually caused by *Streptococcus pyogenes* and *Staphylococcus aureus.*
- *Haemophilus influenzae* type b is uncommon but still needs to be considered in non-immunised children under 5 years. It is often accompanied by bacteraemia or meningitis, or both.
- It may be associated with deeper involvement including necrotising fasciitis, osteomyelitis and septic arthritis.

Management

- Cultures of blood, skin aspirate or skin biopsy – they are positive in about 25% of cases.
- Benzylpenicillin 50 mg/kg (max 3 g) i.v. 6 hourly, or (if a bite or injury) flucloxacillin 50 mg/kg (max 2 g) i.v. 6 hourly.
- Parenteral therapy is needed if there is fever, rapid progression, lymphangitis or lymphadenitis. Non-immunised children under 5 years with facial cellulitis should be treated with cefotaxime 50 mg/kg (max 2 g) i.v. 6 hourly *and* flucloxacillin 50 mg/kg (max 2 g) i.v. 6 hourly.

PURPURIC RASHES

Consider viral infections, meningococcal sepsis, platelet disorders, vasculitis, drug reactions and trauma.

Enteroviral infection

Scattered petechiae can be seen in children who have fever from common enteroviral infections. These children are usually well. If in doubt, or if the child appears unwell, investigate (full blood examination (FBE), blood cultures) and consider treatment for septicaemia.

Septicaemia

Suspect septicaemia (usually meningococcal) in a child with recent onset of fever and lethargy. Skin lesions may be erythematous macules progressing to extensive purple purpura. If in doubt, take blood cultures, give antibiotics and arrange admission (see also Medical Emergencies, chapter 1).

Leukaemia

Suspect leukaemia in a child with generalised petechiae or purpura in the absence of trauma. Look for tiredness or pallor. Obtain an urgent full blood examination (see Haematologic Conditions and Oncology, chapter 25).

Henoch–Schoenlein purpura

See also Rheumatologic Conditions, chapter 33.

Non-itchy, painless macules, papules or urticarial lesions with purpuric centres occur in a symmetrical distribution mainly on the buttocks and ankles, occasionally on the legs, arms and elsewhere. There may be associated abdominal pain, arthralgia or haematuria. Renal involve-ment leading to chronic renal failure is rare, but can occur irrespective of the severity of the rash and other symptoms, and may be delayed until weeks or months after the onset of the illness.

Child abuse

Twisting, compression, pinching and hitting can all cause petechial or purpuric lesions (see Child Abuse and Neglect, chapter 11). Look for bruises of bizarre shapes and different ages, evidence of bony fractures, and an abnormal affect.

Idiopathic thrombocytopenic purpura (ITP)

See also Haematologic Conditions and Oncology, chapter 25.

Bruises, petechiae or purpuric lesions appear over a period of days or weeks, mainly in sites of frequent mild trauma. The child is otherwise well. Full blood examination will show a low platelet count.

Trauma and vasomotor straining

In some ethnic groups it is common to treat a febrile or unwell child by rubbing or suctioning the skin with a variety of implements. This produces bizarre circular and linear patterns of petechiae that can alarm the unwary.

Petechiae can appear around the head and neck in normal children after coughing or vomiting. Restraining a small child for a procedure such as a lumbar puncture can also lead to the development of petechiae on the upper body.

BLUE OR BLACK RASHES

Consider vascular malformations, haemangiomas, Mongolian spots, blue naevi and melanoma.

Vascular malformations

- These can be blue, red, purple or skin coloured. They are developmental defects and do not resolve.

- Such malformations can involve any mix of capillaries (e.g. port-wine stain), veins, arteries (e.g. arteriovenous malformation) and lymphatics (e.g. cystic hygroma).
- Extensive malformations can be associated with soft tissue or bony hypertrophy, bone erosion, haemorrhage, infection and platelet trapping.
- Management requires a multidisciplinary approach using expertise from surgical, paediatric, dermatological and radiologic fields.

Haemangiomas
Clinical features

Superficial haemangiomas begin as macular erythematous lesions and become soft, partly compressible, sharply defined, red or purple swellings that can occur anywhere on the body. Deeper haemangiomas may appear as blue or skin-coloured swellings. Most (but not all) haemangiomas are not present at birth; they grow for several months and resolve fully over several years.

Management

Parents need reassurance about the inherently benign nature of these lesions. Most haemangiomas are best left alone and allowed to involute spontaneously. In some sites, however, haemangiomas can lead to problems such as blindness, destruction of cartilage, respiratory obstruction or death. If any developing haemangioma:

- Is ulcerating and potentially disfiguring
- Is on the eyelid or adjacent to the globe of the eye
- Deforms structures such as the lip, ear cartilage or nasal cartilage
- Begins as an extensive macule that grows thicker
- Is associated with stridor, thrombocytopenia or multiple lesions, it needs urgent assessment by a clinician experienced in this field (within days, not weeks) for possible treatment with steroids, vascular laser, surgery or interferon.

HYPOPIGMENTED LESIONS

In hypopigmented lesions, look for a fine scale. If it is scaly, consider pityriasis versicolor or pityriasis alba. If it is not scaly, consider pityriasis versicolor, post-inflammatory loss of pigment, halo naevi or vitiligo.

Pityriasis versicolor

- This is common in adolescents, and probably caused by an increased activity of commensal yeasts.
- Multiple oval macules, usually covered with fine scale, appear on the trunk or upper arms. The lesions may appear paler or darker than the surrounding skin.
- Treatment with anti-yeast shampoos is effective. For example, apply selenium sulphide 2% (Selsun shampoo). Leave on for 2 h, if tolerated, rinse, and treat weekly for 4 weeks and then monthly. The recovery takes weeks and relapses are common.

Pityriasis alba

This condition is common in prepubertal children. Single or multiple, poorly demarcated hypopigmented 1–2 cm macules are seen on the face or upper body. Lesions are not itchy but often have a fine scale. Treat with hydrocortisone 1%. Resolution takes weeks.

Vitiligo

This condition is characterised by sharply demarcated, often symmetrical areas of complete pigment loss. Eventual repigmentation in childhood vitiligo is common and is helped by topical steroids. In troublesome cases refer to a specialist for advice regarding treatment (e.g. corrective cosmetics or psoralen therapy).

Post-inflammatory hypo- and hyperpigmentation

This condition occurs particularly in dark-skinned people. Many inflammatory skin disorders may heal but leave diffuse, hypo- or hyperpigmented macules that can persist for months or years. No treatment is satisfactory.

HYPERPIGMENTED LESIONS

If they are flat, consider junctional melanocytic naevi, café-au-lait spots, naevus spilus, pityriasis versicolor and post-inflammatory hyperpigmentation. If raised, consider compound melanocytic nevi, Spitz naevi and warts.

Congenital pigmented naevi

Congenital melanocytic naevi that cover large areas or are likely to cause concern need very early assessment by a skin specialist and plastic surgeon, preferably in the first week of life, for diagnosis, surgery, laser treatment and/or long-term follow up.

Acquired pigmented naevi

- During childhood, most children develop multiple pigmented lesions, which may be freckles, lentigines, naevus spilus, acquired melanocytic naevi or rarely, melanoma.
- Immune-suppressed children and those who have had chemo-therapy need to be watched closely.

ANOGENITAL RASHES

Virtually all anogenital rashes seen in infants that wear nappies are primarily caused by reaction with urine or faeces (irritant napkin dermatitis) or by seborrhoeic dermatitis. Soaps, detergents and second-ary yeast infection may contribute. In older children, threadworms (*Enterobius vermicularis*) are a common cause of an itchy anogenital rash. Look for the worms at night and treat with mebendazole 50 mg (<10 kg), 100 mg (>10 kg) (not in pregnancy or less than 6 months) or pyrantel 10 mg/kg (max 500 mg) once oral. A repeat dose 2 weeks later helps reduce the high rate of reinfestation.

Consider also rare causes such as malabsorption syndromes (diarrhoea, erosive dermatitis and failure to thrive), zinc deficiency (a sharply defined anogenital rash with associated perioral, hand and foot 'eczema'), Langerhans' cell histiocytosis, psoriasis and Crohn's disease.

Irritant napkin dermatitis
Clinical features

This is the most common cause of napkin dermatitis in infants and typically presents as confluent erythema that spares the groin folds. Variant presentations include multiple erosions and ulcers, scaly or glazed erythema, and satellite lesions at the periphery. Satellite lesions are suggestive of Candida infection.

Management

- Keep the area clean and dry. Leave the nappy off whenever possible.
- Gel-based disposable nappies or a non-wettable under-napkin can be helpful. Cloth nappies should be thoroughly washed and rinsed.
- Use topical zinc cream for mild eruptions.
- Add hydrocortisone 1% cream if inflamed. Do not use stronger steroids.
- Antifungal therapy is often not needed even if Candida is present.

Candida napkin dermatitis

This occurs secondary to antibiotic use and irritant napkin dermatitis. Treat with a combination of topical antifungal cream (e.g. clotrimazole 1%) and hydrocortisone 1%.

Perianal streptococcal dermatitis

Streptococcus pyogenes infection.

Clinical features

- A localised, well-demarcated erythema that covers a circular area of 1–2 cm radius around the anus.
- If not treated, it may remain for months.
- May have painful defecation, fissures and constipation.

Management

- Perianal and throat cultures are taken to confirm the presence of *Streptococcus pyogenes*.
- Apply paraffin ointment three times daily to the perianal area for symptomatic relief. Treat with oral antibiotics (phenoxy-methylpenicillin 15 mg/kg (max 500 mg) 6 hourly) for a minimum of 2 weeks. Several weeks of therapy may be required. Intramuscular benzathine penicillin can be used if there are concerns about compliance.
- Keep stools soft with oral liquid paraffin for several weeks.

Lichen sclerosis et atrophicus

This condition presents as an asymptomatic or itchy area of atrophy, with white shiny skin, purpura or telangiectasia, or both, and often in the perivulval region of girls aged 3 years or older. Cases have been misdiagnosed as sexual abuse. Management is with moisturisers and brief courses of moderately potent steroid ointment. About 50% of cases resolve spontaneously.

HAIR PROBLEMS

Consider tinea capitis, alopecia areata, traumatic alopecia, kerion and head lice.

Alopecia areata
Clinical features

Typically one or more oval patches of hair loss develop over a few days. Some hairs may remain within the patches. Occasionally, the hair loss is diffuse. The scalp appears normal and does not show scaling, erythema or scarring. Most cases in childhood resolve spontaneously but progression to total scalp or body hair loss or recurrent alopecia can occur. Regrowth can occur decades later.

Management
- For isolated small patches present for weeks without further progression, no treatment is needed.
- For recent or progressive hair loss, treatment with moderate potency topical steroids for a few weeks may help. In difficult cases, other therapies including contact sensitisation, irritant agents and more potent immunosuppression need to be considered.

Traumatic alopecia
Clinical features

This condition is usually caused by rubbing (as on the occiput of many babies), cosmetic practices (e.g. tight braiding) or hair pulling as a habit (trichotillomania). Trichotillomania may be largely nocturnal and parents are often unaware of it. The affected areas are usually angular and on the anterior or lateral scalp. The areas contain hairs of different lengths and are never completely bald.

Management
- Recognition of the problem and a careful explanation to the family is often sufficient.

- Trichotillomania in younger children does not usually indicate that significant psychological problems are present. It is a habit similar to thumb-sucking or nail-biting and a low-key approach similar to that used in those conditions is appropriate.

Tinea capitis
Clinical features

In Australia, tinea capitis is usually caused by *Microsporum canis* contracted from cats or dogs. It is characterised by patches of hair loss with some short, lustreless, bent hairs a few millimetres in length. Redness and scaling are present in the patch. Hair loss without any of these features is not likely to be fungal.

Management

Confirm the diagnosis, if possible, by greenish fluorescence of the hair shafts with Wood's light (not present with some fungi) or by microscopy and culture of hair and scale. Treatment usually comprises griseofulvin orally 10–15 mg/kg (max 0.5–1 g) daily for 4–6 weeks or until non-fluorescent. Pulse therapy (1 week treatment, 3 weeks off, then repeat) with newer antifungals (terbinafine, itraconazole) is just as effective. Children may attend school provided that they are being treated.

Kerion (inflammatory ringworm)

This represents an inflammatory scarring immune response to tinea. It is an erythematous, tender, boggy swelling that discharges pus from multiple points. The swellings appear fluctuant but skin incision should be avoided. Treatment is with oral antifungals, often with antibiotics for secondary infection, and a brief course of oral steroids to suppress the immune response. Other inflammatory granulomas can mimic kerions.

Head lice
Clinical features

Infestation of the scalp with *Pediculus capitis* is associated with itching. Eggs (nits) can be seen attached to the hairs just above the scalp surface. Epidemics of head lice regularly sweep through primary schools in all areas.

Management

- Suitable treatments include pyrethrin 0.165% (e.g. Pyrifoam), maldison 0.5% and permethrin 1% (e.g. Nix and Lyclear cream rinse).

- Wash the hair with soap and water. Thoroughly moisten the hair with the treatment and leave for 10 min. Rinse well and comb out with a fine-toothed comb. Reapply 1 week later to kill any eggs that have subsequently hatched.
- Reinfestation is common. A regular physical inspection and combing of the hair is as important as chemical treatment.

NAIL PROBLEMS

Congenitally abnormal nails are usually atrophic and can be the presenting feature of rare inherited conditions such as ectodermal dysplasias, dyskeratosis congenita, pachyonychia congenita, congenital malalignment of the great toenails and the nail–patella syndrome.

Acquired nail disease is usually a result of fungal infection, psoriasis, ingrown toenails or 20-nail dystrophy. It may also be seen in association with diseases such as alopecia areata and lichen planus. Nail-biting and picking can lead to marked deformity of involved nails.

Tinea unguium (onychomycosis)
Clinical features

- Dermatophyte infection may affect one or more nails.
- White or yellow patches develop at the distal and lateral nail edges. The rest of the nail may become discoloured, friable and deformed with accumulation of subungual debris.
- Tinea is often also present on the adjacent skin.

Management

- Always confirm the diagnosis by microscopy and culture of nail clippings.
- In mild cases, treatment with physical debridement and anti-fungal nail lacquer (e.g. amiolfarone) may be effective.
- Most cases require oral therapy for months – oral griseofulvin 10–20 mg/kg (max 1 g) or griseofulvin ultramicrosize 5.5 mg/kg (max 330 mg). Both terbinafine and itraconazole are also effective.

CHAPTER 19
DIABETES AND HYPOGLYCAEMIA

Glynis Price
George Werther

DIABETES MELLITUS

Diagnosis

Diagnosis is made by either:

- Random blood glucose >11 mmol/L,
  or
- Fasting blood glucose >7 mmol/L,

plus typical symptoms of polyuria, polydypsia and weight loss.

Transient hyperglycaemia

Transient elevation of blood glucose and glycosuria (and possibly ketonuria) may occur in children with an intercurrent illness or with therapy such as glucocorticoids. The risk of later developing diabetes mellitus is about 3%, but it rises to approximately 30% if these findings are picked up in an otherwise well child. An HbA1c and diabetes-related autoimmune markers (antibodies against insulin, glutamic acid decarboxylase (GAD) and islet cells) should be ordered and the child's condition discussed with a paediatric endocrinologist or Diabetes Unit for possible admission for observation.

DIABETIC KETOACIDOSIS (DKA)

This is the form of presentation in >30% of newly diagnosed diabetes in childhood and adolescence.

Definition

Hyperglycaemia >14 mmol/L, metabolic acidosis (pH <7.3 or bicarbonate <15 mmol/L) and hyperketonaemia or moderate to severe ketonuria.

Causes

These include delayed diagnosis of insulin-dependent diabetes mellitus (IDDM), omission of insulin (especially in adolescents with recurrent DKA), acute stress (infection, trauma, psychological) and poor management of intercurrent illness.

History

- Typical symptoms include polyuria, polydipsia, loss of weight and lethargy. They are usually of 1–3 weeks' duration.
- There is occasionally a family history of diabetes or other auto-immune disease.
- Precipitating events.

Examination

Examination to determine:

- The extent of dehydration (*note*: this is usually overestimated):
  - Mild (<3%) – not detectable clinically.
  - Moderate (6%) – reduced skin turgor, poor capillary return and Kussmaul respiration.
  - Severe (≥7%) – poor perfusion, tachycardia and low blood pressure.
- Level of consciousness.
- Body temperature – hypothermia is common.
- The presence of a precipitating cause; e.g. infection.

Investigations

Blood

- Blood glucose level.
- Plasma urea and electrolytes. *Note*: Do not use a capillary specimen for K^+ assessment due to haemolysis. *Note*: To identify hypernatraemia, compensate for the dilutional effect of hyperglycaemia by calculating the adjusted sodium value:

$$\text{Adjusted } Na^+ = \text{plasma } Na^+ + 0.3 \times (\text{plasma glucose} - 5.5)$$
$$\qquad\qquad\qquad (\text{mmol/L}) \qquad\qquad (\text{mmol/L})$$

- Serum osmolality (measure or calculated),

$$\text{Serum osmolality} = Na^+ \times 2 + \text{glucose} + \text{urea}$$
$$\qquad\qquad\qquad (\text{mmol/L}) \quad (\text{mmol/L}) \quad (\text{mmol/L})$$

- Blood gas (capillary or arterial) for acid–base assessment.
- Insulin and GAD antibodies (islet cell antibodies in some centres). This is optional.

Urine

- Test for ketonuria and glycosuria.
- Test for proteinuria, pyuria and nitrites (these may indicate infection).

Other

- Consider blood culture, a chest X-ray or other tests for infection if clinically appropriate.

Management

This depends on severity of presentation.

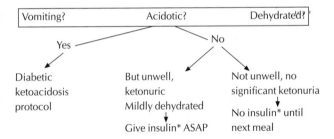

* Use quick-acting insulin; e.g. Actrapid, at 0.25 unit/kg per dose, s.c. Use half the dose if the child is <4 years or if there is only trace or no ketonuria present. If <2 h before next meal, wait until then.

Repeat insulin dose 6 hourly, 30 min before meals, *until normoglycaemia and negative ketonuria are achieved*. Note: a meal at midnight must be given while on 6-hourly insulin injections.

Encourage good fluid intake (e.g. water or any non-sugar-containing fluid). Normal diet according to appetite, but excluding quick sugars (the diet should be adjusted later by a dietitian). Standard meal times plus snacks mid-morning, mid-afternoon and at bedtime (20:00 h).

When normoglycaemia and negative ketonuria are achieved change insulin to a twice-daily mixture of short and intermediate acting insulin, usually at 1 unit/kg per day. However, this may need modification. It should be administered as: 2/3 in the morning, 1/3 at night, 2/3 of each dose intermediate acting, 1/3 as short acting. Occasionally, older adolescents go on to a basal bolus regimen: 30–40% intermediate-acting insulin given at 22:00 h; rest is given as short-acting insulin in three equal doses before meals.

Intravenous therapy
Fluids

- Treat shock if it is present. Use normal saline at 20 mL/kg. This can be repeated as boluses of 10–20 mL/kg until perfusion is re-established.
- Give replacement fluids evenly over 48 h (See Table 19.1). Replacement fluids = deficit + maintenance fluids.

Table 19.1 Intravenous fluid rates in diabetic ketoacidosis (mL/h)*

Bodyweight (kg)	Degree of dehydration		Bodyweight (kg)	Degree of dehydration	
	3%	6%		3%	6%
5	24	27	38	101	125
7	33	38	40	104	129
8	38	43	42	107	133
10	48	54	44	110	137
12	53	60	46	113	141
14	58	67	48	116	146
16	64	74	50	119	150
18	70	80	52	122	154
20	75	87	54	124	158
22	78	91	56	127	162
24	80	95	58	130	167
26	83	100	60	133	171
28	86	104	62	136	175
30	89	108	64	139	179
32	92	112	66	142	183
34	95	116	68	145	187
36	98	120	70	148	191

* Includes deficit and maintenance fluid needs for 48 h. Patients with greater degrees of dehydration should initially be resuscitated until perfusion is adequate. Further fluid management should be discussed with a paediatric diabetes or intensive care unit.

- Deficit = 10 × the percentage of dehydration × bodyweight in kg.
- Maintenance = 100 mL/kg per day for the first 10 kg; add 50 mL/kg for the next 10 kg, and 25 mL/kg thereafter. (Remember to double maintenance value if calculating replacement for 48 h).
- Use 0.9% saline for the first 12 h, then change to 0.45% saline.
- Add potassium chloride (KCl) to the saline at the time of starting the insulin infusion.
- Add 40 mmol/L if weight is <30 kg, 60 mmol/L if weight is >30 kg. *Note:* This may have to be increased if the patient is very acidotic at presentation.
- Add dextrose to intravenous fluids when the blood sugar level drops below 10–12 mmol/L. Five per cent dextrose in saline is usually sufficient but you may have to increase this percentage. (Each 10 mL of 50% dextrose added to 500 mL of any solution adds 1% dextrose.)

Insulin infusion

- Commence after treatment of shock, and simultaneously with addition of KCl to intravenous fluid.
- Use unmodified Actrapid–Novo Nordisk™ or Humulin R-Lilly™ 1 unit/mL via a syringe pump, sideline and three-way tap. Run at 0.1 units/kg per h, or at 0.05 units/kg per h if the blood glucose is <15 mmol/L or if the patient has had insulin within 4 h.
- Reduce the insulin dose to 0.05 units/kg per h when the blood glucose is <10–12 mmol/L, and when giving 0.45% saline/5% dextrose and the patient is improving metabolically. If still acidotic but blood glucose is less than about 10 mmol/L, increase dextrose in the infusate to 7.5–10% and maintain an insulin rate of 0.1 unit/kg per h.
- Change to s.c. insulin when the patient is stable, preferably before meal time. Stop i.v. insulin 30 min after the first s.c. insulin injection.

Bicarbonate

- This is generally not to be used because of risks of hypokalaemia, cerebral acidosis and altered oxygen affinity of haemoglobin.
- In exceptional cases of severe acidosis, it may be given as 50% of calculated deficit (0.3 × bodyweight in kg × base deficit) in mmol over 30 min.

General care

- If the patient is unconscious he or she should be treated in an intensive care unit with careful maintenance of the airway.
- Patient should remain nil orally until alert and stable.
- Nurse the patient in a head-up position and in good light.
- Clinical monitoring should include:
  — Strict fluid balance, vital signs, conscious state, pupil size and light response.
  — Note any *headache* or *altered behaviour that may indicate impending cerebral oedema.*
- Biochemical monitoring should include:
  — 2–4 hourly laboratory blood glucose levels (with hourly bedside glucometer readings), serum sodium (adjusted for hyperglycaemia), potassium, chloride and serum osmolality.
  — *Beware of falling adjusted sodium levels as glucose declines – hyponatraemia may herald cerebral oedema.*
  — If the sodium level falls, consider decreasing the rate of fluid administration to replace over 72–96 h.

COMPLICATIONS OF DKA

Cerebral oedema

This is an uncommon (0.5–3%) but extremely serious complication of diabetic ketoacidosis in children, usually occurring 6–12 h after commencement of therapy. This condition is usually fatal. If the patient survives there may be profound neurological impairment.

Risk factors

- Newly diagnosed diabetes.
- Excessive fluid rehydration, particularly with hypotonic fluids.
- Severe initial acidosis.
- Hyponatraemia or hypernatraemia, and negative sodium trend during the therapy. *Note:* With appropriate therapy the serum sodium should remain stable or rise slightly as blood glucose falls. If the adjusted serum sodium falls during resuscitation, this may be a sign of excess fluid administration and may be associated with the development of cerebral oedema. If this

occurs, decrease the rate of fluid administration to replace over 72–96 h.

Signs

- *Early*: Negative sodium trend, headache, behaviour change (sudden irritability, depression of conscious state) and incontinence.
- *Late*: bradycardia, elevated blood pressure and depressed respiration.

Treatment

This is a medical emergency.

- Administer 20% mannitol i.v. as a bolus dose at 0.25–0.5 g/kg (1.25–2.5 mL/kg of 20%). This can be repeated if the response is inadequate.
- Nurse the patient in a head-up position, maintain the airway, restrict fluids.
- Transfer to an intensive care unit for intubation, intermittent positive pressure ventilation and further management.
- *Do not delay treatment for radiological confirmation – diagnosis is clinical.*

Hypoglycaemia

- Use 25% dextrose at 2 mL/kg i.v. over 3 min.
- Increase the concentration of glucose in the infusate. Only if the patient is metabolically much improved and looking well, consider decreasing the insulin infusion rate.

Hypokalaemia

Monitor frequently and adjust potassium concentration in the infusate. Children at particular risk of this complication are those who are very acidotic or have low potassium levels at presentation.

HYPOGLYCAEMIA IN CHILDREN WITH IDDM

Common causes

- Missed meal/snack.
- Vigorous exercise (can be during exercise or hours afterwards).
- Alcohol.
- Too much insulin.

Management

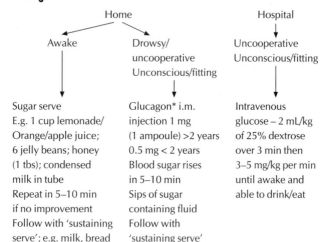

```
                        Home                          Hospital
                      ↙      ↘                          ↓
              Awake        Drowsy/                  Uncooperative
                          uncooperative            Unconscious/fitting
                          Unconscious/fitting
                ↓              ↓                          ↓
```

Awake	Drowsy/uncooperative Unconscious/fitting	Uncooperative Unconscious/fitting
Sugar serve	Glucagon* i.m.	Intravenous
E.g. 1 cup lemonade/	injection 1 mg	glucose – 2 mL/kg
Orange/apple juice;	(1 ampoule) >2 years	of 25% dextrose
6 jelly beans; honey	0.5 mg < 2 years	over 3 min then
(1 tbs); condensed	Blood sugar rises	3–5 mg/kg per min
milk in tube	in 5–10 min	until awake and
Repeat in 5–10 min	Sips of sugar	able to drink/eat
if no improvement	containing fluid	
Follow with 'sustaining	Follow with	
serve'; e.g. milk, bread	'sustaining serve'	

* *Note*: Glucagon can cause headache/vomiting

SICK DAY MANAGEMENT DURING INTERCURRENT ILLNESS IN THE DIABETIC CHILD

Principles

- Frequent testing of blood sugar and urine ketones.
- The meal plan may temporarily be dropped – replace with fluids and easily digested carbohydrates.
- Ensure good fluid intake – alternate sugar and non-sugar-containing fluids depending on blood sugar levels (BSL)s (water is best if BSLs are high).
- Insulin doses usually need to be increased; never omit insulin.
- Keep in touch with medical staff.

Management

	1	2	3
Blood sugar level (BSL)	High (>15 mmol/L)	High	Normal/low
Urine ketones	0–trace	> 1+	0–trace
Vomiting	+/–	Absent to very occasional	+/–
Danger		DKA	Hypoglycaemia
Fluids	Ensure good intake (to thirst); normal meal plan	Increase intake ++; can drop normal meal plan	Ensure good intake
Insulin	Increase normal insulin dose by 10%	Give rapid-acting insulin at 10–20% of total daily dose*. Repeat 4 hourly (2 hourly if 3–4+ ketones or mild vomiting present)	Reduce normal insulin by 10–25%. May drop intermediate insulin if giving quick insulin 4–6 hourly
Testing BSLs and urine ketones	4–6 hourly	2–4 hourly	2–4 hourly
Further action	If ketones increasing → 2	No improvement → admission	If BSL low→ sugar-containing fluid; if high or ketones developing → 1/2

* Total daily dose = sum of all insulin given per 24 h
If total dose < 5 units, use 1 unit increments.

MANAGEMENT OF CHILDREN WITH DIABETES UNDERGOING SURGERY

The main aims are to prevent hypoglycaemia before, during and after surgery, and to provide sufficient insulin to prevent the development of ketoacidosis.

Factors that must be considered are:
- Time of surgery.
- Duration of surgery.
- Urgency of surgery.

Minor elective morning surgery
- Admit the child on the previous evening.
- Aim for the patient to be first on the operating list.
- Administer normal food and insulin until midnight on the night before surgery.
- At 06.00 h perform blood glucose. If blood glucose is <10 mmol/L give lemonade or sugar-containing clear fluid at 5–10 mL/kg (max = 200 mL) and inform the anaesthetist.
- Monitor blood glucose every 2 h and immediately before surgery. If blood glucose is less than 6 mmol/L insert intravenous line and give i.v. glucose.
- Give short acting insulin equal to 1/10th of the total daily insulin dose (short and intermediate acting) at the usual time.
- An intravenous line with glucose will be inserted in the operating theatre (if not required pre-operatively).
- Perform regular blood glucose every 2–4 h postoperatively, and adjust the i.v. glucose infusion as necessary. Give extra insulin 0.25 units/kg every 4–6 h to keep glucose between 5 and 10 mmol/L.
- When the patient can tolerate oral fluids stop the intravenous infusion and resume the normal insulin regimen.

Minor elective afternoon surgery
- Continue normal food and insulin until midnight on the night before surgery.
- Provide a light breakfast at the usual time.

- Give short acting insulin equal to 1/10th of the total daily insulin dose half an hour before breakfast.
- Monitor blood glucose every 2 h. (Commence i.v. glucose if BSL is <6 mmol/L, otherwise i.v. glucose can be commenced in theatre.)
- Give additional insulin at the same dose at 12.00 h.
- Adopt same regimen as above postoperatively.

Minor surgery/short anaesthetic

- Intravenous glucose may not be necessary, provided that the oral intake can be resumed soon after surgery and that the pre-operative blood glucose concentration does not fall below 6 mmol/L. If in doubt, it is safer to follow the routines outlined above.

Emergency and major surgery

- Urgent clinical and biochemical assessment as for diabetic ketoacidosis.
- Rehydrate and start i.v. insulin as required.
- Maintain i.v. 0.45% saline with 5% dextrose and insulin infusion at 0.05–0.1 units/kg per h pre- and postoperatively until the patient is able to resume oral feeding.

HYPOGLYCAEMIA

Definition

A blood sugar level of <2.5 mmol/L. If suspected clinically and on a glucose reflectance meter, it must be confirmed with a true blood glucose measurement in the laboratory.

Causes

See Table 19.2.

The two most common causes of hypoglycaemia beyond the neonatal period are:

- Hyperinsulinism in the first 2 years. This usually results in persistent, severe hypoglycaemia and may lead to permanent brain damage, as the brain depends on glucose in the first 2–3 years of life.

Table 19.2 Neonatal/childhood hypoglycaemia: Causes

Transient neonatal:	–↓ Substrate/enzyme function – prem/SGA*
	  – RDS**
	–↑ Glucose utilisation – hyperinsulinism –
	  • Beckwith–Wiedeman
	  • IDM***
	  • Rh disease
	  – sepsis	

Persistent Neonatal Recurrent Childhood:	–↑ Glucose utilisation Ketone –ve	Hyperinsulinism Salicylates Sepsis
	–↓ Hepatic glucose production Ketone +ve +/–↑ Lactate#	Glycogen storage disease# Gluconeogenic defect# Galactosaemia Fructose intolerance Inborn errors of amino acid metabolism – maple syrup urine Severe liver disease – Reye's syndrome
	–↓ Production of alternative fuels ketone –ve	Fatty acid oxidation defects – medium chain acyl coA dehydrogenase def. Ketogenesis defects
	– Hormonal deficiency ketone +ve	Cortisol – 1° – 2° to ACTH deficiency Growth Hormone
	– Drugs ketone +ve/–ve	Alcohol Salicylates Propranolol Valproate Oral hypoglycaemics

* SGA, small for gestational age.
** RDS, respiratory distress syndrome.
*** IDM, infant of a diabetic mother.

- Ketotic hypoglycaemia (accelerated starvation) beyond the first 2 years. This is the most likely cause of hypoglycaemia in children over 2 years of age. These children are often small for their age and were small for their gestational age. Poor oral intake or vomiting in the 24 h before the hypoglycaemic episode is common. An early morning seizure in a child should suggest the diagnosis. The cause is unclear, and this entity may simply be one end of the normal spectrum. Natural history is for spontaneous remission by 8–10 years.

Signs and symptoms
Infantile/neonatal

- Apnoea/tachypnoea/cyanotic spell.
- Hypotonia, poor crying and feeding.
- Irritability, tremor and seizures.

Childhood

- Catecholamine mediated: hunger, pallor, sweating, tremor and tachycardia.
- Neuroglycopenic effects: altered conscious state, abnormal behaviour and seizure.

Relevant history

- Gestational duration and birthweight.
- Previous episodes.
- Relationship to meals/feeds and duration of fasting.
- Age at onset of hypoglycaemia.
- Family history of neonatal deaths and affected relatives.
- Drugs – alcohol and insulin.
- Intercurrent illness.

Specific examination features

- Growth parameters (height, weight and head circumference). Overgrowth may suggest hyperinsulinism; underweight ketotic hypoglycaemia.
- Midline defects (e.g. cleft lip, central incisor and micropenis) may suggest hypopituitarism.
- Muscle bulk, power and tone (glycogen storage disease).
- Hepatomegaly (e.g. glycogen storage disease and galactosaemia).
- Jaundice (e.g. galactosaemia).

- Cataracts (e.g. galactosaemia).
- Unusual odours (e.g. ketones and maple syrup) suggesting metabolic disease.
- Ambiguous genitalia (congenital adrenal hyperplasia with adrenal crisis).

Investigation

Before i.v. glucose is given (and usually before the true blood glucose is available), blood and urinary samples *at the time of hypoglycaemia must* be obtained as these are essential for diagnosis.

Samples to be taken:

Blood

Venous blood is adequate except for the acid–base status. At least 5 mL, but preferably 8–10 mL of blood should be taken. Distribute as follows (minimum amounts of blood needed are given in parentheses):

- Glucose and lactate: fluoride oxalate tube (1 mL).
- Insulin, cortisol, growth hormone: plain tube (2–4 mL).
- Ammonia: heparinised tube (1 mL).
- Ketones and free fatty acids: fluoride oxalate (BLF) tube (1 mL).
- Amino acids, electrolytes: heparinised tube (1–2 mL) – if enough blood is available.
- Acid–base: a capillary sample.
- Blood drops to be applied to a Guthrie test card (for acyl-carnitine profile).

Urine

- Ward test for ketones, glucose and reducing substances.
- 10–20 mL for amino acids and organic acids.

Sets of the required tubes, labelled 'Hypoglycaemia Kit' are available in the Royal Children's Hospital emergency department and specimens *should be taken and returned on wet ice as soon as possible* to the laboratory.

Please do not discard any blood or urine taken at time of hypoglycaemia – send any excess to the laboratory marked 'excess – store'.

Management

- Neonate: 2–3 mL/kg of 10% dextrose, followed by an infusion of dextrose (5–10 mg/kg per min). *Note:* 10% dextrose at 0.1 mL/kg per min will supply 10 mg/kg per min.
- Older children: 1–2 mL/kg of 25% dextrose, then 3–5 mg/kg per min until stable.

CHAPTER 20
ENDOCRINE CONDITIONS

Garry Warne
Fergus Cameron

SHORT STATURE

Five questions need to be asked:

- Is the child really short?
- Is the child short in relation to other children the same age (i.e. below the third centile)?
- Is the child unexpectedly short for his or her family? Measure the child and, wherever possible, both biological parents. Plot all three heights on appropriate height centile charts, and compare the centiles (see Appendix 2). The child's height centile should approximate the mean of the parents' centiles.
- Is the child growing slowly? Ask for any previous height measurements and plot them on the centile chart. If no previous measurements are available, ask to see the child again at 3-month intervals and, after 6 months, calculate the height velocity and check this against a growth velocity (GV) chart. GV can be reliably calculated from measurements taken over not less than 6–12 months.

   In normal children GV tends to fluctuate, and only a consistently low GV will lead to a falling off in height centile. The criterion for further investigation in a short child is a GV below the 25th centile.
- If the child's growth really is slow, what is the reason?

Physiological
Constitutional delay in maturation

This is a common (and often familial) normal variant. Characteristically, growth slows at about the age of 2 years, producing a fall in the height centile. Thereafter, growth is parallel to the third centile, but the prepubertal decline in growth is exaggerated and the onset of the growth spurt is later than average. Bone age is delayed. The final height is likely to be in keeping with the height of other family members.

Familial short stature

Several adult family members are short. Skeletal proportions and GV are normal. Bone age is equivalent to the chronological age.

Note: Some children from short families also have constitutional delay in maturation.

Organic

Organic causes of growth retardation are classified in Table 20.1.

Diagnosis

- Clues to the diagnosis may emerge from the history and the child's general appearance. Measure the skeletal proportions (span/height and upper/lower segment ratios). The span should be within a few centimetres of height at all ages.
- *The lower segment should be >1/2 the height beyond the age of 8 years.*
- Some serious medical conditions (e.g. chronic renal failure, coeliac disease and Crohn's disease) may present with slow growth as the only abnormal sign.

Investigations

At the initial stage check the bone age. If the GV is <25th centile for bone age then:

- Thyroid function tests (TFTs).
- Chromosomes in all girls (regardless of appearance).
- Haemoglobin and erythrocyte sedimentation rate (ESR) (Crohn's).
- Consider testing for coeliac disease.
- Renal function.
- Serum calcium phosphate and alkaline phosphatase.
- Skeletal survey (if disproportionate).
- Growth hormone (GH) studies: (i) exercise (random serum GH values are meaningless); and (ii) a glucagon stimulation test (the current definitive test).

Table 20.1 Organic causes of short stature

	Examples	Clues to diagnosis
Intra-uterine	Russell–Silver syndrome	Birth length <third centile for gestational age
Skeletal	Bone dysplasia (e.g. achondroplasia) Spinal irradiation	Skeletal dysproportion (short limbs) Low lower : upper segment ratio
Nutritional	Rickets Calorie–protein malnutrition (world no. 1) Malabsorption (e.g. coeliac disease) Chronic illness (e.g. renal failure, Crohn's disease)	History of poor nutrition Low weight-for-height (not if chronic) Abdominal distension Anaemia, high ESR
Iatrogenic	Corticosteroid therapy	Cushingoid features
Chromosomal and genetic	Turner's, Down's, Prader–Willi, Noonan's, Cornelia de Lange, Rubinstein–Taybi syndromes Inborn errors of metabolism: storage disorders (MPS†, Gaucher's) Organic/amino acidopathies (e.g. MMA*, MSUD**)	Specific dysmorphic features Peculiar odour Metabolic acidosis
Endocrine	Hypothyroidism, Cushing's disease, growth hormone deficiency	Height centile > weight centile (i.e. short and plump) Associated examination findings

† MPS, mucopolysaccharidosis
* MMA, methylmalonic aciduria
** MSUD, maple syrup urine disease

Growth hormone therapy

Recombinant human GH is government controlled in Australia because it costs an average of $20 000–$30 000 per year per child. To qualify, children must meet certain criteria:

- The height is below the first centile.
- The GV is below the 25th centile for bone age.
- The bone age is under 13.5 for girls, or under 15.5 for boys.

- They must be free of any condition known not to respond to GH (e.g. high-dose steroid therapy or thalassaemia) or that could be worsened by GH therapy (e.g. insulin-dependent diabetes mellitus (IDDM), Fanconi anaemia or active malignancy).

Good responses are seen in GH deficiency or Turner's syndrome.

The dose is Somatropin 14–22 U/m^2 per week divided into 6–7 doses/week.

TALL STATURE

Aetiology
- Familial.
- Precocious puberty.
- Hyperthyroidism.
- Syndromes: Marfan, Klinefelter, triple X, homocystinuria and Sotos.
- Pituitary gigantism (juvenile acromegaly).

Treatment
High-dose oestrogen is sometimes used in selected very tall girls to accelerate epiphyseal maturation and reduce the final height. The ideal time to start is just after the appearance of the first pubertal changes.

Tall boys may be similarly treated with testosterone.

HYPOTHYROIDISM

Hypothyroidism may be congenital or acquired.

Congenital hypothyroidism
- The incidence is 1 : 3200 births.
- Most cases are detected by neonatal screening (high thyroid-stimulating hormone, TSH). Confirmation of the diagnosis on whole blood TFT is essential.
- Technetium scanning shows that most cases have either an absent or ectopic (sublingual) thyroid. Enzyme deficiencies associated with goitre are found in about 10% of cases.

- Thyroxine therapy (8–12 µg/kg bodyweight per day) must be started as early as possible – before 2 weeks.

Clinical features

- Jaundice.
- Large anterior fontanelle, persistent posterior fontanelle.
- Coarse features.
- Dry skin.
- Supra-orbital oedema.
- Umbilical hernia.
- Harsh cry.
- Slow feeding.
- Distal femoral epiphysis that is not ossified.

Acquired hypothyroidism

Acquired hypothyroidism is called primary when the thyroid gland it-self is abnormal (e.g. ectopic thyroid dysgenesis, auto-immune chronic lymphocytic thyroiditis and dyshormonogenesis) and secondary when the abnormality is a deficiency in pituitary TSH. Helpful investigations include: serum TSH, thyroid auto-antibodies and technetium thyroid scan.

Clinical features

- Growth retardation.
- Constipation.
- Cold intolerance.
- Goitre.
- Dry cool skin.
- Prolonged ankle jerk relaxation time.

Referral to a paediatric endocrine clinic is important for the management of hypothyroidism.

HYPERTHYROIDISM

Hyperthyroidism is almost always due to Graves' disease. Six times as many girls are affected as boys, most commonly during puberty. A family history of thyroid disease (hyper- or hypothyroidism) is common. Family members may also have one of the following: IDDM, vitiligo, pernicious anaemia, Addison's disease or premature gonadal failure.

Clinical features

- Goitre (nearly all).
- Weight loss; heat intolerance; tiredness.
- Warm sweaty hands; tremor; tachycardia.
- Irritability; restlessness.
- Proximal muscle weakness and wasting; accelerated ankle jerk relaxation time.
- Lid lag; exophthalmos.
- Accelerated growth.

Investigations

TFT, TSH receptor antibodies, bone age (usually advanced).

Management

- Antithyroid drugs (carbimazole 0.4 mg/kg (max 30 mg/day) 8–12 hourly, orally for 2 weeks and 0.1 mg/kg (max 5 mg) 8–24 hourly; propylthiouracil 50 mg/m² 8 hourly), interrupted every 2–3 years until remission occurs.
- Subtotal thyroidectomy is recommended if the disease is still active by the age of 19–20, or if the patient is unable to take antithyroid drugs.
- The use of radioactive iodine in children and adolescents is controversial and we do not advocate it.

DELAYED PUBERTY

Delayed puberty is defined as the absence of pubertal changes: over 14 years for girls and over 15 years for boys (see Appendix 2 for pubertal stages charts/diagrams).

Aetiology

With normal or low-serum gonadotrophins

- Constitutional delay (usually familial) is the most common cause. It is associated with slow growth and a delayed bone age.
- Chronic illness/poor nutrition (e.g. cystic fibrosis, thalassaemia, juvenile chronic arthritis and Crohn's disease).
- Endocrine causes: hypopituitarism (gonadotrophin, and possibly GH and other hormonal deficiencies), Kallmann syndrome

(isolated gonadotrophin deficiency with anosmia), hypothyroidism and hyperprolactinaemia consider prolactinoma.

With elevated serum gonadotrophins

This signifies primary gonadal failure, which may be due to:

- A genetic abnormality associated with gonadal dysgenesis (Turner, Klinefelter and Noonan syndromes).
- Anorchia.
- Gonadal destruction secondary to vascular damage, irradiation, infection, torsion or autoimmune disease.

Investigations

- Serum follicle-stimulating hormone (FSH), luteinising hormone (LH), testosterone or oestradiol; serum prolactin; other pituitary function tests (e.g. GH studies), as indicated by growth.
- Full blood examination, ESR.
- Urea, creatinine, serum proteins.
- TFT.
- Chromosomes.
- Bone age.

Treatment

A referral should be made to a paediatric endocrinologist who may use testosterone 100–500 mg i.m. every 2–4 weeks in boys, or oestradiol (oral contraceptive pill) in girls. GH therapy may be offered to girls with Turner's syndrome.

PRECOCIOUS PUBERTY

Precocious puberty is defined as the onset of pubertal changes under 8 years in girls and under 9.5 years in boys. For pubertal staging, refer to Appendix 2.

Aetiology

Gonadotrophin dependent ('central' or 'true')

- True precocious puberty is more common in girls than boys, and girls are less likely to have an underlying pathological cause than boys.

- Girls with this disorder have accelerated growth, development of both pubic hair and breasts, and the vaginal mucosa has a pale, shell-pink colour with increased mucus secretion.
- Boys with true precocious puberty have enlargement of both testes, as well as accelerated linear and genital growth.
- The commonest pathological cause is hypothalamic hamartoma. Practically all intracranial pathologies (malformation, trauma, tumour, infection and haemorrhage) are associated with an increased prevalence of precocious puberty.
- Investigations are designed to demonstrate the premature activity in the hypothalamo–pituitary–gonadal axis, and to exclude intracranial pathology.

Gonadotrophin independent (or 'pseudo')

- Congenital adrenal hyperplasia.
- Adrenal, testicular or ovarian neoplasms.
- Tumours that secrete non-pituitary gonadotrophin such as chorionic gonadotrophin (hCG).
- McCune–Albright syndrome.
- Familial male precocious puberty.

Investigation

- Serum FSH and LH.
- Gonadal steroid (testosterone or oestradiol).
- Bone age.
- Magnetic resonance imaging (MRI) head, if increased FSH or LH.

Treatment

A referral should be made to a paediatric endocrinologist, who may use medroxyprogesterone acetate, cyproterone acetate or a luteinising hormone releasing hormone superagonist. Not all cases require treatment.

Conditions resembling precocious puberty
Premature thelarche

- Isolated breast development is common in girls under 2 years of age (8–10%) and can be expected to regress spontaneously in most cases.
- Simple observation is sufficient.

Premature adrenarche

- The isolated appearance of pubic hair (usually in a girl) under the age of 8 years may occur as a variant of the norm, but it may also signify non-classical congenital adrenal hyperplasia.
- Appropriate investigations are bone age, basal serum dehydro-epiandrosterone sulphate (DHEA-S), androstenedione, testosterone and 17-hydroxyprogesterone (17-OHP). The measurement of 17-OHP at 30 and 60 min after intramuscular Synacthen (synthetic adrenocorticotrophic hormone) is recommended to diagnose non-classical congenital adrenal hyperplasia.
- Referral to a paediatric endocrinologist is recommended.

PUBERTAL GYNAECOMASTIA

- In true gynaecomastia there will be a palpable disc of breast tissue; this is to be distinguished from adiposity of the breast area.
- Breast development occurs transiently in many boys mid-way through puberty and is physiological.
- If associated with testicular volumes <6 mL, Klinefelter's syndrome must be excluded by a chromosomal analysis.
- Adrenal and gonadal tumours can cause gynaecomastia, but this is rare.
- Many drugs, notably cimetidine, digoxin, spironolactone and even i.m. testosterone, can induce breast development, as can heavy marijuana use.
- Prepubertal gynaecomastia also occurs, but in most cases no cause can be found.

Treatment

There is no medical treatment. Refer boys with significant breast enlargement to a plastic or general surgeon for subareolar mastectomy.

OBESITY

See also Infant and Child Nutrition, chapter 7 and Table 20.2.

Table 20.2 Endocrine causes of obesity

Cause	Clinical features	Screening investigation
Cushing's disease	Growth retardation, hypertension, hirsutism, striae, typical facial changes, bruising	24 h urinary-free cortisol
Hypothyroidism	Growth retardation, tiredness, constipation, cold intolerance, dry skin	Thyroid function tests (TFT)
Growth hormone (GH) deficiency	Growth retardation	GH studies
Prader–Willi syndrome	Neonatal hypotonia, growth retardation, developmental delay, hyperphagia, hypogonadism, typical facial appearance, small hands and feet	Specific DNA test

Nutritional obesity is associated with growth acceleration and advancement of bone age. Endocrine obesity is associated with growth retardation and a delay in bone age.

AMBIGUOUS GENITALIA

An underlying endocrine or genetic cause should be sought in:
- Any infant with ambiguous genitalia.
- Boys with perineal hypospadias.
- Boys with any combination of the following: micropenis, hypospadias, short stature, dysmorphic features or undescended testis.
- Girls with inguinal herniae containing gonads.

Note: Clitoral enlargement of any degree is abnormal.

Aetiology

In decreasing order of frequency:
- Gonadal dysgenesis.
- Congenital adrenal hyperplasia.
- Androgen insensitivity syndrome.
- Testosterone biosynthetic defects.

Investigations

- Pelvic ultrasound.
- Serum 17-hydroxy progesterone and 24 h urine steroid profile.
- Chromosomes.
- Electrolytes, urea and blood glucose.

Management

- Refer urgently to an experienced paediatric endocrinologist or surgeon.
- Inform the parents about the problem and show them the genitalia; tell them that the infant appears otherwise healthy, and that the true sex will be ascertained within a few days. Do not attempt to predict the child's sex.
- Offer emotional support (refer to a social worker or an experienced Mental Health professional).
- Transfer the baby to a tertiary-referral centre without delay.
- Avoid offering unsubstantiated opinions about the sex of the baby.
- Call a meeting of all nursery staff and discuss policy about communication with the parents about the baby. Keep detailed notes about communication with the parents.

ADRENAL DISEASES—ADRENAL HYPOFUNCTION

Primary adrenal insufficiency
X-linked adrenoleukodystrophy

- This is the commonest cause of primary adrenal insufficiency in school-age boys. Look for:
    - Hyperpigmentation of the skin (ACTH-mediated), tiredness, nausea, anorexia and weight loss.
    - Adrenal features usually preceded by the development of a neurological disability (e.g. memory loss, sleep disturbance or ataxia).
    - Test blood and skin fibroblasts for very long-chain fatty acids.
    - Dietary modification and bone marrow transplantation may be helpful in cases with normal MRI.

Autoimmune destruction (Addison's disease)

- This is usually part of the autoimmune polyglandular syndrome (in combination with either chronic mucocutaneous candidiasis, primary hypoparathyroidism, or both).

Congenital adrenal hyperplasia

- — 21-Hydroxylase deficiency.
- — Other rare types.
- — Other features (e.g. ambiguous genitalia and precocious sexual development) are more striking than those due to adrenal insufficiency.

Investigations

- Serum electrolytes (low sodium and high potassium).
- Simultaneous serum cortisol and plasma ACTH.
- Specific investigations if congenital adrenal hyperplasia (CAH) is suspected.

Treatment

- Hydrocortisone 20 mg/m^2 BSA per day in divided doses.
- Fludrocortisone 0.05–0.2 mg daily, orally.
- Steroid cover for stress (see Appendix 4).

'Secondary' adrenal insufficiency (due to ACTH deficiency)

- This is not usually associated with salt-wasting.
- There is no hyperpigmentation of the skin.
- Treat with hydrocortisone alone; fludrocortisone is unnecessary.
- Steroid cover for stress (see Appendix 4).

ADRENAL HYPERFUNCTION

Adrenocortical tumours

- This may manifest as Cushing's syndrome, virilisation, hypertension, abdominal mass or pain.
- These tumours are very rare.

Adrenocortical hyperplasia

- This is usually secondary to a pituitary adenoma secreting ACTH.
- The primary micronodular form (genetic cause) is seen rarely.

Adrenal medullary tumours

- Neuroblastoma in very young children.
- Phaeochromocytoma leading to hypertension in older children (*Note:* usually part of genetic multiple endocrine neoplasia Type 2 syndrome; may be bilateral and familial).

Investigations

- c-ret oncogene mutational analysis.
- 24 h urinary catecholamines and calcitonin studies.

DISORDERS OF CALCIUM METABOLISM

Table 20.3 Differential diagnosis and investigation of hypocalcaemia

Age	Differential diagnoses	Initial investigations
Neonate	• Prematurity/IUGR/asphyxia • Gestational diabetes • Hypoparathyroidism • Phosphate loading (milk formulas with high phosphorus) • Magnesium deficiency	• Total/ionised calcium • Albumin • Magnesium • Phosphate • Parathyroid hormone (PTH)
Childhood	• Hypoparathyroidism • Vitamin D deficiency • Chronic renal failure • Magnesium deficiency • Nutritional deficiency • Pancreatitis • Critical illness • Organic acidaemia	• Total/ionised calcium • Albumin • Magnesium • Phosphate • PTH • 1, 25$(OH)_2$VitD, 25(OH)VitD • Wrist/knee X-rays • Urea and electrolytes/ creatinine • Lipase • Alkaline phosphatase (ALP)

Table 20.4 Differential diagnosis and investigation of hypercalcaemia

Age	Differential diagnoses	Initial investigations
Neonate	• Iatrogenic • Hyperparathyroidism (primary or secondary) • Subcutaneous fat necrosis • Bartter's syndrome • Infantile hyophosphatasia • Williams syndrome • Familial benign hypocalciuric hypercalcaemia • Idiopathic	• Total/ionised calcium • Albumin • Magnesium • Phosphate • PTH • Urinary phosphoethanolamine • 1, 25(OH)$_2$Vitamin D • Alkaline phosphatase (ALP)
Childhood	• Hyperparathyroidism • Familial benign hypocalciuric hypercalcaemia • Hypervitaminosis D (nutritional, inflammatory disease) • Immobilisation • Neoplasia • Drugs (thiazides, lithium, alkalis) • Hyperthyroidism	• Total/ionised calcium • Albumin • Magnesium • Phosphate • PTH • Urinary phosphoethanolamine • 1, 25(OH)$_2$Vitamin D • Chest X-ray • Thyroid function tests (TFTs)

Treatment of severe hypercalcaemia

- Rehydration.
- Bisphosphonates.
- Calcitonin.

CHAPTER 21

EAR, NOSE AND THROAT CONDITIONS

Robert Berkowitz
Mike South

OTITIS MEDIA

This term covers a spectrum of conditions, which are characterised by the presence of fluid in the middle ear, as recognised by tympanic membrane appearance or by a demonstration of tympanic membrane immobility (by either pneumatic otoscopy or tympanometry). Clinically, otitis media presents as either: (i) acute suppurative otitis media; or (ii) otitis media with effusion.

Acute suppurative otitis media (ASOM)

This condition is characterised by both:

- Middle ear effusion.
- Features of inflammation that are either:
  — localised (e.g. ear pain) *or*
  — generalised (e.g. fever, irritability) and where no other cause is apparent (or develops) to explain these generalised features of inflammation.

The degree of redness of the tympanic membrane is relatively unhelpful in deciding whether or not bacterial infection is present. ASOM is frequently over-diagnosed.

The causative organism is usually *Streptococcus pneumoniae*, non-typable *Haemophilus influenzae* or *Moraxella catarrhalis*. ASOM is often preceded by a viral upper respiratory tract infection.

Be cautious of accepting ASOM as the sole diagnosis in an unwell infant with a fever. There may be a coexistent serious bacterial infection. Consider a septic work-up or very careful observation.

Management
Initial management

Antibiotics confer only a modest benefit in most cases of ASOM. Acute symptoms resolve in 60% of cases without antibiotics within 24 h. Antibiotics do not reduce the later incidence of recurrent ASOM or chronic otitis media with effusion (see below). In children over 2 years who are only mildly unwell it is reasonable to wait 24–48 h before commencing antibiotics if the clinical features have not resolved in this time.

Amoxycillin 15 mg/kg (max 500 mg) orally, 8 hourly for 5 days is recommended. For true cases of penicillin allergy, erythromycin 15 mg/kg (max 500 mg) orally, 8 hourly may be used. When ASOM is associated with acute tympanic membrane perforation, drainage of the middle ear is often incomplete as the perforation heals rapidly, and the standard criteria for the use of antibiotics are applicable. There is no benefit in adding topical antibiotics.

Whether antibiotics are prescribed or not, a key part of the treatment is adequate analgesia. Give paracetamol 15 mg/kg 4 hourly (max 90 mg/kg per 24 h) as needed.

Follow up

The key features of ASOM, inflammation and middle-ear effusion, need to be followed up separately. Review in 48 h if there is no resolution of the symptoms of inflammation.

Possible explanations include:
- The wrong diagnosis (most commonly a viral upper respiratory tract infection).
- A failure to take the medication (either the antibiotics were not given or they were vomited).
- An inappropriate antibiotic was prescribed (switch to amoxycillin with clavulanic acid 15 mg/kg (max 500 mg) orally, 8 hourly).
- The antibiotic itself is responsible for the child remaining unwell.
- A suppurative complication of ASOM has developed (e.g. mastoiditis).

If the appropriate medical treatment has been unsuccessful, acute drainage of the ear (myringotomy) with or without insertion of a tympanostomy tube may need to be considered. Refer to a paediatric ear, nose and throat surgeon.

Follow up of the middle-ear effusion should be based on a knowledge of the expected persistence of fluid following an ASOM. There is persistent middle-ear effusion in 70% of cases at 2 weeks, 40% at 1 month, 20% at 2 months and 10% at 3 months. A check at 3 months is therefore recommended.

Otitis media with effusion (OME)

This presents as a persistent middle-ear effusion without clinical features of inflammation.

Management

The need for active management, either medical or surgical, depends on the severity and duration of symptoms, including hearing impairment.

OME tends to resolve spontaneously in time. For symptomatic cases that have not resolved in 3 months, a prolonged course of antibiotics (amoxycillin 15 mg/kg (max 500 mg) 8 hourly for 3 weeks) will result in a resolution of a significant proportion.

Where OME is associated with recurrent ASOM, prophylactic antibiotics can help to prevent further episodes of ASOM and thereby allow the middle-ear effusion to resolve spontaneously. However, this must be balanced against the risk of inducing resistant organisms and the potential morbidity of long-term antibiotic use. No other medications are of practical benefit.

Insertion of tympanostomy tubes does not cure the underlying Eustachian tube dysfunction responsible for OME, but only temporarily removes the symptoms. If OME is symptomatic and is likely to be present for a significant period of time in the future, insertion of tympanostomy tubes should be considered. Adenoidectomy may be beneficial in addition (by removing a reservoir of infection from the nasopharynx), but it adds significant morbidity to an otherwise very minor procedure.

The prerequisites for tympanostomy tubes are:

- Middle-ear effusion present for at least 3 months and appears likely to persist long term. This is important because 90% of effusions will resolve within the first 3 months and early treatment is therefore unnecessary.
- Symptoms must be present: either recurrent ASOM or functionally significant hearing loss (e.g. speech delay, behavioural disturbance or poor school performance).

OME and ASOM are often related to upper respiratory tract infections and are therefore more common over the winter months. Where OME has been present for 3 months at the end of winter, it may be appropriate to delay inserting tubes in the expectation that there may be a resolution with the onset of warmer weather.

The benefits of the temporary alleviation of symptoms of OME by the insertion of tympanostomy tubes need to be balanced against the disadvantages:

- The need for general anaesthesia and surgery.
- Tubes usually remain *in situ* for only 6–9 months (although longer-stay tubes are available) and the reinsertion rate of tubes is approximately 25%.
- There is a tympanic membrane perforation rate of approximately 1% per year when the tube is *in situ*.
- Otorrhoea occurs in up to 25% of cases; it is often associated with an upper respiratory tract infection. It may also occur because of external contamination (e.g. swimming or bathing without ear protection).

In a child with tympanostomy tubes, discharging ears should be treated by ear toilet and topical antibiotics. Discharge refractory to treatment can be managed by 3% hydrogen peroxide ear washes; however, the possibility of an underlying immunodeficiency or cholesteatoma should be considered and the child should be reviewed by an ENT surgeon.

OTITIS EXTERNA

Clinical features

The features of this condition are the inflammation of the ear canal (which includes the tympanic membrane) and pre-auricular tenderness. Tympanic membrane mobility on pneumatic otoscopy rules out otitis media.

Management

Regular ear toilet and topical antibiotics are required. Where the ear canal is very oedematous, an ear wick should be inserted and moistened frequently with topical antibiotics to maintain patency of the ear canal.

Hospital admission for administration of (anti-Pseudomonas) intravenous antibiotics may be necessary when ear pain is severe and not relieved by regular analgesics, or where cellulitis has extended beyond the ear canal. See Antimicrobial guidelines.

ACUTE PHARYNGITIS/TONSILLITIS

The child with a fever and sore throat is a common presenting problem, but the areas of controversy are in making the correct diagnosis and following up with the appropriate use of antibiotics.

Some facts

- Most sore throats are due to a viral infection.
- The only clinically important bacterial pathogen is group A *β-haemolytic streptococcus* (GAS).
- GAS is found in around 20–30% of older children presenting with an acute sore throat.
- GAS colonises the throat in some normal children (up to 1 in 5).
- Distinguishing colonisation from acute infection is a major problem. A child with a sore throat may be colonised with GAS and therefore have a positive throat swab, yet the cause of this episode may be a viral infection.
- GAS is very uncommon as the cause of a sore throat in children under 4 years of age and antibiotics are generally unnecessary.

- GAS is more likely if the child has tenderness of the tonsillar cervical lymph nodes, inflammation of the tonsils and the rest of the pharynx (pharyngotonsillitis), or a generalised erythematous (scarlatiniform) rash.
- The presence of tonsillar exudate is not helpful in distinguishing viral infection from GAS.
- GAS is less likely if the child also has coryza or cough.
- If an antibiotic is to be prescribed, this should be penicillin (usually oral phenoxymethylpenicillin 30 mg/kg (max 1 g) 12 hourly for a full 10-day course. Erythromycin 15 mg/kg (max 500 mg) 8 hourly or roxithromycin 2.5 mg/kg (max 150 mg) 12 hourly may be used for children with true penicillin allergy. Amoxycillin should not be used.
- Penicillin does lead to a more rapid resolution of symptoms but only to a modest degree. Treated patients recover an average of only 8 h earlier. Penicillin probably reduces the incidence of rare suppurative complications (e.g. quinsy). Penicillin probably reduces the risk of subsequent rheumatic carditis. In low-risk populations (e.g. Caucasian Australians) this is in any case a very rare problem.
- The early use of penicillin may increase the risk of future recurrent GAS tonsillitis because the child may have insufficient time to develop a lasting immune response.

Practical management

Children who probably don't need antibiotics are those aged less than 4 years and/or those with associated cough or coryza.

Children who probably do need antibiotics are those aged over 8 with marked pharyngotonsillitis, tender tonsillar cervical nodes, and without cough and coryza. Give oral phenoxymethylpenicillin 30 mg/kg (max 1 g) 12 hourly for 10 days.

In between these two ends of the clinical spectrum, the decision will need to be individualised on the relative risk factors. Remember to include in the decision-making process the costs, adverse effects and promotion of bacterial resistance associated with use of antibiotics. At present, in our community, antibiotics are over-used in children with sore throats. A lower threshold for use of penicillin is appropriate for certain higher risk groups (e.g. Australian Aborigines).

Infectious mononucleosis is a relatively common cause in older children and often becomes apparent when there is no response to penicillin, other characteristic features develop (e.g. generalised lymphadenopathy, mild jaundice and rashes) and there is a more prolonged course of the condition.

Recurrent acute pharyngitis/tonsillitis

Recurrent sore throats are a normal part of growing up for very many children. True recurrent GAS pharyngotonsillitis is much less common but often over-diagnosed.

A variety of strategies have been used to reduce recurrences:
- The use of another antibiotic to attempt eradication of GAS (e.g. erythromycin, a cephalosporin and clindamycin).
- The use of low-dose prophylaxis with penicillin.
- The treatment of culture-positive family members.
- Tonsillectomy.

None of these is universally effective in preventing recurrent episodes and each has its own disadvantages.

Tonsillectomy (with or without adenoidectomy) probably works by removing a reservoir of GAS infection. It should be considered if the pattern of infection – i.e. frequency, severity, and duration of infections – is such that significant morbidity is expected to continue for a prolonged and unacceptable period of time. Children with suspected recurrent GAS pharyngotonsillitis should have a throat swab taken during an acute episode to aid in treatment decisions.

OBSTRUCTIVE ADENOTONSILLAR HYPERTROPHY

Pathophysiology

Upper airway obstruction occurs when there is an imbalance between the neuromuscular control, which supports the airways, and the negative inspiratory pressure, which tends to collapse the airways. The site of obstruction is generally in the oropharynx at the level of the tonsil, and tonsillectomy therefore is beneficial in relieving upper airways obstruction. Removal of the adenoids improves the nasal airway and thereby decreases the negative pressure generated during inspiration.

Indications for surgery

Involution of the adenoids and tonsils will occur with time, and is accompanied by the resolution of obstructive symptoms. With this in mind, the indications for surgical management depend on the severity of the symptoms, which can be classified as follows:

- Snoring alone: this does not require surgical management.
- Sleep disturbance characterised by laboured respiration, restlessness, and waking at night with daytime somnolence or chronic mouth breathing by day.
- Observed episodes of apnoea while asleep.
- Complications of obstructive sleep apnoea (OSA), which include failure to thrive, significant hypoxia and *cor pulmonale*.

If the adenoids alone are enlarged then adenoidectomy (which is associated with much less morbidity than adenotonsillectomy) is sufficient, but if the tonsils are also enlarged then adenotonsillectomy is required. However, the decision to proceed with surgery depends on the level of discomfort being experienced. Obstructive sleep apnoea (OSA) usually requires adenotonsillectomy unless there is no significant lymphoid tissue enlargement (as may be the case in children with neuromuscular disorders or craniofacial anomalies). Adenotonsillectomy is clearly mandatory for children with complications of OSA.

PERIORBITAL AND ORBITAL CELLULITIS

Periorbital (preseptal cellulitis) refers to infection in the soft tissues of the eyelids, while orbital cellulitis occurs when infection is present around and behind the globe of the eye. Orbital cellulitis is a medical emergency and should be treated with the same level of urgency as meningitis or a brain abscess. The potential for loss of vision and suppurative intracranial complications is significant.

Infection in the tissues around the eye may spread from the upper respiratory tract. In older children it is often associated with sinus infection (especially in the ethmoid sinuses). It may also spread from purulent conjunctivitis, dacrocystitis, or gain entry via local trauma or insect bite.

Periorbital cellulitis

It is important to distinguish this condition from a *periorbital allergic reaction*. A well child, who has no fever, and who has eyelid swelling without much redness, tenderness and local warmth, is quite likely to have an allergic reaction to an allergen that has been blown or rubbed into the eye, or to an insect bite. An oral antihistamine may be used. The child should be reviewed if the swelling does not settle in a few hours or if signs of inflammation develop. In this case no specific radiological imaging is required.

If the condition is *mild*, amoxycillin/clavulanate 22.5 mg/kg (max 875 mg) p.o., 12 hourly, *otherwise* admit for i.v. therapy; i.e. flucloxacillin 50 mg/kg (max 2 g) 6 hourly. If *severe* or under 5 years and not Hib immunised, add cefotaxime 50 mg/kg (max 2 g) intravenously 6 hourly. See also Antimicrobial guidelines.

Orbital cellulitis

This is an emergency and is differentiated from periorbital cellulitis by the presence of:
- Chemosis
- Proptosis
- Ophthalmoplegia
- Decreased visual acuity
- Systemic symptoms.

If the features of orbital cellulitis are present, a CT scan is required to determine whether or not the sinusitis is complicated by abscess formation. This is most commonly a subperiosteal abscess, which requires surgical drainage usually by an external ethmoidectomy approach. If no abscess is present, treatment is by intravenous antibiotics alone; however, CT scanning may need to be repeated if there is a progression of symptoms and signs, or if there is a lack of improvement following medical treatment.

Intravenous antibiotic therapy is required; i.e. flucloxacillin 50 mg/kg (max 2 g) 4–6 hourly and cefotaxime 50 mg/kg (max 2 g) 6 hourly. See also Antimicrobial guidelines.

ENT and ophthalmological consultation should be sought urgently in suspected orbital cellulitis.

EPISTAXIS

This is usually due to bleeding from the anterior nasoseptal vessels. Acute bleeding usually settles with local pressure, but occasionally the application of a cotton wool pledget soaked with a topical decongestant is necessary.

Recurrent bleeding can be treated by the application of an antibiotic ointment if there is significant nasal crusting present, or by cautery if enlarged blood vessels are seen. Nasal cautery can be performed as an office procedure following the application of a topical anaesthetic and decongestant (e.g. Cophenylcaine spray comprising lignocaine and phenylephrine), using a silver nitrate stick. Only one side should be cauterised at a time, and local trauma to the nose should be avoided for 2 weeks to allow healing to occur without further bleeding. Epistaxis is very unlikely to be due to a nasal tumour or a previously undiagnosed coagulopathy, but further evaluation is necessary if there are suggestive symptoms or signs present.

TRAUMA

Nasal trauma

Treatment is required for either cosmesis or septal haematoma.

- *Cosmesis.* A nasal deformity due to a displaced nasal fracture should be reduced within 7–10 days of injury. The presence of a bony deformity due to a nasal fracture is best determined at about 5 days following the injury once the soft tissue swelling has resolved. The decision to reduce the nasal fracture is based on clinical grounds and radiology is unhelpful.
- *Septal haematoma.* This can occur after nasal trauma and it does not matter if a fracture is present or not. It invariably leads to septal abscess formation with cartilage destruction and nasal collapse. A septal haematoma presents with nasal obstruction associated with a bulge of the septum that can be confirmed by palpating with an instrument (e.g. wax curette) following the application of a topical anaesthetic. Treatment involves incision

and drainage, nasal packing to prevent recurrence, and anti-staphylococcal antibiotics.

Oral/oropharyngeal trauma

These invariably occur after a fall with a stick or similar object in the mouth, and may sometimes be associated with a significant injury.

Hospital admission and further evaluation may be required in the following situations:

- The child unable to feed.
- The upper airway is obstructed.
- There is a significant laceration, requiring debridement, closure or both.
- There is a significant retropharyngeal injury.
- There is a suspicion of injury to the internal carotid artery.

Any involvement of the retropharynx may not be obvious by oral examination, particularly for injuries through the soft palate. The retropharynx is ideally examined by flexible nasopharyngoscopy. In addition, a lateral cervical spine X-ray is required to rule out the presence of gas in the soft tissues, the presence of a foreign body, and any associated cervical spine injury. Widening of the retropharynx may also be demonstrated, but this may be misleading unless the radiological features are confirmed by nasopharyngoscopy. A significant retropharyngeal injury requires intravenous antibiotics and a period of nasogastric feeding to prevent abscess formation.

The internal carotid artery lies posterolateral to the tonsil. An injury to this region may be associated with injury to the internal carotid artery whether the trauma is blunt or sharp. While internal carotid artery injuries are rare, they are usually due to a blunt trauma that causes intimal disruption and progressive thrombosis presenting with neurological signs over a period of about 24 h. Where an internal carotid artery injury is suspected, the patient should be admitted for observation and consideration given to angiography.

Aural trauma

Trauma to the external auditory canal is usually associated with bleeding, but it is an insignificant injury and requires no treatment. The tympanic membrane can be perforated by direct trauma or a pressure wave (e.g. a slap across the ear or diving). Acute tympanic membrane perforations usually heal within weeks and do not require acute intervention. Topical antibiotics, however, are recommended for water-related injuries. Direct trauma may rarely cause ossicular disruption, facial paralysis or inner ear damage (with complete deafness and vertigo).

FOREIGN BODIES

The first attempt at foreign body removal is always the easiest and should be performed by an experienced clinician with the appropriate instruments and good illumination. Failure of the initial removal may lead to the need for an otherwise unnecessary general anaesthetic.

Ear

Foreign bodies in the external auditory canal are best removed by a hook-shaped instrument, which is passed behind the foreign body and is then used to pull it out. Grasping instruments, such as forceps, should not be used as they invariably lead to the foreign body being displaced further medially. Suction may occasionally be useful.

Nose

The technique for the removal of nasal foreign bodies is the same as for foreign bodies in the external auditory canal. A topical anaesthetic (e.g. Cophenylcaine) should, however, be applied prior to the attempted removal. The risk of inhalation of a nasal foreign body is minimal and therefore acute removal should be deferred until appropriate personnel and equipment are available.

Fish bone in pharynx

A fish bone usually lodges in the tonsil or base of the tongue and therefore can be seen on oral examination and removed following the prior application of a topical anaesthetic. If the fish bone cannot be seen during the oral examination, a more thorough examination by nasopharyngoscopy is required. Fish bones rarely reach the oesophagus and therefore oesophageal evaluation is usually unneces-sary. Where a fish bone is not found, despite a suggestive history, the child should be reviewed until symptoms resolve and an examination under general anaesthetic is considered. Although fish bones are radiolucent, radiology may be helpful to detect the presence of complications when symptoms have persisted.

Oesophagus

The vast majority of swallowed foreign bodies pass without difficulty. If a foreign body becomes lodged in the oesophagus, it usually does so in the upper oesophagus, at the level of the cricopharyngeus. Lower oesophageal foreign bodies suggest the presence of underlying oesophageal pathology (e.g. stricture). The likelihood of impaction is dependent on the size and shape of the foreign body. Objects larger than 20 mm are more likely to impact. Broken plastic toys are particularly dangerous, as they often impact, yet their radiolucency may lead to a delay in diagnosis, and they may present with respiratory symptoms some time after ingestion.

If a swallowed object reaches the stomach it will almost always pass without incident. Two types of object, however, may cause problems: (i) long thin objects (e.g. hair pins and locker keys) may impact at the duodenojejunal flexure; and (ii) button batteries, if held up at any point in the alimentary canal, may release alkali, causing local necrosis and perforation. X-rays should be taken if there are symptoms suggestive of oesophageal lodging (e.g. drooling and dysphagia), or if long thin objects or button batteries have been swallowed. X-rays should include the neck, chest and abdomen. Oesophageal foreign bodies impact in the coronal plane, whereas tracheal lodgement occurs in the sagittal plane. Radiolucent foreign bodies may be imaged by barium swallow. If an object is impacted in the oesophagus, arrangements should be made for endoscopic removal.

CHAPTER 22
EYE CONDITIONS

James Elder

IMPORTANT PRINCIPLES

- Always test and record vision as the first part of any eye examination. In infants, observe following and other visual behaviour and listen to the parents' impressions concerning their child's vision.
- A child with a squint is never too young to be assessed. Transient malalignment of the eyes is common up to 6 months of age. A child with a constant squint at any age or any transient squint after 6 months of age should be referred to an ophthalmologist promptly. True squints rarely improve spontaneously.
- Never pad a discharging eye.
- Always pad an eye into which a local anaesthetic has been instilled until the effect of the local anaesthetic has worn off.
- Do not use local steroid drops unless corneal ulceration has been excluded by fluorescein staining. If you do not consult an ophthalmologist only use them for short periods (2 days or less).
- X-ray the orbit (anteroposterior and lateral or CT scan) if an intra-ocular foreign body is suspected from the history, even though the eye may appear normal.
- In cases of photophobia or watery eyes in the first year of life, when there is no significant discharge, consider the possibility of congenital glaucoma.
- All children with a white–red reflex or white masses in the retina must be referred immediately to an ophthalmologist to exclude retinoblastoma.

TRAUMA

Trauma to the eye can take many forms. Physical trauma to the eye and surrounding structures may be blunt or sharp. Trauma can also result from radiation (thermal and electromagnetic) and chemical agents.

Foreign bodies

Foreign bodies on the surface of the eye present with a painful, watery eye. If a foreign body or corneal ulcer is suspected, instil one drop of local anaesthetic to ease the pain and facilitate examination. Suitable local anaesthetics are proxymetacaine 0.5%, amethocaine 0.5 or 1%, or benoxinate 0.4%. Do not use local anaesthetics for the continuing treatment of ocular pain under any circumstance.

Conjunctival foreign bodies are common and are often found on the posterior surface of the upper lid. Therefore, eversion of the lid is essential. Most foreign bodies are easily removed with a moist cotton wool swab. If they are embedded or difficult to remove, refer the patient to the ophthalmologist.

If corneal foreign bodies are not readily removed with a moistened cotton wool swab, refer to an ophthalmologist. Beware of an iris naevus and iris prolapse through a perforating injury of the cornea mimicking a corneal foreign body.

Intraocular foreign bodies are generally high-velocity fragments. Suspect if the history involves an explosion, metal(s) striking on metal, or any other situation that involves high-speed objects (e.g. power tools or a lawn mower). If the history is at all suggestive, even in the absence of local signs, an X-ray of the orbit (AP and lateral) is necessary. If an intraocular foreign body is demonstrated the immediate referral to an ophthalmologist is mandatory.

Eyelid injuries

All eyelid lacerations except the most minor should be repaired as an in-patient procedure. Suspect canalicular injury in all lacerations involving the medial aspect of the eyelids and refer to an ophthalmologist. All lacerations involving the lid margin should be referred to an ophthalmologist.

Hyphaema (blood in the anterior chamber)

This is the result of blunt trauma to the eye. This generally requires admission to hospital. All cases require ophthalmic referral as there is a potential for secondary haemorrhage and loss of vision.

Fracture of the orbital bones

A blow-out fracture through the wall of the orbit is suspected if one or more of the following three cardinal signs are present.

- Restricted movement of the eye, particularly in a vertical plane, with double vision.
- Infra-orbital nerve anaesthesia.
- Enophthalmos – this may be difficult to assess initially because of eyelid haematoma.

Diagnosis is most often clinical. A CT scan is used to demonstrate the fracture of the orbital wall and entrapped orbital tissue (the classic sign is a tear drop 'polyp' hanging from the roof of the maxillary antrum). Refer to an ophthalmologist.

Penetrating injury

This should always be considered in patients with lacerations involving the eyelids, particularly after motor car accidents. Suspect if the pupil is distorted or the iris is prolapsing through the cornea, or pigmented tissue is seen over the sclera. If suspected, protect the eye with a cone or shield that places no pressure on the eyelids or eye and admit. Prevent vomiting with anti-emetic. Refer to an ophthalmologist immediately.

Chemical burns

Irrigate the eye with saline or water copiously for 15 min using an i.v. giving set. The instillation of local anaesthetic will facilitate this. Refer all chemical burns to an ophthalmologist. Most alkali burns will require admission.

Thermal burns

The ocular surface is rarely involved. Check for ulceration with fluorescein staining. Butesin picrate ointment is suitable for use on lid burns. Secondary lid swelling may result in corneal exposure and ocular lubricants are then required.

THE ACUTE RED EYE

Common causes of the acute red eye are conjunctivitis, corneal ulceration, corneal or conjunctival foreign bodies (see above), and less common causes are pre-septal and orbital cellulitis. Table 22.1 gives a brief outline of the presenting features of red, sticky and watery eyes, which have a large number of causes and whose clinical presentations may overlap.

Conjunctivitis

Aetiology
- Bacterial – generally pus is present.
- Viral – generally there is watery discharge.
- Allergic – history of atopy and 'itchy eyes'.

Neonatal conjunctivitis (ophthalmia neonatorum)
Neisseria gonorrhoeae

Acute severe, purulent discharge associated with marked conjunctival and lid oedema (the clinical appearance is of 'pus under pressure'). It occurs within a few days of birth. This is an ocular emergency because of the risk of corneal perforation.

- *Diagnosis.* Urgent Gram stain for Gram-negative intracellular diplococci and direct culture to appropriate culture media.
- *Treatment.* In uncomplicated cases (i.e. without evidence of sepsis), a single i.m. dose of ceftriaxone 50 mg/kg (max 125 mg) is sufficient. If complicated by sepsis or pre-septal cellulitis, admit and give i.v. cefotaxime 50 mg/kg (max 2 g) 6 hourly. In all cases local measures such as ocular lavage and topical antibiotics (chloramphenicol or neomycin) may be of help.
- Investigate and treat the mother and partner.

Chlamydia

This condition causes about 30% of sticky eyes in the neonatal period. Fails to respond to routine topical antibiotics. If left untreated, there is a risk of pneumonitis.

Table 22.1 The causes of red, watery and sticky eyes

Problem	Symptoms	Signs
Neonatal conjunctivitis (ophthalmia neonatorum)	Severe pain	Moderate epiphora Copious discharge Moderate to severe erythema
Congenital nasolacrimal duct obstruction	Painless	Mild to moderate epiphora Mild to copious discharge Minimal erythema
Infantile glaucoma	Photophobia	Moderate epiphora No discharge Minimal erythema Enlarged and cloudy cornea
Viral conjunctivitis	Moderate discomfort	Moderate epiphora Mild discharge Mild to moderate erythema
Bacterial conjunctivitis	Moderate to severe discomfort	Moderate epiphora Copious discharge Moderate to severe erythema
Allergic conjunctivitis	Itch often prominent	Mild to moderate epiphora Stringy discharge Mild erythema
Chemical conjunctivitis	Intense pain	Severe epiphora Mild discharge Moderate to severe erythema
Corneal abrasion	Intense pain	Moderate epiphora No discharge Variable erythema Fluorescein staining
Foreign body	Intense pain	Moderate epiphora No discharge Variable erythema Variable fluorescein staining
Preseptal cellulitis	Moderate pain	Minimal epiphora Variable discharge Marked erythema and swelling of eyelids – the eye is white
Orbital cellulitis	Severe pain Reduced eye movements	Minimal epiphora Variable discharge Marked erythema and swelling of eyelids – the eye is often inflamed and proptosed

- *Diagnosis*. Giemsa stain of conjunctival scraping for intranuclear inclusions. Also antibodies in tears and immunofluorescent stains of conjunctival scrapes. Consult an ophthalmologist for advice on specimen collection.
- *Treatment*. Oral erythromycin 10 mg/kg 6 hourly and eye toilet.
- Investigate and treat the mother and partner.

Other bacteria

This is generally caused by *Staphylococcus*, *Streptococcus* or diphtheroids. Culture and treat with neomycin or chloramphenicol eye drops. A rapid clinical response is anticipated.

Blocked nasolacrimal duct

A mucopurulent discharge with a watery eye. On waking the discharge is worse and conjunctiva is not inflamed (see Watering Eyes, p. 320).

Chemical

A purulent discharge with lid oedema seen within 24 h of the instillation of silver nitrate prophylaxis. The treatment is frequent lavage and topical neomycin.

Conjunctivitis in older children

Management of this condition depends on the aetiology.

Bacterial

Chloramphenicol eye drops: 2 hourly by day and ointment at night.

Viral

This condition usually clears spontaneously. If it is unclear whether the infection is viral or bacterial, Neomycin eye drops may be given.

Herpes simplex conjunctivitis

Suspect if the child has lid vesicles. Check for corneal ulceration and treat with 4 hourly aciclovir ointment. Refer to an ophthalmologist.

Allergic

In mild cases use astringent (phenylephrine 0.125% or naphazoline 0.1%). In moderate cases use topical antihistamine (antazoline 0.5%). In severe cases refer to the ophthalmologist. Topical steroid or sodium cromoglycate should only be given under the supervision of an ophthalmologist.

Corneal ulceration

Aetiology
- Trauma (with or without a foreign body).
- Herpes simplex (dendritic ulcer).

Diagnosis
- The symptoms are pain, photophobia, lacrimation and blepharospasm.
- Fluorescein stain after the instillation of a local anaesthetic.

Treatment
- If traumatic: Chloramphenicol ointment (1%) and pad. Review in 24 h. If the condition has not healed in 48 h, refer to an ophthalmologist. If it has healed, continue chloramphenicol ointment twice daily for 1 week.
- Herpes simplex: Aciclovir eye ointment (1 cm inside of the lower conjunctival sac) five times a day for 14 days, and refer to an ophthalmologist.

PRE-SEPTAL (PERIORBITAL) AND ORBITAL CELLULITIS

See also Ear, Nose and Throat Conditions, chapter 21.

Both conditions present with erythematous, swollen lids in a febrile, unwell child. In pre-septal cellulitis the lid swelling frequently prevents the eye from opening. The lids must be separated (a Desmarres' lid retractor may be used) to exclude proptosis and the limitation of eye movement. These are important signs of orbital cellulitis, which are commonly associated with sinusitis. Proptosis may be so severe that it prevents lid closure and corneal exposure may result. Bilateral orbital (or pre-septal) cellulitis may be associated with cavernous sinus thrombosis.

Treatment

All cases require admission and intravenous antibiotics. See Antimicrobial guidelines. Refer all cases of suspected orbital cellulitis to an ophthalmologist and ear, nose and throat surgeon. These children require an urgent CT scan to identify the orbital collection of pus and sinus pathology. An orbital abscess often requires urgent drainage by an ENT surgeon. A delay in the diagnosis of orbital cellulitis may result in permanent loss of vision.

WATERING EYES

Watery eyes are common in children and are the result of poor tear drainage or the over-production of tears. The latter is usually the result of eye irritation and causes include foreign bodies, corneal ulcer, conjunctivitis and infantile glaucoma (these are discussed elsewhere).

Nasolacrimal duct obstruction is the commonest cause of watery eyes and discharge that persists after the first 2 weeks of life. The discharge is worse on waking and the conjunctiva is not inflamed. It usually resolves spontaneously, due to an opening of the lower end of the nasolacrimal duct. Local eye toilet fails to control the discharge and if the infection is troublesome, topical neomycin eye drops may be given (avoid repeated courses of chloramphenicol). If the discharge and watering have not settled by 12 months of age, refer to an ophthalmologist for probing.

STRABISMUS OR SQUINT (TURNED EYE)

Refer all children with squint or suspected squint to the eye clinic. This will allow amblyopia to be detected early, and perhaps prevented, and will enable any underlying pathology such as retinoblastoma or cataract to be detected. Examine the red reflex of all children suspected to have a squint, if the reflex is abnormal (very dull or white) urgent referral to an ophthalmologist to exclude the cataract or retinoblastoma is required.

A child does not 'grow out of' a squint. However, babies in the first few months of life may have an intermittent squint, especially when feeding. If the parents report a squint, the child should be referred to the eye clinic. All children with a first-degree relative with a squint should be seen by an ophthalmologist at about $3-3^1/2$ years of age, even if there is no squint as they may have a refractive error alone.

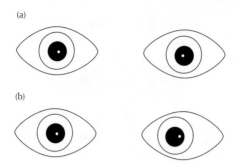

(a)

(b)

Fig. 22.1 Corneal light reflex. Shine a light at the child's eyes and observe the reflection. (a) Eyes are straight and the corneal light reflex is symmetrical. (*Note*: it is displaced slightly to the nasal side of the centre in each eye.) (b) Left convergent strabismus. The reflection from the deviated eye is displaced laterally.

A pseudo-strabismus (pseudo-squint) is due to a broad nasal bridge or epicanthic folds, or both. This results in the appearance of a squint, but corneal light reflexes are central and there is no movement on cover testing (see Figs 22.1 and 22.2). Only make the diagnosis of pseudo-strabismus if absolutely certain. Refer doubtful cases to an ophthalmologist.

EYELID LUMPS AND PTOSIS

Styes are acute bacterial infections of an eyelash follicle. They are red and tender and at the eyelid margin. Removing the lash directly related to the stye will often result in discharge of pus and hasten the resolution of a stye. Local antibiotics are sometimes indicated and systemic antibiotics are rarely needed.

A chalazion is an obstructed tarsal (or meibomian) gland. These glands are situated within the substance of the eyelid and thus a chalazion will present as a lump within the eyelid rather than at the margin like a stye. There may be no associated symptoms. Redness associated with a chalazion is usually the result of sterile inflammation

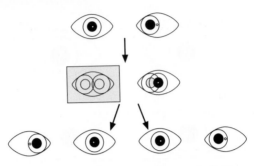

Fig. 22.2 The cover test. The child's attention is attracted with a toy. The eye that appears not to be deviating is covered. The uncovered eye is then observed for movement. If there is a convergent squint, the eye will move outwards (top and middle). The uncovered eye should also be observed when the cover is removed from the fellow eye. In an alternating squint there will be no movement of the uncovered eye and the previously covered eye will now be deviated (bottom left). In non-alternating or constant squint (vision is usually reduced in the deviating eye), there will be a rapid return to the original situation (bottom right). If no movement is detected, the test should be repeated but cover the other eye first.

due to a leakage of the contents of the chalazion rather than a bacterial infection. Thus local or systemic antibiotics seldom influence the natural history of these lesions. Warm compresses may hasten resolution. If the chalazion is persistent (more than 6 months), large or causes discomfort, incision and drainage under a general anaesthetic may be indicated.

Ptosis is a droopy or lowered upper eyelid. In children it is usually the result of a minor and isolated anomaly in the development of the levator muscle. It may be unilateral or bilateral, and it is sometimes inherited in a dominant manner. If the lowered eyelid obstructs the pupil in a young child, visual loss will occur secondary to amblyopia. Urgent referral to an ophthalmologist is appropriate in such cases. In more minor degrees of ptosis, surgical intervention is for cosmesis and is less urgent.

RARE BUT IMPORTANT EYE CONDITIONS

Iritis

Acute iritis is very rare in children and presents with an acute red eye similar to the symptoms for a corneal ulcer. The pupil is small and does not react well to light. Refer to an ophthalmologist. Consider iritis in children with juvenile chronic arthritis (JCA). This form of iritis is chronic and painless.

Infantile glaucoma

The presenting features are:

- A hazy cornea
- An enlarged cornea
- Watery eyes
- Photophobia.

This is a rare condition, but early recognition is vital. Prompt surgery offers a chance of cure and preservation of vision. All infants with suspected glaucoma require urgent referral to an ophthalmologist for examination under anaesthesia to measure corneal diameter, optic disc cupping and intraocular pressure.

Congenital cataracts

Congenital cataracts are rare, but early detection and removal with subsequent optical correction (contact lenses or spectacles) offers a good chance of visual preservation. All newborn infants should have their red reflexes examined prior to discharge from hospital. Check the red reflexes and fundi in any infant with poor visual performance (fixation and following). Nystagmus is a late sign for congenital cataracts. Any child suspected of having a congenital cataract must be referred urgently. A unilateral cataract will often present as a squint.

Retinoblastoma

This is a rare childhood cancer of the retina and presents with squint, a white pupil (cat's eye reflex), poor vision or a family history of the tumour. Prompt recognition is vital to maximise the possibility of preserving vision. Untreated this is a fatal disorder. If suspected refer urgently to an ophthalmologist.

CHAPTER 23

GASTROINTESTINAL CONDITIONS

Tony Catto-Smith
Lionel Lubitz

ACUTE INFECTIOUS DIARRHOEA

See also Infections Diseases, chapter 26.

Dehydration is the most important complication of acute infectious diarrhoea.

Differential diagnosis of vomiting and diarrhoea

It is important that children who present with the acute onset of vomiting, diarrhoea and fever are repeatedly re-evaluated, even after admission to a hospital gastroenteritis ward. Other causes to be considered include (but are not restricted to):

- Appendicitis
- Intussusception
- Malrotation
- Urinary tract infection
- Otitis media
- Meningitis.

Assessment of dehydration

- Recent change in bodyweight provides the most accurate indication of the degree of fluid depletion. This underscores the importance of accurate weights as a part of clinical assessment.
- Starvation produces no more than 1% of bodyweight loss per day. Any change in excess of this is due to water loss.
- Signs of ketosis such as Kussmaul breathing and typical ketotic breath are the best clinical indicators of moderate to severe dehydration.

For practical clinical purposes, the state of hydration should be evaluated as:

- No, or mild dehydration (<4% bodyweight loss)
- Moderate dehydration (4–6%)
- Severe dehydration (≥7%).

Note: These percentages are approximate and given only as a guide.

Management
General comments

Treatment is aimed at restoring and maintaining water and *electrolyte balance and normal nutrition.*

The important general principles are:
- Continued breast-feeding in infants
- The use of oral rehydration
- The feeding of hungry children
- Drug avoidance: *antibiotics, anti-emetics and antidiarrhoeals have no place in the treatment of most cases of childhood gastroenteritis.*

Oral rehydration

- *Breast-feeding*: continue through the illness, supplemented if necessary with an oral rehydration solution by cup, bottle or nasogastric tube.
- *Artificial feeding*: commercially available oral rehydration solutions will greatly enhance the absorption of water from the small bowel, and can be used to rehydrate children with even moderately severe dehydration, provided they are not shocked.
- *Vomiting* is not a contraindication to oral rehydration. It is best to give small amounts of fluid frequently.
- *Oral rehydration* encourages early return of appetite.

Solutions

Sachets containing glucose and electrolyte powder are commercially available and can be added to water as required (e.g. Gastrolyte). They contain glucose, sodium, potassium, chloride and citrate, and should be used to *correct dehydration.*

Readily available solutions of sugar in water (without salt) can be prepared at home and used for the maintenance of hydration in mild or moderate diarrhoea without dehydration. These include:

- Sucrose (table sugar): one teaspoon in 200 mL water
- Cordials: 1 part to 16 parts of water
- Lemonade: 1 part to 6 parts of water
- Fruit juice: 1 part to 6 parts of water.

Do not use undiluted or low-calorie lemonade or fruit juice.

Parent education

The most important message for parents is that *children with diarrhoea need to drink more fluid more often* (because water loss is the main cause of morbidity and mortality).

Fluid is best given in small volumes and frequently. The easiest and safest method is as free water, which may be flavoured with appropriately diluted cordials or juices. Where diarrhoea becomes significant, electrolyte loss is of increasing concern and it is important to provide an electrolyte source such as a glucose–electrolyte rehydration preparation, or food.

Although home-made solutions and oral rehydration powder are important in the management of childhood gastroenteritis in the home, they are potentially dangerous if made up incorrectly.

Specific treatment guidelines

Indications for admission

- In cases of severe illness.
- Where there is moderate or severe dehydration.
- For young babies (<6 months old).
- High-risk patients (e.g. ileostomy, short gut, cyanotic heart disease, chronic renal disease or metabolic disorders).
- If the diagnosis is in doubt.
- If the family is unable to cope.

No dehydration

- Children with no clinical features of dehydration can usually be managed as out-patients.
- Breast-feeding should be continued on demand, and formula-fed infants should be given their normal feeds with extra water.

Vomiting babies will tolerate half-strength feeds better than full-strength feeds.

- Children with mild to moderate diarrhoea can continue on their normal diet with extra water. This can be given as water, cordial, diluted fruit juice or diluted lemonade.
- If the child refuses to eat, food may be stopped for up to 24 h; however, *starvation* beyond this may delay recovery.

Mild dehydration

- These children may have a history of diarrhoea and vomiting with an inadequate oral intake. Urine is usually concentrated but skin turgor and mucous membranes may appear normal.
- Children who are dehydrated need to be provided with water and electrolytes to replace their deficits, and they need an ongoing amount of fluid for *maintenance* requirements.
- For practical purposes, the *deficit* is best determined by using a calculation based on the percentage of bodyweight. Recent accurate bodyweights are, however, rarely available.

The rehydration and maintenance fluid volumes for 24 h should be translated into an easily understood message (e.g. 50 mL every 30 min). Ideally, an oral rehydration solution such as Gastrolyte should be given, but this can be alternated with other appropriately diluted fluids that may be more palatable, such as cordials. It is not usually necessary to admit these children, although a *review within 8–12 h is advisable.*

Note: Persistent vomiting makes oral rehydration difficult. The best strategy is for frequent, but much smaller volumes, and then to build up as vomiting subsides.

Moderate to severe dehydration

- The clinical assessment of the percentage dehydration is at best approximate.
- Moderate dehydration (4–6%) may be accompanied by dry mucous membranes, sunken eyes and mild oliguria.
- Clinical signs of increased degrees of dehydration (≥7%) are more exaggerated, with evidence of ketosis, acidotic breathing, decreased skin turgor and impaired peripheral perfusion.
- Most children who are moderately dehydrated can be rehydrated orally, even if they are vomiting. Children who are

Table 23.1 Recommended hourly oral or nasogastric rehydration rate for children

Weight (kg)	Maintenance (mL/h)	Moderate dehydration (4–6%) (mL/h)		Severe dehydration (≥7%) (mL/h)	
		1st 6 h	Next 18 h	1st 6 h	Next 18 h
5	20	45	35	70	35
10	35	85	55	135	55
15	50	125	70	200	70
20	60	140	80	220	80
30	70	190	95	300	95
40	80	250	110	400	110
50	90	300	120	500	120

The daily water requirement is relatively high in neonates (150 mL/kg), reducing to 100 mL/kg in older infants and 80 mL/kg per day between 1 and 5 years.

not shocked should be given a trial of oral rehydration, using adequate volumes of a physiologically balanced fluid by mouth or via a nasogastric tube.

The aim is to rehydrate them quickly. A useful rule of thumb for rehydration is to provide a total fluid intake over the first 6 h of between 50 mL/kg (in older children) and 100 mL/kg (for infants). Thereafter give maintenance fluids or as desired (see Table 23.1).

If the child is tired or cannot keep up with fluid losses, a nasogastric tube should be inserted. Small amounts of fluid should be given frequently, and the child should be reassessed after 4–6 h. Breast-feeding should be resumed as soon as oral rehydration is complete, or before if this takes longer than 6 h.

Severe dehydration with shock

Children who are shocked need immediate resuscitation with intravenous fluids.

Intravenous therapy
Indications

- Severe dehydration with shock.
- Failed oral or nasogastric rehydration.
- Gastroenteritis complicated by another problem; e.g. ileostomy or cyanotic congenital heart disease (relative indication).

Resuscitation fluid

If the child is shocked, give 20 mL/kg of colloid solution (e.g. 5% albumin, Haemaccel) or 0.9% saline as quickly as possible to treat circulatory failure. This should be repeated in boluses of 10–20 mL/kg if there are still signs of shock.

Replacement and maintenance fluid

- The use of 0.45% saline in 4% dextrose with 20 mmol/L of potassium chloride is usually adequate. Sodium bicarbonate is added if there is persistent acidosis (acidosis will usually correct itself as the patient is rehydrated).
- Aim to replace the deficit over 24 h if the serum sodium is normal (see Hypernatraemic dehydration below). The maintenance requirement is approximately 4 mL/kg per h up to 10 kg.

For example:
- A 10 kg child is 10% dehydrated.
- They have a deficit of 1000 mL = 40 mL/h for 24 h.
- A maintenance of 4 mL/kg per h = 40 mL per h.
- Use a total of 80 mL/h for the first 24 h, then 40 mL per h.

An oral rehydration solution and breast milk should be offered once the circulation has been restored. It may be possible to remove the drip after a few hours. Appetite is restored more quickly in children who are given oral fluids.

Weight should be monitored 6 hourly in hospitalised patients.

Biochemical investigations

Electrolyte and acid–base studies are not required routinely. Indications are:
- Prolonged diarrhoea with severe dehydration
- Disturbance of the conscious state or convulsions
- Any child aged <3 months
- Any child requiring intravenous fluid.

Special circumstances

Clinical signs of dehydration provide at best an approximation of the degree of dehydration. Assessment is further complicated in patients who have significant *plasma sodium imbalance*, those who are *malnourished* and those who are *obese*.

Hypernatraemic dehydration (Na>150 mmol/L)

Because of osmotic shifts, *these children may actually be more dehydrated than they clinically appear*. They are at great risk of severe neurological sequelae if rehydration is not carried out appropriately. Rehydration must be slow. Repeated aliquots of 10 mL/kg colloid solution should be given quickly to restore the circulation if the child is shocked, but the remainder of the *deficit should be replaced over at least 48 h* if intravenous fluid is used. As long as rehydration is slow, the intravenous fluid used does not need to have a high sodium concentration. A suitable solution is 0.45% saline in 4% dextrose with 20 mmol/L potassium chloride and 10 mL/L 10% calcium gluconate. Oral replacement should be over at least 24 h.

Consultation with an intensive care unit is recommended for these patients. Serum electrolytes should be measured frequently. As a guideline, serum sodium should not fall faster than 1 mmol/L per h (on average).

Hyponatraemic dehydration (Na<130 mmol/L)

Severe hyponatraemia causing fitting or coma requires consultation with an intensive care unit. Beware of iatrogenic hyponatraemia from fluid (hypotonic) overload.

Malnutrition

Malnourished children may be *less* dehydrated than the clinical examination would suggest. Such infants may be depleted of magnesium and potassium. Obese infants may be *more* dehydrated than the clinical signs indicate.

Drug therapy

Antidiarrhoeal agents and *anti-emetics* are not recommended for children with gastroenteritis. They can have potentially dangerous side effects. *Antibiotics* have a limited role; they are occasionally required in neonates, severely ill infants, severe shigellosis or for prolonged symptomatic *Campylobacter* infection.

SUGAR INTOLERANCE

Lactose intolerance

After infectious diarrhoea, infants may have a temporary lactose intolerance. Up to 50% of formula-fed babies less than 6 months old with infectious diarrhoea requiring admission to hospital are unable to tolerate normal amounts of lactose for at least a week. Lactose intolerance may occasionally persist for some weeks.

Clinical features of sugar intolerance are:
- Persistently fluid stools
- Excessive flatus
- Excoriation of the buttocks.

Typically, these infants appear otherwise well.

Diagnosis

Collect the stool fluid in napkins lined with plastic. Dilute five drops of stool fluid with 10 drops of water. Add a Clinitest tablet. A colour reaction corresponding to 0.75% or more reducing substances indicates that sugar intolerance is present and is probably the main cause of continuing diarrhoea.

Management

Breast-fed babies rarely have clinically significant lactose intolerance, and breast-feeding should be continued unless the diarrhoea is persistent and the baby is failing to thrive.

Formula-fed babies should have their feed changed to a full strength lactose-free formula, such as Delact or Digestelac. After 3–4 weeks the usual formula may be reintroduced by substituting for the lactose-free milk in increasing proportions over 2–3 days.

Note: A clinical response after change to soy formula may indicate either post-infectious lactose intolerance or allergy to cow milk protein.

Monosaccharide intolerance

Infrequently, infants with severe bowel damage secondary to gastroenteritis may be unable to absorb normal amounts of monosaccharide such as glucose or fructose. Diarrhoea will continue even with a lactose-free formula. Monosaccharide intolerance requires consultation with a gastroenterologist.

CHRONIC DIARRHOEA

An increase in stool frequency or fluid content are often of concern to parents, but do not necessarily imply significant organic disease, although this needs to be excluded. In every child who presents with chronic diarrhoea, the decision must be made as to whether further investigation is required.

The algorithm in Fig. 23.1 outlines an approach to the child with chronic diarrhoea.

Toddler diarrhoea

- This is a clinical syndrome characterised by chronic diarrhoea often with undigested food in the stools of a child who is otherwise well, gaining weight and growing satisfactorily. Stools may contain mucus and are passed between three and six times a day; they are often looser towards the end of the day.
- Its onset is usually between 8 and 20 months of age.
- There is often a family history of functional bowel disease, such as irritable bowel syndrome.
- The treatment consists of reassurance and explanation. No specific drug or dietary therapy has been shown to be of value in toddler diarrhoea. Some toddlers on a high-fructose intake (i.e. 'apple juice' diarrhoea) may have diarrhoea that responds to dietary change.

COELIAC DISEASE

Coeliac disease may present with a history of diarrhoea or of failure to thrive, but an increasing number are recognised through serological screening of asymptomatic groups with a high risk, such as affected siblings and diabetics. Antigliadin and antiendomysial antibodies and assays for tissue transglutaminase are very useful as screening assays, but they are neither 100% sensitive or specific. An abnormal serological result should always be followed by an histological confirmation of

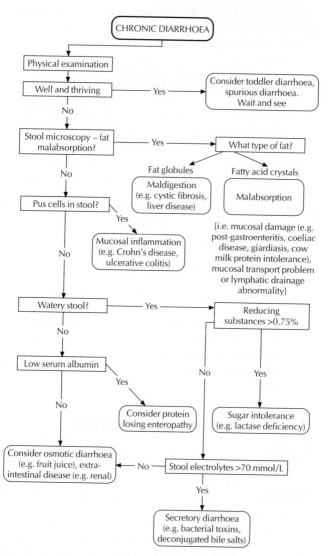

Fig. 23.1 Investigation of chronic diarrhoea

villous atrophy. The need for subsequent biopsies will be dictated by whether the patient was asymptomatic, and according to age (if <2 years) and clinical response to a gluten-free diet.

COW MILK PROTEIN INTOLERANCE (CMPI)

Symptoms related to the ingestion of food or milk may be induced by any one of several components (see also Allergy and Immunology, chapter 14). These may be due to immune or non-immune effects.

Allergic responses to cow milk protein may result in a rapid or delayed onset of symptoms. Rapid onset responses are less common, often characterised by the sudden onset of vomiting, and rarely by acute anaphylaxis. Delayed onset responses may be more difficult to diagnose, and present with diarrhoea, malabsorption or failure to thrive, and occasionally intestinal loss of protein or blood.

- CMPI can only be diagnosed with a complete and thorough history, and with *unequivocal reproducible reactions to elimination and challenge.*
- Blood tests and skin testing may help, but they are not substitutes for clinical assessment.
- After a definitive diagnosis is established, cow milk protein should be removed from the diet and replaced with either soy, a hydrolysed or an elemental formula.
- Most food allergies in infants improve or resolve with increasing age.

CHRONIC INTESTINAL INFECTION

Giardiasis
See Infectious Diseases, chapter 26.

Nematodes
See Infectious Diseases, chapter 26.

RECTAL BLEEDING

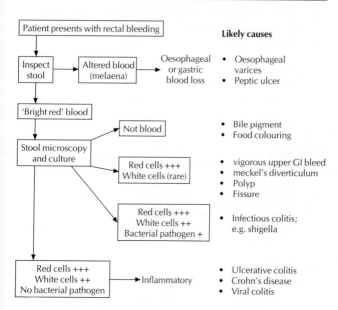

Fig. 23.2 Algorithm – an approach to lower gastrointestinal blood loss

INFLAMMATORY BOWEL DISEASE

- Crohn's disease is increasingly common in both children and adults.
- In childhood, it should be suspected if there is unexplained diarrhoea (with or without blood), malaise, weight loss or abdominal pain.
- Laboratory parameters suggesting active disease include anaemia, thrombocytosis, raised ESR and low albumin.
- Evaluation and management should be made with the aid of a paediatric gastroenterologist.

CONSTIPATION

Constipation is common in childhood and it is usually associated with abnormalities in control of defecation and occasionally with delayed colonic transit.

Although it is important to consider organic causes of constipation such as Hirschsprung's disease, these are rare.

Painful defecation or blood on the surface of the stools suggests the presence of an *anal fissure*. Children past the toddler age with severe constipation may also develop faecal soiling.

Examination

- Abdominal palpation will usually reveal abnormal amounts of firm faeces.
- The anus should be inspected for a fissure.
- Rectal examination may be required.
- The tone of the anal sphincter and the presence of anal stenosis should be assessed.

Investigations

Investigations are rarely helpful, but an abdominal X-ray may be useful to determine the extent of faecal retention.

Hirschsprung's disease is a rare cause of constipation. Rectal biopsy is unnecessary unless the onset of symptoms dates back to early infancy or there is some other clinical indication (such as considerable abdominal distension or failure to thrive).

Management

- The aim of treatment is to empty the colon and to prevent re-accumulation of abnormal amounts of faeces by regular toileting and with the use of laxatives.
- Rectal disimpaction may be required initially.
- *Babies*: an adequate fluid intake with prune juice, high-residue cereals and vegetables may be effective. If not, lactulose (5 mL/day) is usually effective and safe.
- *Older children*: a short course of laxatives with the establishment of a *regular toileting regimen* is usually effective.

In general, the laxative dose should be effective in achieving the passage of at least one soft but formed stool each day. It is often useful and more effective to combine a faecal softener (e.g. paraffin oil) with a stimulant laxative (e.g. senna). The laxative dose should be gradually reduced with the aim of eventually weaning the patient. The longer constipation has been a problem, the longer it takes to achieve this aim. *A common mistake is to give intermittent short courses of treatment that do not allow an adequate readjustment of colonic size and sensation.* When an anal fissure is present, stools should be kept soft with a softening agent.

ENCOPRESIS

Encopresis is defined as the involuntary passage of formed or semi-formed stools into the underwear on a regular basis. It is a distressing symptom to the child and family alike.

The majority of children with encopresis have significant faecal retention. Chronic faecal retention is associated with rectal dilatation and insensitivity to the normal urge to pass stool. This is why a structured toileting program with regular laxatives is a most important aspect of management.

Investigation
A plain abdominal X-ray is often helpful to document the nature and extent of faecal retention, and as a baseline for further treatment.

Management
- The first stage of therapy is to clear the bowel of faeces. An initial clean out with suppositories (e.g. Durolax), given twice a day for up to 2 days is usually effective in rectal disimpaction.
- This should coincide with the commencement of maintenance laxative treatment (e.g. senokot one tablet/day and flavoured paraffin oil 15 mL/day). The dosage should be individualised to produce a daily soft stool without significant abdominal discomfort.
- Regular toileting two to three times daily is essential, with the child being comfortably seated on the toilet for at least 10 min and asked to push during this time. A footstool is often helpful.

- Close follow up is essential with the assistance of behavioural techniques such as a star chart diary to reward regular sitting and successful defaecation in the toilet.
- A good, normal diet with regular meals, adequate fluids and exercise should be encouraged. The aim of treatment is to institute good dietary and toileting habits so that the problem does not recur, and then gradually wean the child from medications.
- The treatment regimen should be maintained for a minimum of 6 months to ensure a resolution of the megacolon.

Children with encopresis may demonstrate secondary adjustment difficulties. This usually improves with the resolution of soiling. Sometimes it is clear that disordered family dynamics exist or that there are emotional factors beyond those that one would expect given the symptoms. In these instances there should be careful evaluation of the child and the family, either by the paediatrician or by a referral to a psychologist, psychiatrist or family therapist.

GASTRO-OESOPHAGEAL REFLUX

Oesophageal reflux of gastric contents occurs normally and is more frequent after meals. It is regarded as pathological if associated with frequent regurgitation or if it results in clinically significant adverse sequelae. The number of reflux episodes is normally increased in infants compared with older children.

Reflux of gastric acid with heartburn may result in episodic irritability, but this is usually associated with obvious regurgitation and is rarely 'silent'. Although gastro-oesophageal reflux can cause infant distress, it is important to consider other possible causes. Both infant distress and frequent regurgitation are common in the first 6 months of life. Coexistence does not prove cause and effect. Twenty-four hour oesophageal pH monitoring can be useful to correlate any episodes of reflux with irritability.

It is important to recognise that vomiting in infants may result from other causes, such as urinary tract infection. These need to be excluded.

Complications

- *Peptic oesophagitis*: this is usually correlated with an increase in the number and duration of reflux episodes. Blood-flecked vomitus and anaemia may result.
- *Peptic strictures*: these are well recognised in childhood and present with dysphagia.
- *Failure to thrive*: severe cases of gastro-oesophageal reflux may cause the loss of calories and anorexia.
- *Pulmonary complications*: recurrent or persistent cough and wheeze may be present and can occur without marked vomiting. These symptoms may result from aspiration of refluxed material (inhalation pneumonia) or through reflex bronchospasm. This mode of presentation requires a high degree of clinical suspicion.

Specialist advice should be sought if complications are present.

Management

Regurgitation of gastric contents is common in infancy. In most cases this 'possetting' does not result in any adverse sequelae and the most appropriate therapy is parental reassurance. 'Physiological' gastro-oesophageal reflux with regurgitation usually resolves by the age of 9–15 months.

Simple measures

In the absence of signs of significant oesophagitis, aspiration or growth failure the following should be suggested:

- The avoidance of excessive handling.
- *Posturing* after feeds: the infant should be placed in a cot in the head-up position at or near 30°, preferably on their side. (Although nursing in the prone position has been recommended in the past, there is now evidence that this increases the risk of sudden infant death.)
- *Thickening* of feeds: use a proprietary thickening agent or a pre-thickened formula if formula fed.

Medication

Note: Medications are not indicated in otherwise healthy, thriving infants with frequent regurgitation.

- Mylanta may offer relief from symptoms of heartburn (0.5–1.0 mL/kg per dose given three to four times a day). There are some concerns about its long-term use because of its mineral content.
- In more severe cases, prokinetic agents such as cisapride (0.2 mg/kg per dose given three to four times a day before meals) will reduce the frequency of reflux episodes and improve gastric emptying. Cisapride should not be given concurrently with drugs such as erythromycin, which impair its metabolism, as there is a risk of cardiac dysrhythmia.
- H2 receptor antagonists such as ranitidine (2–3 mg/kg per dose given two to three times a day before meals) will reduce gastric acidity.

There may be a role for a brief empirical trial of antireflux therapy in infants in whom it is thought that reflux is the cause of their distressed behaviour. However, these agents are not without risk and should not be prescribed for prolonged periods without evidence to substantiate the severity of reflux.

Surgery

Fundoplication is indicated for reflux with complications when medical therapy has failed or is inappropriate.

RECURRENT ABDOMINAL PAIN

Recurrent abdominal pain affects about 10% of school-age children. There is usually no specific identifiable cause, and it is only infrequently the result of emotional problems. Recent evidence suggests there may be a subgroup with migrainous abdominal pain (associated with pallor and family history). Emotional factors, lifestyle and temperamental characteristics can modulate the child's response to pain, irrespective of its cause.

Assessment

- It is essential to take a careful history, including psychosocial details. It may be helpful to interview the parents alone, the child alone and the family together.
- A thorough physical examination is essential.

- Urine microscopy and culture and a plain abdominal X-ray if bowel habit suggests constipation are appropriate baseline investigations.

Management

- The two major causes in childhood are constipation and dysfunctional pain.
- The treatment of underlying constipation is essential, and the management of non-organic issues need to be taken up if necessary.
- 'Dysfunctional' pain may be related to a variation in the perception of visceral sensation in the absence of an identifiable organic cause. A detailed consultation and reassurance is often all that is required.
- The diagnosis of psychogenic recurrent abdominal pain cannot be made simply in the absence of positive findings for an organic disorder. Positive evidence of emotional maladjustment is separately required. If present it should be managed appropriately.

LIVER DISEASE

Biliary atresia

Although rare, biliary atresia is important to diagnose early, as the success of treatment depends on the timing of surgery. This condition should be suspected in any infant who has white or grey stools in the first few months of life. Jaundice may be mild in the first 1–2 months. *Prompt and early specialist referral is vital.*

Hepatitis

See also Infectious Diseases, chapter 26.

Hepatitis may be either infectious or non-infectious. If no viral aetiology is found in a child with hepatitis (particularly adolescent females), auto-immune and other causes of hepatitis should be considered. Auto-immune hepatitis in childhood usually responds well to corticosteroid therapy, but may have a rapid and fatal course if untreated. Hepatitis C is infrequent in children, but in the past it has been most commonly acquired through blood product transfusions.

CHAPTER 24

GYNAECOLOGIC CONDITIONS

Sonia Grover

PREPUBESCENT PROBLEMS

Vulvovaginitis

This is the commonest gynaecologic problem in childhood, usually occurring in girls aged between 2 and 8 years. The vaginal skin in childhood is thin and atrophic. Overgrowth of mixed bowel flora occurs in this environment and the resultant discharge can be an irritant to the vulval area, which is also atrophic. The moist environment between the opposed skin surfaces may also be exacerbated by urine dribbling, particularly in the obese young girl.

Presentation

- Erythema/irritation of the labia and perineal skin.
- Itch and dysuria may also be present.
- There is an offensive vaginal discharge.

Management

Investigations are usually not required. If urinary symptoms present check the urine (mid-stream urine (MSU)) to exclude UTI.

Management consists of:
- Explaining and reassuring parents.
- Vinegar ($\frac{1}{2}$ cup white vinegar in a shallow bath) or the use of a simple barrier, or both, and soothing cream to the labial area (e.g. zinc–castor oil or nappy rash cream).
- Toileting/hygiene advice: avoid potential irritants such as soaps and bubble bath.

Rarely, if the problem persists, further action may be required. The natural history is for recurrences to occur up until the age when oestrogenisation begins.

- If a heavy discharge persists or marked skin inflammation is present, take swabs from the perineum in case of an overgrowth of one organism (e.g. group A Streptococcus) and treat it with the appropriate antibiotics (usual culture findings are mixed coliforms).

- Do not take vaginal swabs as it is painful and distressing. If swabs for culture are required, introital area swabs will do.
- If itch/irritation is the main complaint, consider pinworms.
- If eczema occurs elsewhere on the body, this can be superimposed on the irritation. Combined treatment of the vulvovaginitis (as above) and hydrocortisone may be indicated.
- Foreign bodies are a potential cause for a persistent, unresolving, often blood-stained discharge. An examination under anaesthesia with vaginoscopy is required to exclude this.
- Keep the possibility of sexual abuse in mind.

Thrush is very uncommon in this age group unless there has been significant antibiotic use. (Thrush thrives in an oestrogenised environment, not in the atrophic setting.)

Vaginal pessaries should never be prescribed to this age group.

Labial adhesions

Labial adhesions are seen in infancy through to about 8 years, although they may occasionally persist up to 9 or 10 years. The adhesion is not congenital, but it is acquired from a secondary adherence of the atrophic surfaces of the labia minora, presumably as a result of irritation. Labial adhesions in children do not need to be divided as long as the child is able to void, and any nappy rash or vulvovaginitis is managed as described above. Parents should be reassured that the labia will separate when oestrogenisation occurs as the child grows. Although it is possible to divide the adhesions with lateral traction this is frequently distressing for the child and the parents, and unnecessary. There is a considerable recurrence rate after this approach.

MENSTRUAL PROBLEMS

Dysmenorrhoea
Clinical features

- Cramping lower abdominal pain, lower back pain and pain radiating to the anterior aspects of the thighs with menses (these may begin a few days before menstruation).

- Associated symptoms such as nausea, vomiting, change in bowel actions (usually softer bowel actions or diarrhoea, but occasionally constipation), headaches and general lethargy may occur. These symptoms should be looked for as they support the diagnosis of a prostaglandin-induced dysmenorrhoea. Occasionally these symptoms, occurring in an intermittent pattern, may begin a few months prior to menarche.
- Stress will often precipitate more severe episodes of dysmenorrhoea.
- Vaginal examination is not performed if the young woman is not sexually active. Occasionally in young women who are using tampons a vaginal examination may be possible, but alternatives such as a pelvic ultrasound examination should provide all the required information (e.g. obstructive congenital anomalies and ovarian cysts).

Management

- General measures: assess and manage other adolescent issues (see Adolescent Health, chapter 8), and encourage exercise.
- Antiprostaglandins (e.g. mefenamic acid 10 mg/kg (max 500 mg) orally, 8 hourly; naproxen 5–10 mg/kg (max 500 mg) orally, 12–24 hourly; ibuprofen 2.5–10 mg/kg (max 600 mg) orally, 6–8 hourly) ideally should be commenced prior to the onset of any symptoms. The failure to respond to one type of antiprostaglandin warrants the trial of an alternative type.
- If the menstrual cycle is too irregular for prophylactic use of antiprostaglandins, the menstrual cycle may need to be regulated with hormonal treatment. The oral contraceptive pill (OCP) can also be used for dysmenorrhoea. This may be the first-line treatment in a sexually active teenager.
- Non-responsive or worsening dysmenorrhoea will require investigation. Pelvic ultrasound can usually identify an obstructive congenital anomaly and detect significant endometriosis (i.e. an endometrioma).
- Diagnostic laparoscopy may identify mild endometriosis. However, the value of treating this with specific hormonal therapy or operative laser diathermy is unclear from both the short-term and long-term perspective. Therefore, this operative investigation should be withheld until optimal management with antiprostaglandin

therapy or OCP, or both, has been tried and failed, and other adolescent issues explored.

Amenorrhoea

Primary

See delayed puberty, Endocrine Conditions, chapter 20.

Secondary

Consider the following diagnoses:

- Pregnancy
- Weight loss/anorexia nervosa
- Strenuous exercise
- Stress (e.g. exams, social–family or travel)
- *Polycystic ovaries*: associated problems of hirsutism and obesity are usually present. These patients often have irregular, infrequent periods rather than amenorrhoea. Investigations can help confirm or support the diagnosis, but they are not essential (e.g. follicle-stimulating hormone, luteinising hormone and pelvic ultrasound). Amenorrhoea itself does not need treatment but associated problems may require intervention (e.g. obesity – dietary/nutritional, exercise; hirsutism – the oral contraceptive pill, particularly Diane 35™, which contains cyproterone acetate, an antiandrogen). The use of hormonal treatment to cause withdrawal bleeds has the advantage of making periods lighter and more regular, rather than infrequent and heavy.

Metrostaxis (severe heavy loss)

Check the Hb and clotting profile; exclude pregnancy. Metrostaxis in the young woman having her first or second period usually requires oestrogen therapy (Fig. 24.1). As with women with established menstrual cycles, the young woman who has been menstruating for some time will usually respond to progestogen therapy (Fig. 24.2).

Ongoing management

The treatment should be continued for at least 3–6 months before a trial without hormonal therapy should be considered. The alternatives are:

- Cyclical progesterones (norethisterone 5 mg daily or twice daily for 14 or 21 days/month).
- The oral contraceptive pill.

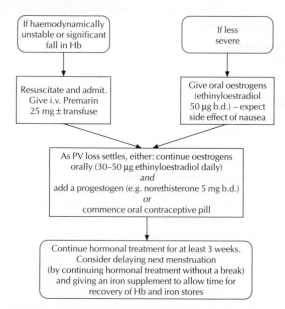

Fig. 24.1 Heavy loss at first or second period

Either of these approaches would also be appropriate for the management of the adolescent with menorrhagia.

Non-steroidal medications are also very effective in reducing menstrual loss.

PELVIC PAIN: GYNAECOLOGICAL CAUSES

Midcycle pain (Mittelschmerz)

This occurs in midcycle; therefore, it can often be diagnosed on history.

Ovarian cysts

Most ovarian cysts detected from a scan will be normal follicles and the reassurance that these are physiological and represent healthy functioning ovaries is important. Presume that all cysts less than 6 cm are physiological unless specific features are present to suggest

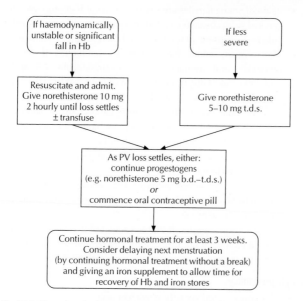

Fig. 24.2 Heavy loss in the young woman who has been menstruating for some time

otherwise. Repeating a scan 4–6 weeks later to prove the resolution of cysts less than 6 cm can prevent operative intervention.

Torsion of the ovary is very uncommon, but it usually occurs in the presence of an ovarian cyst. The history is of a sudden onset of severe pain with associated nausea, vomiting and dizziness. A diagnostic laparoscopy is the best way of excluding this condition, although if an immediate ultrasound can be performed and the ovaries are normal the diagnosis is most unlikely.

Pelvic inflammatory disease (PID)

- This only occurs in females who have been sexually active.
- A history of dyspareunia, discharge and fever may be associated with the pelvic pain.
- Chlamydial PID may cause endometritis with intermenstrual bleeding, menorrhagia or metrostaxis.

- As these young females are sexually active it is appropriate that cervical swabs be taken, including specific swabs for chlamydia culture, or utilising urine or cervical LCR testing for chlamydia.
- Management: admit for intravenous antibiotics if febrile; otherwise oral antibiotics (e.g. metronidazole 7.5 mg/kg (max 800 mg) orally, 8 hourly; amoxycillin 10–25 mg/kg (max 500–1000 mg) orally, 8 hourly; and doxycycline 2 mg/kg (max 100 mg) orally daily). *Note:* If gonococcal disease is a significant risk in the community, appropriate antibiotics are ceftriaxone 250 mg (in 1% lignocaine), i.m. stat plus doxycycline (for 14 days) or amoxycillin–clavulanate (dose as for amoxycillin) plus doxycycline (14 days).
- In the sexually active teenager Papanicolaou (PAP) smears should be taken annually, commencing approximately 6 months after intercourse began.
- Discuss contraception. If PID is suspected it generally implies that condoms are not being used. Discuss the benefits of condoms for protection against sexually transmitted diseases (STDs).

Ectopic pregnancy

- This concerns the sexually active teenager.
- A recent 'period' does not exclude this diagnosis.
- The use of contraception does not exclude this diagnosis. Suspicion is increased if an intra-uterine device (IUD) is used (although unlikely in a teenager), and decreased with the use of the oral contraceptive pill.
- Perform a pregnancy test and organise a pelvic ultrasound unless the clinical situation (i.e. shock) necessitates immediate resuscitation and surgical intervention.
- Contraception and PAP smear need to be discussed.

Congenital obstructive anomalies

- May cause acute onset pain or progressively increasing dysmenorrhoea (if there is unilateral obstruction) or progressively increasing pelvic pain without menstruation (if there is complete obstruction).
- Pelvic mass may be palpable. Perineal examination may reveal an imperforate hymen.
- Pelvic ultrasound or other imaging techniques will help clarify the anatomy.

- Associated renal agenesis on the side of the obstructed genital tract may occur.

BREAST PROBLEMS

- The asymmetrical development of the breast bud may lead to a presentation with a 'breast lump'. Biopsy at this early stage is contraindicated. Reassure during the time of breast growth and development. Growth that is initially asymmetric may correct itself.
- Persistent unequal breast size can cause considerable embarrassment and distress to the teenager, and referral to a specialist (usually a plastic surgeon with an interest in breast surgery) may be appropriate. Eventually, surgical correction may be required, but this would not be undertaken until growth has ceased.

CONTRACEPTION: BEST OPTIONS FOR YOUNG WOMEN

There is the need to explore other issues that are pertinent to adolescence and health risk behaviours (see HEADSS approach, Adolescent Health, chapter 8).

Condoms

Condoms offer the advantage of protection from STDs, as well as fairly good contraception. They may not be a reliable form of contraception if alcohol and drug-taking are issues.

Oral contraceptive pill (OCP)

Contraindications

- There is a history of thromboembolic disease.
- Liver disease is present.
- Oestrogen-dependent tumours are present.

Short-term side effects

- Nausea.
- Breakthrough bleeding (this should resolve with continuing usage).
- Migraines.

Types

- Sequential pills (e.g. Triquilar and Triphasil): these are generally the first choice.
- Constant dose (e.g. Microgynon 30ED and Nordette): for the patient who suffers erratic, heavy periods, premenstrual moodiness or irregular lifestyle routines (there is a slightly greater leeway in the time of taking such pills).
- Higher oestrogen content: if using anticonvulsants or if there is persistent breakthrough bleeding.
- Depo Provera: a 150 mg, 3-monthly injection. This often causes irregular bleeding initially but amenorrhoea after 6–9 months' usage. This is a very reliable form of contraception. Long-term usage in teenagers may have some impact on bone density.

Intra-uterine contraceptive (IUD) devices and diaphragms are generally not appropriate for young women.

The progesterone-only pill is also generally not appropriate – it needs to be taken at the same time every day to be effective, and it is less reliable than the combination OCP.

Emergency contraception: the morning-after pill

- It can be used up to 72 h after unprotected intercourse.
- Contraindications are as for OCP.
- Administer two 'pill' tablets immediately and another two pills 12 h later.
- 'Pill' tablets should comprise any OCP that contains 50 μg of ethinyl oestradiol and 125 μg of levonorgestrel (e.g. Nordiol and Microgynon 50).
- As nausea and vomiting may occur, administer an oral anti-emetic (e.g. metoclopramide 10 mg) 30 min before the 'pill' tablets.

This treatment is effective (>90%), but it does not provide continuing contraception. Discuss and plan ongoing contraception and PAP smears, and plan follow-up strategies to ensure that the emergency treatment has worked.

CHAPTER 25

HAEMATOLOGIC CONDITIONS AND ONCOLOGY
Peter Smith
Michael South

THE PALE CHILD

The initial investigation is a full blood count and film. Further investigations are determined by the blood film appearance. Remember that there is a variation in the lower limit of normal haemoglobin (Hb) at different ages (see Reference ranges, Appendix 1).

Where possible, treatment is deferred until a definitive diagnosis is made. Transfusion is avoided in nutritional anaemias if possible.

IRON DEFICIENCY ANAEMIA

Iron deficiency is common among Australian children. However, it is often subclinical, and only leads to anaemia in the small proportion with a more severe deficiency. Iron deficiency may be present in 10–30% of children in the high-risk groups. Iron deficiency may lead to reduced cognitive and psychomotor performance, even in the absence of anaemia.

Malabsorption and gastrointestinal bleeding (except in association with cow milk) are rare causes of iron deficiency in childhood. Most cases are dietary.

Suspect iron deficiency in the at-risk groups (see Table 25.1); take a careful history including diet.

Suspect iron deficiency anaemia if there is pallor (but remember this physical sign is only reliably detected when the Hb is <70–80 g/L), listlessness and irritability. Eating or chewing unusual items (geophagia and pica) are rare features. Severe anaemia may cause cardiac failure.

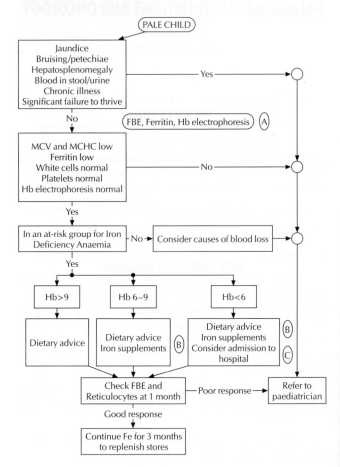

Fig. 25.1 The approach to take for the pale child

(A) Consider haemoglobinopathy in children of African, Mediter-
     ranean, Southeast Asian and Arabic descent, especially if
     there is a family history, or a normal ferritin and/or anaemia,
     resistant to iron therapy. Order Hb electrophoresis if iron stores
     are normal.

(B) Supplemental iron is best given as a ferrous gluconate mixture (the daily dose = 1 mL/kg of the 300 mg/5 mL preparation), and should be continued for 3 months after the Hb has returned to normal to replenish stores. The stools may become black/grey. Dietary advice must always be given. *An iron overdose can be fatal, and supplements should be stored in a locked cabinet.*

(C) Parenteral iron supplementation is rarely indicated in children. A blood transfusion is also rarely indicated. It may be used if a very anaemic child requires urgent surgery, or if significant cardiac failure is present. A transfusion should be slow and aimed only to raise the Hb to 60–80 g/L (see Calculating the blood transfusion volume page 359).

Table 25.1 High-risk groups for iron deficiency

Group	Additional risk factors	Mechanisms
<6 months of age	Prematurity Low birthweight Multiple births Maternal iron deficiency	Inadequate stores
6–24 months of age	Exclusive breast feeding after 6 months Delayed introduction of iron-containing solids Excessive cow milk	Inadequate intake Cow milk may cause microscopic gut blood loss
Adolescents	Females Poor diet	Menstruation Rapid growth spurt
Aborigines Migrant families Socially disadvantaged Vegetarians/fad diets	Poor diet Excessive cow milk	Inadequate intake

Prevention of iron deficiency

- Introduce iron-containing solids from 4 to 6 months.
- Avoid cow milk in the first 12 months (small amounts allowed in, e.g. custards and cereals).

- Avoid the excessive intake of cow milk up to 24 months.
- Ensure that formulas (if used) and cereals are iron fortified.
- Consider supplementation in high-risk groups (e.g. prematurity).

Good sources of iron for children

See also Infant and Child Nutrition, chapter 7.

- Infant milk formulas.
- Fortified breakfast cereals.
- Meat (including red meat, chicken and fish).
- Green vegetables (especially legumes, e.g. peas and beans).
- Dried beans and fruit.
- Egg yolk.

Note: Foods high in Vitamin C, including citrus fruit, strawberries, cauliflower and broccoli, will increase iron absorption from non-meat sources.

Investigation and management

In most patients two investigations usually suffice: the full blood examination (FBE) and serum ferritin.

Note: Ferritin is an acute phase reactant and may be misleadingly normal/high during an intercurrent illness. In mild iron deficiency, the FBE is normal but the ferritin is reduced, which demonstrates low iron stores. Dietary advice is usually all that is needed in this group.

In iron deficiency anaemia the ferritin, Hb, mean corpuscular volume (MCV) and mean corpuscular Hb concentration (MCHC) are low (see Appendix 1). Remember that iron deficiency anaemia caused by a poor diet may be associated with other macro- or micronutrient deficiencies.

THALASSAEMIA MAJOR

Transfusion

The patient is transfused to a high normal Hb level using packed cells, which are frequently depleted of white cells, to maintain the Hb above 100 g/L.

Desferrioxamine

This is usually given with each unit of blood transfused. A dose of 0.5 g is used. Subcutaneous infusions administered by a constant infusion pump are given overnight for 5–6 days/week once serum ferritin levels exceed 1000 µg/L.

Immunisation

Pneumococcal, meningococcal and *Haemophilus influenzae* type b immunisation (ideally pre-splenectomy) and penicillin prophylaxis (12.5 mg/kg twice daily indefinitely) is given to all patients who have had a splenectomy.

SICKLE CELL DISEASE

Patients may present with a crisis that may be haemolytic, infarctive, aplastic or splenic sequestration. Splenic sequestration is a medical emergency, the child presenting with hypovolaemic shock, anaemia and acute splenic enlargement. Most patients in crisis require admission. Consultation with the clinical haematologist is essential in the management of these patients.

DRUG-INDUCED HAEMOLYSIS

This may present at any age, including the newborn period, with anaemia, jaundice or both. The FBE will show a normocytic, normochromic anaemia. Characteristic features on the blood film include a reticulocytosis, spherocytes and/or fragmented red cells.

Drugs that produce haemolysis when taken by subjects with erythrocyte glucose-6-phosphate dehydrogenase deficiency or haemoglobin H disease include:

- Antimalarials: chloroquine; primaquine; quinacrine; quinine
- Antipyretics and analgesics: acetylsalicylic acid; quinidine
- Nitrofurans: nitrofurantoin; nitrofurazone
- Sulphones: sulphamethoxazole
- Other drugs: aminosalicylic acid; chloramphenicol; dimercaprol (BAL); methylene blue; naphthalene; phenylhydrazine;

probenecid; trinitrotoluene; Vitamin K (water-soluble analogues; Synkavit).

Fava beans (broad beans) may also produce haemolysis in patients with this deficiency.

COAGULATION DISORDERS

Investigation of a child with a suspected bleeding disorder

When investigating a child with a suspected disorder the following tests can be used:

- A platelet count
- Activated partial thromboplastin time (APTT)
- Prothrombin time (PT)/international normalised ratio (INR)
- Fibrinogen.

Special tests to identify a specific disorder

These may be arranged depending on the results of tests listed above and after discussion with a haematologist. Such tests might include specific coagulation and function assays, a von Willebrand Factor assay or platelet function studies.

HAEMOPHILIA A (FACTOR VIII DEFICIENCY)

Management of bleeding

Factor VIII dose (desired levels of Factor VIII to control haemorrhage)

In general, 1 unit of Factor VIII raises Factor VIII levels by 2%. Thus 15 units/kg will increase Factor VIII by 30% and 25 units/kg by 50%.

Most bleeding can be controlled with a single dose calculated to increase the Factor VIII level to 30–50%. *Note:* a minor head injury can become serious: the Factor VIII level should be raised to 100% and the child admitted for observation.

Recombinant human Factor VIII (Kogenate/Recombinate) has recently become available; it is used for all patients without previous exposure to human derived Factor VIII.

Patients with Factor VIII inhibitors are now treated with recombinant Factor VIIa (NOVOSEVEN™). The usual dose is 90–100 µg/kg repeated in 2 h.

Mouth bleeding

Use tranexamic acid tablets. For children <25 kg: 250 mg, three times daily; 25–35 kg: 500 mg, three times daily; 35–50 kg: 750 mg, three times daily; >50 kg: 1 g, three times daily.

General measures

These are applicable to all congenital bleeding disorders.
- Analgesia. Do not give aspirin. Avoid narcotic analgesics.
- Do not give intramuscular injections.
- The splinting of limbs reduces pain.

Consult with a haematologist about the need for joint aspiration. Beware of the risk of Volkmann's ischaemic contracture in forearm bleeds, and of femoral nerve palsies with retroperitoneal bleeds tracking underneath the inguinal ligament.

VON WILLEBRAND DISEASE

This responds to cryoprecipitate, or, less predictably, to Factor VIII. Many patients respond to desmopressin. The half-life of von Willebrand's Factor is approximately 4 h, but Factor VIII levels continue to be increased for 48–72 h after the infusion of cryoprecipitate. Further doses are given if bleeding recurs.

CHRISTMAS DISEASE – HAEMOPHILIA B (FACTOR IX DEFICIENCY)

This is treated with Factor IX concentrate (MONOFIX™).
- Requirements: as in haemophilia.
- Dose: in general 1 unit Factor IX/kg increases the Factor IX level by 1.6%.
- Frequency: injections at 24 h intervals (the half-life for Factor IX is 24 h).

RARE BLEEDING DISORDERS

When the diagnosis of the disorder is in doubt, treat with fresh frozen plasma (20 mL/kg) +/– platelets until the precise defect is known.

IDIOPATHIC THROMBOCYTOPENIC PURPURA (ITP)

In young children this usually presents with bruising and petechiae, following an apparent viral infection. The gradual onset in an older child, particularly a female over 10 years of age, suggests a higher chance of chronic disease. With the acute form, more than 80% of those afflicted undergo spontaneous remission within 8 weeks.

Management

- If the clinical presentation and FBE/blood film suggest classical ITP (i.e. no pallor, hepatosplenomegaly or lymphadenopathy; no anaemia, leucopenia or blasts), a bone marrow biopsy is not necessary.
- Careful observation without specific treatment may be appropriate in many cases. If the patient and family have been seen by a paediatrician, and are assessed as having a good understanding of the necessary precautions, and adequate follow up is assured, admission may not be required. However, if there are any concerns regarding parental education/reassurance, it is often helpful to have the child in hospital for 24 h.
- The indications for treatment, as well as the best form of treatment for children with acute ITP, remain controversial. Without active treatment, most patients' platelet counts will return to a level at which normal activity can be recommenced within 4–6 weeks. Patients with active bleeding (e.g. mucosal and gastrointestinal) should receive treatment to increase their platelet count rapidly. Some authorities also recommend treating patients with a platelet count $<10 \times 10^9$ /L and a florid petechial rash (especially mucosal petechiae).
- When treatment is indicated, the choice lies between corticosteroids (prednisolone 4 mg/kg per day for 2 weeks, then tapered) or high-dose i.v. immunoglobulin (normal human

immunoglobulin (INTRAGAM) 1 g/kg over 8–12 h, once, or daily for 2 days).

- Splenectomy is reserved for patients with severe chronic thrombocytopenia and should be accompanied by the usual precautions (see Thalassaemia major, above). Consultation with a paediatric haematologist is recommended.

USE OF BLOOD COMPONENTS

Many forms of anaemia do not require a transfusion. Removal of the cause of the anaemia and replacement of the deficiency will frequently produce a rapid rise in the Hb and avoid the need for a transfusion. Irradiated blood products (red cells and platelets) should be used for immunocompromised patients and those on chemotherapy.

Whole blood

Indicated for patients with dual problems of a symptomatic oxygen carrying capacity combined with hypovolaemia; e.g. during acute blood loss.

Red blood cells (RBC)

Used in preference to whole blood for the treatment of anaemia. RBC are especially indicated for cardiac failure, renal disease, liver disease and autoimmune haemolytic anaemia.

Leucocyte-depleted cells

For patients with recurrent febrile non-haemolytic transfusion reactions with demonstrated leucocyte or platelet antibodies and for the prevention of cytomegalovirus transmission in selected patients.

Calculating the blood transfusion volume

This assumes a haematocrit of 33% for whole blood and 66% for packed cells.

- Whole blood (mL) = wt (kg) × Hb rise required (g/L) × 6.
- Packed cells (mL) = wt (kg) × Hb rise required (g/L) × 3.

Table 25.2 outlines many of the possible reactions to blood transfusions.

Table 25.2 Reactions to blood transfusions

Type	Symptoms and signs	Treatment	Prevention
Pyrogenic	Pyrexia, rigors, anxiety and restlessness	Slow rate of flow Antihistamines	If not better in 30 min, discontinue transfusion
Allergic	Usually pyrexia and rigors, urticaria, facial and laryngeal oedema, dyspnoea cyanosis and peripheral collapse	Discontinue transfusion Adrenaline Antihistamines Hydrocortisone, i.v.	Prophylactic antihistamines Use appropriate leucocyte-poor or washed cells
Haemolytic	Pyrexia, rigors, lumbar pain, pain in vein, jaundice, haemoglobinuria, haemoglobinaemia, oliguria later	Discontinue transfusion Obtain expert advice Check all labels Take blood samples Save urine	Careful grouping and cross-matching Care in storing blood Check labels prior to transfusion
Infected blood	Pyrexia, pain in limbs and chest, pallor, dyspnoea headache, shock	Discontinue transfusion Save donor blood Treat shock Antibiotics	Care in collecting Storage of blood at correct temperature Observation of expiry time
Circulatory	Pulmonary oedema, dyspnoea, headache, venous distension, heaviness in limbs Possibly pyrexia and rigors	Slow rate of flow Diuretic (frusemide) Digoxin Venesection if extreme	Use of packed cells Give all fluids very slowly If in doubt, give frusemide

Platelets

Indicated for bleeding associated with thrombocytopenia or platelet function disorders, especially in leukaemia and aplastic anaemia. Dose: 4–6 units/m^2.

The normal life-span for platelets is 10 days, but the effective life-span of transfused platelets may be greatly shortened in the presence of bleeding or infection. A transfusion may be required every 1 or 2 days for the control of bleeding or more frequently if there are clinical indications.

Platelets must be stored at room temperature and may be transfused through a leucocyte reduction filter specifically designed for platelets.

Coagulation factors (see Coagulation disorders, above)

- Recombinant Factor VIII.
- Cryoprecipitate.
- Factor IX concentrate (see Factor IX deficiency, above).

Fresh frozen plasma

Each pack contains approximately 200 mL. The required dose is 10–20 mL/kg.

Indications

- Emergency therapy of congenital bleeding disorders.
- Congenital bleeding disorders that are not responsive to cryoprecipitate or Factor IX concentrate.
- Post-extracorporeal circulation.

Albumin

Contents

- 20% albumin in 10 or 100 mL of buffered solution.
  - Sodium: 46–58 mmol/L.
  - The use is restricted to hypoproteinaemia.
- 5% albumin in 50 or 500 mL of buffered solution.
  - Sodium: 140 mmol/L.
  - This solution may be used to expand blood volume in shock.

Immunoglobulins

Normal gamma-globulin

This is obtained from pooled serum. Indications:

- *Hypogammaglobulinaemia.* Loading dose of 400–600 mg/kg is given. This may be repeated if IgG levels remain low. Maintenance doses are given every 4 weeks to maintain IgG levels above the fifth percentile. A dose adjustment should be made in consultation with an immunologist. Major reactions to pH-modified i.v. globulin are not common. Consult with an immunologist if these occur.
- *Infectious hepatitis contacts.* 0.2 mL/kg, i.m. (max 5 mL).
- *Measles contacts.* 0.2 mL/kg, i.m. in children <12 months and 0.5 mL/kg, i.m. for immunocompromised children (max 15 mL; split dose and give in two separate sites).

Hyperimmune gamma-globulins

Varieties currently available are:

- Anti-Rh (D) for prophylaxis of Rh haemolytic disease in the newborn.
- Tetanus for both prophylaxis and therapy (see Procedures, chapter 3).
- Varicella (zoster immune globulin) for the prevention of chicken-pox when it may be life-threatening; e.g. in immune deficiency states. Must be given within 96 h of exposure. The dose to administer is 2 mL (0–5 years), 4 mL (6–12 years) and 6 mL (adult).

ONCOLOGY

The management of paediatric cancers is a specialised field within the discipline of paediatrics and is best undertaken under the supervision of a specialist in a paediatric tertiary referral centre.

Presentations of childhood malignancies

The possibility of a malignancy should be considered in children presenting with any of the following symptoms and signs:

- Combinations of pallor, bruising, petechiae, fever and bone pain
- Lymphadenopathy – marked or persistent/progressive
- Hepatosplenomegaly
- Any unusual mass
- Persisting, severe headache associated with vomiting or visual disturbance
- Ataxia or other neurological signs
- Unexplained weight loss.

These children should be referred to a centre of paediatric expertise for investigation and management.

Emergencies in acute leukaemia

Complications of acute leukaemia or its treatment are the immediate cause of most early deaths rather than the leukaemia itself. It is important that they be recognised early and treated vigorously to ensure the patient's survival.

The most likely complications are infection, haemorrhage, toxic drug reactions, hyperuricaemia and other metabolic disturbances.

- Cultures are taken and appropriate broad-spectrum intravenous antibiotics are used to treat the infection.
- Platelets and blood transfusions are used to treat haemorrhage.
- Adequate hydration, allopurinol 10 mg/kg (max 600 mg) daily in two to three divided doses, biochemical monitoring and attention to fluid balance are used to prevent/treat hyperuricaemia.

Febrile neutropenia

Any child receiving chemotherapy who has a fever must be considered likely to be neutropenic and should have a white cell count performed. If the child's total neutrophil count is less than 0.5×10^9 /L then blood and urine cultures should be taken. Broad-spectrum intravenous antibiotics should be given to prevent overwhelming septicaemia. Pipericillin 50 mg/kg (max 2 g) 6 hourly and gentamicin 2.5 mg/kg (max 80 mg) 8 hourly in children with liquid tumours. Ceftazidime 37.5 mg/kg (max 2 g) 12 hourly should be used in children with solid tumours.

Nausea and vomiting

Nausea and vomiting are well-described complications of chemo-therapy. The use of new-generation anti-emetics will ameliorate this problem for most children.

For children receiving intensive chemotherapy agents, such as *cis*-platinum, cyclophosphamide, ifosfamide or high-dose anthracyclines, it is better to use a new-generation anti-emetic such as ondansetron 0.15 mg/kg (max 8 mg) 8 hourly prophylactically.

For children receiving a less emetogenic program, such as a stand-ard acute lymphoblastic leukaemia (ALL) induction, a trial of an agent such as metoclopramide 0.12 mg/kg (max 10–15 mg) is recommended.

Constipation

Constipation is a common side effect of vincristine when used regularly, such as in an ALL induction. Children who have gone more than 2 days without a bowel motion should be given an aperient. Enemas should be avoided.

Pain

See also Pain Management in Children, chapter 4.

It is important to do as much as possible to minimise pain and distress in children with cancer.

- Procedures should be performed after a careful explanation to the parent(s) and child, and after the use of appropriate sedation, analgesia and/or anaesthesia.
- At presentation, the pain of an active disease usually responds to the appropriate major analgesia; e.g. i.v. morphine and the application of the appropriate treatment protocol. The localised pain related to the disease during a relapse will often respond to local palliative radiotherapy. More generalised chronic pain usually requires major analgesia (e.g. with a sustained release of morphine or parenteral morphine), which can be delivered i.v. or s.c. by constant infusion.
- For older children, a patient-controlled device should be considered.
- For severe refractory pain, consultation with a pain clinic, anaesthetist or neurosurgeon may be indicated.

Long-term effects

Before commencing any chemotherapeutic program it is essential to discuss the long-term effects of treatment. These can be classified under the headings of effects on growth, development, fertility and risk of a second neoplasm. The likely long-term effects in a given child will depend on the modalities and intensity of the treatment.

- Radiation treatment given to a young child will invariably inhibit growth of the part irradiated. Similarly, irradiation of gonads will invariably lead to infertility. Cranial radiotherapy may lead to hypothalamic–pituitary dysfunction later in life.
- The effect of chemotherapy on these parameters will also depend on the agents used and the intensity of treatment. Less-intensive treatment with antimetabolites has little effect on growth and development and a minimum effect on fertility. Intensive treatment with alkylating agents is likely to have a more serious effect on fertility. The risk of second malignancies is increased by the use of agents such as radiotherapy, alkylating agents and epipodophyllotoxins.

CHAPTER 26
INFECTIOUS DISEASES

Nigel Curtis
Mike Starr

RATIONAL ANTIMICROBIAL PRESCRIBING

- Unnecessary antibiotic use for viral illnesses is common, and has led to increasing rates of antibiotic resistance among *Streptococcus pneumoniae* and other community-acquired pathogens. Most respiratory tract infections in children, including tonsillitis and otitis media, are self-limiting and do not require antibiotic therapy. Judicious use of antibiotics will decrease antibiotic resistance. If the diagnosis is unclear, it is preferable to perform repeated clinical evaluations and simple laboratory tests than to use empiric antibiotic therapy 'just in case'.
- Antibiotics do not prevent secondary bacterial infection in viral illnesses.
- The use of antibiotics may make definitive diagnosis and subsequent decisions about management more difficult.
- Empiric antibiotic therapy (i.e. not based on specific aetiological diagnosis) should only be prescribed when a *serious* bacterial infection is suspected (e.g. meningitis) *and* it is not safe or possible to obtain definitive culture specimens, or culture results are pending.
- The choice of empiric therapy should be based on the likely aetiology, local antibiotic resistance patterns and individual host factors (e.g. immunocompromise), and should be consistent with local guidelines.
- For mild infections, the safest and best tolerated antibiotic with the narrowest spectrum against the most likely pathogens should be chosen (e.g. trimethoprim for urinary tract infection).
- For serious infections, broad-spectrum agents are chosen until the pathogen and its sensitivity is identified (e.g. cefotaxime for meningitis).

- The temptation to prescribe the newest antibiotic should be resisted. Theoretical benefits based on *in vitro* data do not necessarily translate into greater efficacy. Newer antibiotics are often expensive, with many side effects, and frequently result in resistance or superinfection. The factors used to determine the role of new antibiotics include evidence that the drug has superior clinical efficacy and safety.

ANTIBIOTIC RESISTANCE

Although many bacteria are still susceptible to long-established treatments, antibiotic resistance in some is an increasing problem worldwide. Examples of particular clinical concern include:

- Penicillin (and cephalosporin)-resistant *Streptococcus pneumoniae* (PRP)
- Methicillin (multi-drug)-resistant *Staphylococcus aureus* (MRSA)
- Vancomycin-resistant (glycopeptide intermediate) *Staphylococcus aureus* (GISA)
- Vancomycin-resistant *Enterococcus* (VRE)
- Multi-drug-resistant *Mycobacterium tuberculosis* (MRTB)
- Bacteria that produce inducible β-lactamases (e.g. some *Pseudomonas* spp. and *Enterobacter* spp.) (IBL)
- Bacteria that produce extended-spectrum β-lactamases (e.g. some *Klebsiella* spp.) (ESBL)
- Multi-drug-resistant *Salmonella* spp.

Strategies to deal with infections caused by these organisms include the use of new or broader spectrum antibiotics, or the use of two or more antibiotics concurrently. The choice for empiric therapy becomes increasingly difficult.

FEVER

Fever is the most common presenting symptom in children in the primary care setting. Although there is no universally accepted definition, fever is generally considered to be present if:

- Rectal temperature >38°C
- Oral temperature >37.5°C
- Axillary temperature >37°C.

Although tympanic thermometers provide certain advantages over other thermometers (ease of use, rapid results and convenience), several studies have found that they are not as accurate or sensitive for the detection of fever. This is particularly the case in infants <3 months of age.

Self-limiting viral infections are the most common cause of fever in children. However, the challenge to the clinician is to identify those children with a more serious cause. Fever in children may be classified into three groups:
- Fever with localising signs
- Fever without focus
- Fever of unknown origin.

Fever with localising signs

A careful history and examination will identify the source of infection in most patients. These children should be managed according to the individual condition and its severity.

Fever without focus

In a small number of children presenting with fever, no focus is found. While most will have a viral infection, a more serious illness such as a urinary tract infection (5–8%), occult bacteraemia (3–5%) or meningitis may be present. Infants with rectal temperature >38.9°C have an 8–15% risk of occult bacteraemia.

Most children who present with fever and no identifiable focus appear otherwise well. History should include details about immunisation status, infectious contacts, travel, diet, and contact with animals or insects. A thorough physical examination should be performed, paying particular attention to:
- General appearance: the level of activity and social interaction; peripheral perfusion and colour.
- Vital signs: pulse; respiration; blood pressure.
- Possible clues to source: full fontanelle; neck stiffness; respiratory distress (tachypnoea; grunt; nasal flare; retractions); abnormal chest signs; rhinitis, pharyngitis, otitis or mastoiditis; lymphadenopathy; abdominal distension, tenderness or masses;

hepatosplenomegaly; bone and joint tenderness or swelling; skin rashes, petechiae or purpura, or skin infection.

Patients with unexplained fever with a higher likelihood for serious infection include the following patient groups or conditions:

- Neonates
- Immunocompromise (e.g. congenital immunodeficiency, HIV, neoplasms, cytotoxic drugs and steroids)
- Asplenic children
- Children with central venous or arterial catheters, or other foreign bodies, including shunts
- Multiple congenital abnormalities
- Other specific illnesses (e.g. sickle cell disease, cystic fibrosis or structural cardiac defects (endocarditis))
- Toxic-appearing children (e.g. those with an altered conscious state, decreased peripheral perfusion or blood pressure, or purpuric rash)
- Children under 12 months of age with apparent febrile convulsion (meningitis must be excluded)

These children require admission to hospital, with culture of blood, urine and CSF, and a chest X-ray if indicated. Antimicrobial therapy should be based on the patient's clinical illness and the local epidemiology of potential pathogens and their antibiotic susceptibility.

In the absence of the above risk factors, a well-appearing febrile child (over 3 months of age) without a focus of infection does not require laboratory testing or treatment. There is no evidence that oral or parenteral antibiotics prevent the rare occurrence of focal infections from occult bacteraemia; instead, they result in delayed diagnosis, drug side effects, additional costs and the development of resistant organisms. What is required is a careful clinical assessment, review within the next 24 h and parental education. See Table 26.1 and Box 26.1.

Occult bacteraemia

Some infants with bacteraemia clear the bacteria spontaneously. This is particularly true for pneumococcal bacteraemia. Patients who grow *Streptococcus pneumoniae* in their original blood culture, but who are now well, remain afebrile and have not received antibiotics, do not require further investigation or treatment, as they have cleared the

Box 26.1 Advice for parents about fever

When caring for your child:
- Make the child comfortable; e.g. give tepid baths and dress in light clothing
- Give small, frequent drinks of clear fluid; e.g. water and diluted juice
- Fever does not necessarily require treatment with medication. Finding the cause and treating it is often more important
- Paracetamol should be given only if the child is irritable, miserable or appears to be in pain (15 mg/kg p.o. 4 hourly when required to a max of 90 mg/kg per day)
- Giving paracetamol has not been shown to prevent febrile convulsions
- Do not continue giving regular paracetamol for >48 h without having the child assessed by a doctor
- Aspirin should be avoided

Seek immediate medical attention if there is no improvement in 48 h or if the child:
- Looks 'sick': pale, lethargic and weak
- Suffers severe headache, neck stiffness or light hurting eyes
- Has breathing difficulties
- Refuses to drink anything
- Persistently vomits
- Shows signs of drowsiness
- Suffers pain

organism themselves. Parents should, however, be asked to bring children back for immediate review if they develop further fever within the following 7 days.

Other pathogens such as *Neisseria meningitidis* and *Haemophilus influenzae* type b (now rare with routine Hib immunisation) carry a significantly increased risk of meningitis, and should be treated with appropriate antibiotics (usually a penicillin and a third-generation cephalosporin, respectively). Similarly, *Staphylococcus aureus* bacteraemia should be treated (usually with flucloxacillin) because of the potential risk of bone and joint infection.

Table 26.1 Management of fever without focus

Age	Investigations	Management
<1 month	FBE; blood, urine and CSF cultures; CXR	• Admit • Empiric i.v. benzylpenicillin and gentamicin, *plus* cefotaxime if meningitis is suspected (see Antimicrobial guidelines)
1 to 3 months	As above (CXR may be omitted if no respiratory symptoms or signs present)	• If WCC 5–15 × 10^9 /L with other investigations normal: discharge and review within 12 h, or sooner if deterioration occurs • If child is unwell, or any results are abnormal: admit and consider empiric antibiotics (see Antimicrobial guidelines)
3 months to 3 years *and well*	Consider urine culture (mandatory if <6 months)	• If <6 months and UTI is suspected from dipstick urine testing: admit for i.v. benzylpenicillin and gentamicin (see Antimicrobial guidelines) • Otherwise: discharge and review within 24 h, or sooner if deterioration occurs

3 months to 3 years *and unwell*	FBE; blood, urine and CSF cultures; CXR if respiratory symptoms or signs present	• Admit and start empiric antibiotics:
		  – if CSF normal: i.v. flucloxacillin and gentamicin
		  – if CSF abnormal or unavailable: i.v. cefotaxime (see Antimicrobial guidelines)

Notes:
• Fever = rectal temperature >38°C (>38.9°C over 3 months of age)
• FBE = full blood examination, including film; CSF = cerebrospinal fluid; WCC = white cell count; CXR = chest X-ray
• Urine specimens should be obtained by suprapubic aspiration or catheter drainage. Bag specimens are useless in this context
• Lumbar puncture should not be performed in a child with impaired conscious state or focal neurological signs (See Medical Emergencies, chapter 1)
• Ceftriaxone can be substituted for cefotaxime (see Antimicrobial guidelines)

Partially treated bacterial infection

Patients presenting with fever who have received prior antibiotics should be assessed with a high index of suspicion. Although the child may have a viral illness, partial treatment with antibiotics may mask the typical clinical presentation of a serious bacterial infection, such as meningitis. A full septic screen should be considered in most cases even if the child looks well.

Fever of unknown origin (FUO)

This is defined as prolonged fever (2 weeks or longer is the commonest definition) for which history, examination and routine tests have failed to reveal a cause. In general, FUO in children has a poorer prognosis than fever without focus, as it is more likely to be due to chronic, non-infectious conditions, such as juvenile chronic arthritis and other collagen vascular diseases, inflammatory bowel disease or malignancy. Infectious causes include systemic viral syndromes (such as infectious mononucleosis), upper or lower respiratory infections (e.g. sinusitis), urinary tract infection, central nervous system (CNS) infection, bone infection, tuberculosis, abscess (e.g. parameningeal, intra-abdominal), endocarditis and enteric infections (e.g. typhoid fever). The term FUO is often *incorrectly* applied to patients who are suffering a series of simple viral infections.

Febrile neutropenia

See Haematologic Conditions and Oncology, chapter 25.

KAWASAKI DISEASE

Kawasaki disease is a systemic vasculitis that predominantly affects children under 5 years of age. Although the specific aetiological agent remains unknown, it is believed that Kawasaki disease is caused by an infectious agent (although it is not transmitted from person to person).

Diagnosis is often delayed because the features are similar to those of many viral exanthems. The diagnostic criteria for Kawasaki disease are:
- Fever for 5 days or more; plus
- Four of the following five conditions:
  — Polymorphous rash
  — Bilateral (non-purulent) conjunctivitis

- — Mucous membrane changes; e.g. reddened or dry cracked lips, strawberry tongue, or a diffuse redness of oral or pharyngeal mucosa
- — Peripheral changes; e.g. erythema of the palms or soles, oedema of the hands or feet, and *in convalescence* desquamation
- — Cervical lymphadenopathy (larger than 15 mm in diameter, usually unilateral, single, non-purulent and painful)
- • Exclusion of diseases with a similar presentation: staphylococcal infection (e.g. scalded skin syndrome and toxic shock syndrome), streptococcal infection (e.g. scarlet fever and toxic shock-like syndrome, *not just isolation from throat*), measles, other viral exanthems, leptospirosis, rickettsial disease, Steven's Johnson syndrome, drug reaction and juvenile rheumatoid arthritis.

The diagnostic features of Kawasaki disease can occur sequentially and may not all be present at the same time. Moreover, it is recognised that some patients with Kawasaki disease do not develop sufficient features to fulfil the formal diagnostic criteria. Clinical vigilance and recognition of this possibility are necessary to recognise these 'incomplete' or 'atypical' cases. Other relatively common features include arthritis, diarrhoea and vomiting, coryza and cough.

Laboratory features may include neutrophilia, raised ESR and CRP, mild normochromic, normocytic anaemia, raised transaminases, hypoalbuminaemia; and marked thrombocytosis in the second week.

Up to 30% of untreated children develop coronary artery involvement, with dilation or aneurysm formation. These can occur up to 6–8 weeks after the onset of the illness. Echocardiography should therefore be performed at least twice: at the initial presentation and, if negative, again at 6–8 weeks.

Management includes early administration of intravenous immunoglobulin (IVIG) (2 g/kg over 10 h; preferably within the first 10 days of the illness) and aspirin (3–5 mg/kg once a day (anti-platelet dose) for at least 6–8 weeks). There is no evidence that using high (anti-inflammatory) dose aspirin decreases the risk of aneurysm development. Paracetamol can be used for symptomatic relief.

Treatment with IVIG is highly effective in preventing the potentially devastating complication of coronary artery involvement. Treatment should still be undertaken in patients presenting after 10 days of illness if they have evidence of ongoing inflammation (fever, raised acute phase markers).

CERVICAL LYMPHADENITIS

This is usually caused by an infection or inflammation of the lymph nodes. Malignancy is much less common.

The infectious causes are:

1 Acute bilateral lymphadenitis
   — Viral upper respiratory tract infections
   — Systemic viral infections (e.g. Epstein–Barr virus (EBV) and cytomegalovirus (CMV))

2 Acute unilateral lymphadenitis
   — Group A streptococcus or *Staphylococcus aureus*: 40–80% of acute unilateral lymphadenitis; occurs at 1–4 years of age; fever, tenderness, overlying erythema; may be associated with cellulitis
   — Anaerobic bacteria: older children with dental caries or periodontal disease
   — Group B streptococcus (neonates)

3 Subacute/chronic unilateral lymphadenitis
   — *Bartonella henselae* (cat-scratch disease): occurs about 2 weeks after a scratch or lick from a kitten or dog, usually involves axillary nodes (tender)
   — *Mycobacterium avium* complex (formerly known as MAIS): occurs at 1–4 years of age, painless, skin is purplish, patient afebrile
   — *Toxoplasma gondii*: fatigue, myalgia, there may be other involved nodes
   — *Mycobacterium tuberculosis*: usually a contact history, affects older children; systemic symptoms.

GROUP A STREPTOCOCCAL INFECTIONS

Group A beta haemolytic streptococci (GABHS) cause a variety of infections including pharyngotonsillitis (see Ear, Nose and Throat

Conditions, chapter 21), impetigo, scarlet fever, otitis media, glomer-ulonephritis and rheumatic fever. GABHS infection usually occurs in school-age children.

Scarlet fever

Transmission	Droplet, direct contact
Incubation period	2–5 days
Infectious period	10–21 days (24–48 h, if adequate treatment)
Clinical features	*Prodrome*: sudden onset high fever, vomiting, malaise, headache, and abdominal pain.
	Rash: appears within 2 h of prodrome, diffuse red flush involving torso and skin folds, blanches, circumoral pallor, strawberry tongue (initially white, then red day 4–5), pharyngotonsillitis, tender cervical / submaxillary nodes.
Complications	Otitis media; rheumatic fever; glomerulonephritis.
Diagnosis	Culture of throat swab may confirm clinical impression.
Treatment	Phenoxymethylpenicillin (Penicillin V) 250 mg p.o. (under 10 years), 500 mg p.o. (over 10 years) 12 hourly for 10 days.
Control of case	Exclude from school until treated for longer than 24 h.

Impetigo

See Dermatologic Conditions, chapter 18.

MYCOPLASMA PNEUMONIAE INFECTION

Transmission	Droplet
Incubation period	1–4 weeks
Infectious period	Unknown, likely to be many months; it typically infects all members of a family over a period of weeks/months.
Clinical syndromes	*Pneumonia*: malaise, fever, headache, non-productive cough for 3–4 weeks (may become productive); 10% have rash (usually maculopapular); bilateral, diffuse infiltrates on chest X-ray; bronchitis, pharyngitis, otitis media.

	CNS manifestations (uncommon): aseptic meningitis, meningoencephalitis, encephalitis, polyradiculitis/ Guillain–Barré syndrome, acute cerebellar ataxia, cranial nerve neuropathy, transverse myelitis, acute disseminated encephalomyelitis and choreoathetosis.
Complications	Idiopathic thrombocytopaenic purpura.
Diagnosis	*Serology*: four-fold rise in IgG; IgM alone can be difficult to interpret; polymerase chain reaction (PCR) is available in some laboratories.
Treatment	Roxithromycin 2.5–4 mg/kg (max 150 mg) p.o. 12 hourly for 10 days; role of antibiotics in CNS infections is unclear.

VIRAL INFECTIONS

Cytomegalovirus (CMV)

CMV is a ubiquitous herpesvirus. It persists in latent form after primary infection, and reactivation can occur years later, particularly under conditions of immunosuppression.

Transmission	*Horizontal*: salivary contamination or sexual transmission; blood transfusion/organ transplantation. *Vertical*: transplacental, intrapartum by passage through infected genital tract and postnatal by ingestion of CMV-positive breast milk.
Incubation period	Unknown, infection usually manifests 3 weeks to 3 months after blood transfusion, and 4 weeks to 4 months after tissue transplantation.
Clinical features	Vary with age and immunocompetence of child; asymptomatic infection is most common; *CMV mononucleosis*: cervical lymphadenopathy; hepatosplenomegaly in children, fever in adults. *Note*: clinical signs of CMV infection are shared by graft rejection in transplant patients. Both events peak 30–90 days after transplantation.
Diagnosis	Distinguishing CMV infection from active CMV disease can be difficult. The following tests on

blood, urine, oral secretions or biopsy specimens can help make this distinction: *viral culture* (rapid enhanced tissue culture immunofluorescence), *PCR, antigenaemia assay* (degree of antigenaemia correlates with the severity of CMV disease and is therefore a good means of predicting CMV disease and monitoring disease progression).

Complications	Encephalitis, myocarditis, pneumonia, haemolytic anaemia, thrombocytopenia. Primary CMV infection has been described in conjunction with Guillain–Barré syndrome and other peripheral neuropathies. Pneumonia, retinitis, hepatitis and colitis in immunocompromised.
	Congenital infection: >90% appear normal at birth: CNS sequelae in 10–20% of these (mainly sensorineural hearing loss); 5% present early with petechiae, hepatosplenomegaly, microcephaly and thrombocytopenia.
Treatment	Ganciclovir for active CMV disease in the immunocompromised.

Enterovirus (non-polio)

Coxsackie A, B and echoviruses are important causes of childhood infections, especially in the summer months. These include a wide range of clinical presentations, including non-specific febrile illness, pharyngitis, herpangina, gastroenteritis, aseptic meningitis, encephalitis, myocarditis, pericarditis and several forms of viral exanthem (maculopapular, vesicular, petechial, hand, foot and mouth disease). Infection in agammaglobulinaemic patients can cause particularly severe or persistent meningoencephalitis.

Hand, foot and mouth disease

Cause	Coxsackie A virus (A16)
Transmission	Direct contact/droplet
Incubation period	3–6 days
Infectious period	Until blisters have gone
Clinical features	Vesicles on cheeks, gums, sides of the tongue; papulovesicular lesions of palms, fingers, toes, soles, buttocks, genitals, limbs (may look haemorrhagic); sore throat; fever and anorexia.

Diagnosis	Tests are usually unnecessary as the clinical picture is sufficient for diagnosis.
Control of case	Exclusion is unnecessary (as virus is excreted in faeces for weeks).
Treatment	Symptomatic

Epstein–Barr virus (EBV) (infectious mononucleosis)

Incubation period	30–50 days
Infectious period	Unknown, viral excretion from oropharynx for months.
Clinical features	Fever, malaise, exudative tonsillopharyngitis, generalised lymphadenopathy and hepatosplenomegaly. Highly variable clinical course: acute phase lasts 2–4 weeks and convalescence may take weeks to months.
Diagnosis	Atypical lymphocytes in the peripheral blood. Monospot test in blood for heterophile antibody identifies 90% of cases in older children and adults, but lacks sensitivity in children under 4–5 years of age. Serology is the gold standard.
Complications	Upper airways obstruction; dehydration from poor oral intake (uncommon).
Treatment	Symptomatic: Prednisolone 1 mg/kg (max 50 mg) orally, daily may be considered in cases where hospitalised for airways obstruction. Amoxycillin and ampicillin may cause a florid rash in children with EBV infection.

Herpes simplex virus (HSV)

Manifestations of HSV infection include skin and mucous membrane involvement, gingivostomatitis (predominantly HSV-1), genital herpes (mainly HSV-2), eczema herpeticum (see Dermatologic Conditions, chapter 18), herpetic whitlow and eye involvement. HSV encephalitis is an important treatable condition not to miss (see page 392 and Neuro-logical Conditions, chapter 29). Pneumonia and disseminated infection occur in the immunocompromised. Congenital infection also occurs. Infection can be primary (e.g. gingivostomatitis) or from a reactivation of the latent virus (e.g. cold sores).

Primary herpes gingivostomatitis

Cause	Usually due to HSV-1 in young children
Transmission	Droplet, direct contact
Incubation period	2–14 days
Infectious period	Indeterminate; virus can be excreted for at least 1 week, occasionally months. Shed intermittently in the absence of symptoms for years afterwards.
Clinical features	Fever, irritability, cervical lymphadenopathy, halitosis, diffuse erythema and ulceration within the oral cavity (buccal mucosa, palate, gingiva and tongue) and mucocutaneous junction. Duration is 7–14 days.
Diagnosis	Immunofluorescence or culture of vesicular scrapings.
Complications	Poor oral intake; autoinoculation resulting in herpetic whitlow, keratitis or genital herpes; eczema herpeticum; dissemination (particularly in immunocompromised).
Treatment	Symptomatic, analgesia (rectal paracetamol), fluids (oral/nasogastric or intravenous) and a soft diet. Aciclovir should be given only if immunocompromised.

HSV in pregnancy

Primary infection during the first 20 weeks of gestation is associated with an increased risk of spontaneous abortion, stillbirth and congenital malformations. Beyond 20 weeks, premature labour and growth retardation are more common.

Neonatal HSV

Transmission	*Intrapartum* (70–85%): perinatal acquisition from maternal genital tract; usually presents day 5 to 19. *Postnatal* (10%): usually presents day 5 to 19. *Intrauterine* (5%): transplacental; usually presents within 48 h of birth.

- Transmission is 10 times more likely to occur with primary than with recurrent infection, both of which may be asymptomatic in women.

- More than 70% of women who give birth to infants with neonatal HSV infection give no history of genital HSV in themselves or their partners.
- The risk to a baby of an asymptomatic woman with a history of recurrent genital herpes is <3%.

Clinical features   Neonatal infection presents in three ways:

- *Localised skin, eye and/or mouth ('SEM') disease* (45%). Onset 7 to 14 days. Death is rare; 30% or more eventually develop evidence of neurological impairment.
- *Central nervous system disease* (50%). Onset 14 to 21 days. Encephalitis or a more disseminated disease. Mortality is 15%; 50–60% of survivors have psychomotor retardation, with or without microcephaly, spasticity, blindness, etc.
- *Disseminated disease* (20%). Onset 5 to 10 days. Involves any organ but primarily liver and adrenals; encephalitis in 70% or more. Presentation includes irritability, seizures, respiratory distress, jaundice, coagulopathy, shock and characteristic vesicular rash. *Note:* about 20% of babies never have skin lesions. Mortality is 50–60% (in spite of treatment), and neurological sequelae in 40%.

Diagnosis   Viral isolation from neonatal vesicular fluid, mouth or conjunctival swabs, stool, urine, leucocytes and maternal genital tract swabs. HSV antigen detection by immunofluorescence. Serology is not always helpful, as maternally acquired IgG confounds interpretation in the neonate, and IgM may not be produced until 2 weeks after the onset of illness. Detection of viral DNA by PCR. Changes on EEG, CT and MRI may all provide supporting evidence of HSV infection.

Complications   Overall mortality (following treatment) is 15–20%, and 40–50% of infants have some neurological impairment.

| Treatment | Aciclovir 10–20 mg/kg i.v. 8 hourly (see Antimicrobial guidelines). |
| Prevention | Twenty per cent of newborns will be infected even if delivered by Caesarean section. |

HSV encephalitis

See page 392 and Neurologic Conditions, chapter 29.

Human herpes virus 6 (HHV-6) (roseola infantum)

Ninety-five per cent of children are infected with HHV-6 by the age of 2 years. Up to 30% will present with the clinical features of roseola. HHV-7 has also been shown to be the cause in a small number of children. HHV-6 infection may also present as an acute febrile illness without a rash.

Transmission	Direct contact/droplet (asymptomatically shed)
Incubation period	9–10 days
Infectious period	Unknown (greatest during period of the rash)
Clinical features	Fever, occipital lymphadenopathy; then rapid defervescence corresponding with appearance of a red, maculopapular rash over trunk and arms for 1–2 days. *Note:* many children are started on antibiotics for the fever, and then misdiagnosed as having a drug reaction when the rash appears.
Diagnosis	Does not usually alter management, but serology may be performed.
Complications	Febrile convulsions (HHV-6 is thought to be the cause of up to one-third of febrile convulsions in children under 2 years of age), aseptic meningitis, encephalitis (rare), hepatitis.
Treatment	Symptomatic

Measles virus (rubeola)

As a result of widespread measles immunisation, this disease is now seen infrequently. However, outbreaks continue to occur in most parts of the world.

Cause	Measles virus (paramyxovirus)
Transmission	Droplet, direct contact
Incubation period	7–14 days (14 days to the appearance of a rash)

Infectious period	1–2 days before the onset of symptoms to 4 days after the onset of the rash.
Clinical features	*Prodrome*: fever, conjunctivitis, coryza, cough and Koplik's spots (white spots on a bright red buccal mucosa).
	Rash: appears 3–4 days later; erythematous and blotchy; starts at hairline and moves down the body, then becomes confluent; lasts 4–7 days; may desquamate in the second week.
Diagnosis	Serology (IgM is usually detectable 1–2 days after onset of rash), nasopharyngeal aspirate immunofluorescence and culture.
Complications	Otitis media (25%), pneumonia (4%), encephalitis (<0.1%), subacute sclerosing pan encephalitis (SSPE) (1/25 000).
Treatment	Symptomatic. Vitamin A should be considered for young infants with severe measles, the immunocompromised and those with vitamin A deficiency.
Control of case	Exclude from school for at least 5 days from the appearance of the rash.
Contacts	Measles, mumps, rubella (MMR) vaccine should be given within 72 h of exposure to unimmunised children over 6 months of age (needs to be repeated 3 months later for children under 12 months of age). If MMR is contraindicated, or if longer than 72 h since exposure, Normal Immunoglobulin should be given i.m. within 7 days. Exclude from school for 2 weeks if unimmunised.

Parvovirus B19
(erythema infectiosum, slapped cheek disease, fifth disease)

Cause	Parvovirus B19
Transmission	Droplet, direct contact
Incubation period	4–21 days
Infectious period	Highly infectious until rash appears (50% of adults are immune)

Clinical features	Fever in 15–30%; non-specific prodrome.
	The rash has three stages:

- Slapped cheek appearance (1–3 days)
- Maculopapular rash on proximal extensor surfaces, flexor surfaces and trunk; fades over next few days, central clearing, reticular pattern (after 7 days)
- Reticular rash reappears with heat, cold and friction (weeks/months).

Diagnosis	Mainly clinical. PCR on blood and serology.
Complications	Arthritis; aplastic crisis in children with chronic haemolytic anaemia (e.g. sickle cell disease); bone marrow suppression; foetal hydrops.
Treatment	Symptomatic (exclusion inappropriate).

Rubella

Transmission	Droplet, direct contact
Incubation period	14–21 days
Infectious period	5 days before to 7 days after rash
Clinical features	25–50% have no symptoms
	Prodrome: (1–5 days) low-grade fever, malaise, headache, coryza, conjunctivitis (more common in adults), postauricular/occipital/posterior triangle lymphadenopathy precedes rash by 5–10 days.
	Rash: small, fine, discrete pink maculopapules; starts on face, and spreads to chest and upper arms, abdomen and thighs, all within 24 h.
Diagnosis	Serology
Complications	Arthralgia/arthritis, encephalitis, thrombocytopenia, myocarditis.
	Congenital rubella syndrome: more than 25% during 1st trimester; 10–20% have single congenital defect if infection occurs at 16–40 days.
Control of case	Exclude from school for at least 5 days from the onset of the rash.

Contacts	Check serology if pregnant. Immunoglobulin given after exposure in early pregnancy may not prevent infection or viraemia, but may modify risk of abnormalities in the baby.

Varicella zoster virus (VZV) (chickenpox, shingles)

Incubation period	14–16 days (may be as short as 10 days or as long as 21 days). Shorter incubation in the immuno-compromised. Zoster Immune Globulin (ZIG) may prolong incubation to 28 days.
Infectious period	1–2 days before, and until the rash is fully crusted.
Clinical features	Fever, irritability, anorexia and lymphadenopathy The rash develops over the next 3–5 days

- Macular, papular, vesicular and crusted by 5–10 days
- Scalp, face, trunk, mouth, conjunctivae and extremities
- Central crops and itchy

Diagnosis	Immunofluorescence of vesicular scrapings for VZV antigen, or serology.
Complications	Secondary bacterial infection of skin lesions (most commonly *Streptococcus pyogenes* or *Staphylococcus aureus*); neurological (cerebellitis, transverse myelitis, Guillain–Barré syndrome); dissemination (pneumonitis, hepatitis, encephalitis) in patients with abnormal T-cell immunity. *Herpes zoster* ('shingles'), resulting from a reactivation of the latent virus, is more common in children who have had chickenpox in infancy or who have been exposed *in utero*.
Treatment	Aciclovir in patients with impaired T-cell immunity. Aciclovir is *not* indicated in the immunocompetent child. Antibiotics for secondary bacterial skin infection (e.g. flucloxacillin). Aspirin is *contraindicated* because of the association with Reye's syndrome.

Prevention	ZIG within 96 h of exposure (6 mL for adults, 4 mL for children 6–12 years of age, 2 mL for children up to 5 years of age) for the following patient groups in contact with varicella or shingles:

- Immunocompromised children (e.g. HIV, immunosuppressive therapy (including high-dose steroids; 2 mg/kg or more of prednisolone per day), and patients with transplants, lymphoma, leukaemia and severe combined immunodeficiency syndrome).
- Newborn infants whose mothers have varicella within the 5 days before, or 2 days after delivery.
- Hospitalised premature infants with no maternal history of varicella.
- Hospitalised premature infants under 28 weeks gestation or <1000 g, regardless of maternal history.

CENTRAL NERVOUS SYSTEM INFECTIONS

Bacterial meningitis

Bacterial meningitis is a medical emergency.

Clinical features

In infants, the presenting symptoms and signs are non-specific, and they may include only fever, lethargy, irritability or vomiting.

In older children, headache, vomiting, drowsiness, photophobia and neck stiffness may be present. Kernig's sign (inability to extend the knee when the leg is flexed at the hip) and Brudzinski's sign (bending the head forward produces flexion movements of the legs) may be positive.

Diagnosis

Diagnosis is confirmed by lumbar puncture (LP). However, when a child has a significantly depressed conscious state (see Fig. 1.2, Medical

Emergencies, chapter 1), demonstrates focal neurological signs, has had a recent (within 30 min) or prolonged (longer than 20 min) seizure, or has signs of raised intracranial pressure, the LP must be delayed because of the risk of coning. If the LP is deferred or reveals no organism, identification of the pathogen will rely on other methods. These include:

- Blood cultures, which are positive in a high proportion of cases.
- Rapid antigen tests: may be useful to determine the causative organism in a definite case of bacterial meningitis, but should not be used to diagnose or exclude meningitis where the cerebrospinal fluid (CSF) findings are equivocal. They are of limited value due to a high rate of false negative (when the bacterial load is low) and false positive (cross-reacting antigens) tests.
- PCR on blood or CSF for enterovirus and other viruses, TB and *N. meningitidis*.
- Blood smear for Gram stain.
- Skin scraping or aspirate from purpuric lesions, which may reveal meningococci on Gram stain or (less likely) culture.
- Throat swab: this is positive in up to 50% of cases of meningococcal meningitis, even up to 48 h after antibiotics have been started. It is useful in infants and young children in whom carriage rates are low, but not in teenagers and young adults in whom the asymptomatic carriage rate is up to 40%.
- Serology of paired samples for meningococcal outer membrane proteins (specialist centres only).

Antibiotics must be given immediately after the collection of appropriate cultures, but they should not be delayed if the LP is to be deferred. Antibiotics should be rationalised to more specific treatment based on CSF or blood culture results (but not on the basis of a Gram stain or PCR result alone).

Interpretation of cerebrospinal fluid findings

CSF findings should always be interpreted in the light of the clinical setting. In particular, the following should be noted (see Table 26.2):

- CSF microscopy should be performed without delay. Red and white cell lysis begins shortly after collection: neutrophils may decrease by up to one-third after 1 h and by one-half after 3 h (lymphocytes may decrease by about 10% after 2 h).

Table 26.2 Classical cerebrospinal fluid (CSF) findings

	Neutrophils (× 10⁶/L)	Lymphocytes (× 10⁶/L)	Protein (g/L)	Glucose (CSF : blood ratio)
Normal (>1 month of age)	0	≤5	<0.4	≥0.6 (or ≥2.5 mmol/L)
Normal term neonate	Higher than for older infant/child	<20–30	Higher than for older infant/child <1.7	Lower than for older infant/child
Bacterial meningitis	100–10 000 (may be normal)	Usually <100	>1.0 (may be normal)	<0.4 (may be normal)
Viral meningitis	Usually <100	10–1000 (may be normal)	0.4–1 (may be normal)	Usually normal
TB meningitis	Usually <100	50–1000 (may be normal)	1–5 (may be normal)	<0.3 (may be normal)
Encephalitis	Usually <100	<100	0.4–1 (may be normal)	Usually normal
Brain abscess	Usually 5–100		>1 (may be normal)	Usually normal

- Macroscopic appearance of CSF may be misleading: $200-500 \times 10^6$ /L cells are necessary for the CSF to be cloudy to the naked eye.
- In early bacterial meningitis there may be no increase in the CSF cell count.
- The CSF cell count may remain normal in up to 4% of younger infants and up to 17% of neonates with bacterial meningitis.
- The presence of neutrophils in the CSF should always raise concern (except in neonates, see Table 26.2).
- In early viral (typically enteroviral) meningitis, the CSF findings can mimic bacterial meningitis with a neutrophil predominance. This shifts to a lymphocytic picture after 6–8 h.
- In bacterial meningitis there can be a shift to a lymphocytic predominance after 48 h of therapy.
- Listeria infection is associated with a lower neutrophil rise than other causes of bacterial meningitis.
- CSF protein is normal in about 40% of school-age children with bacterial meningitis.
- CSF glucose is normal in about half of school-age children with bacterial meningitis.
- CSF glucose may be decreased in mumps meningitis and lymphocytic choriomeningitis, as well as in bacterial and TB meningitis.
- Gram stain may be negative in up to 60% of cases of bacterial meningitis even without prior antibiotics.
- If the CSF is contaminated with blood (14% of neonatal taps), a ratio of one white blood cell to 500 to 700 red blood cells is allowable, and 0.01 g/L protein for every 1000 red blood cells. However, it is safer to be more cautious and interpret the CSF as if it has *not* been contaminated with blood.
- Antibiotics usually prevent the culture of bacteria from the CSF, but they do not significantly alter the CSF cell count or biochemistry in samples taken early. In 'partially treated meningitis' the CSF should be interpreted like any other CSF.
- It is safer to assume that seizures do *not* cause an increased CSF cell count.
- The interpretation of CSF may be difficult in neonates. Normal values for CSF cell counts and biochemistry differ from those of older infants (typically higher cell count and protein, and lower glucose, particularly in premature neonates).

Antibiotic treatment of meningitis

Age greater than 2 months

The incidence of bacterial meningitis has fallen dramatically since the introduction of conjugated *Haemophilus influenzae* type b (Hib) vaccine. The major pathogens are now *Streptococcus pneumoniae* and *Neisseria meningitidis*. A third-generation cephalosporin is given as initial empiric therapy.

Penicillin (and cephalosporin) resistant pneumococci (PRP) are an increasing problem worldwide. The prevalence of invasive strains that are highly resistant to penicillins or cephalosporins in Melbourne is currently low. Cefotaxime remains the drug of first choice for the empiric treatment of meningitis at RCH. The prevalence of resistant strains is being monitored and this recommendation may change.

In areas with a significantly high incidence of PRP, vancomycin 15 mg/kg (max 500 mg) i.v. 6 hourly should be added to a third-generation cephalosporin as empiric therapy. When vancomycin is not used for the treatment of pneumococcal meningitis, a repeat LP should be performed to detect treatment failure if there is prolonged or secondary fever, or where sensitivity testing indicates the pneumococcal isolate has reduced susceptibility to penicillin.

Initial therapy

Cefotaxime 50 mg/kg (max 2 g) i.v. 6 hourly.

Continued therapy

Antibiotic treatment is adjusted according to the culture and sensitivity results to complete at least a 7–10 day course of therapy; e.g. benzylpenicillin 50 mg/kg (max 3 g) i.v. 4 hourly, amoxycillin 50 mg/kg (max 3 g) i.v. 4 hourly, or continue with cefotaxime (dose as above).

See Table 26.3 (p. 390) for prophylaxis regimens.

Age 1 to 2 months

The organisms responsible for meningitis in this age group can be either neonatal pathogens (e.g. group B streptococcus, *Escherichia coli* and *Listeria monocytogenes*), or those more commonly detected in older children (e.g. *Streptococcus pneumoniae*, *Neisseria meningitidis*, Hib).

Initial therapy

Benzylpenicillin 50 mg/kg (max 3 g) i.v. 4 hourly, cefotaxime 50 mg/kg (max 2 g) i.v. 6 hourly and gentamicin 2.5 mg/kg (max 80 mg) i.v. 8 hourly (see Antibiotic guidelines).

Continued therapy

Treatment is adjusted according to the culture and sensitivity results. Gentamicin is used for its synergistic action with penicillin for the treatment of group B streptococcal and Listeria meningitis. Therapy is continued for 2–3 weeks for these two infections, and for at least 3 weeks in Gram-negative coliform meningitis.

See Table 26.3 (p. 390) for prophylaxis regimens.

Neonatal meningitis

See Neonatal sepsis, Neonatal Paediatrics, chapter 28.

Meningitis associated with shunts, neurosurgery, head trauma and CSF leak

In addition to the organisms discussed above, meningitis in these circumstances can be caused by *Staphylococcus aureus*, *Staphylococcus epidermidis* and Gram-negative bacilli including *Pseudomonas aeruginosa*.

Initial therapy

Vancomycin 15 mg/kg (max 500 mg) i.v. 6 hourly and ceftazidime 50 mg/kg (max 2 g) i.v. 8 hourly.

General measures

After any fluid resuscitation for shock, fluid restriction is an important theoretical principle of management because of the risk of the syndrome of inappropriate antidiuretic hormone secretion (SIADH). A patient who is not in shock, and whose serum sodium is within the normal range, is given 50% of maintenance fluid requirements as initial management. If the patient is hyponatraemic, restrict fluids to insensible losses plus urine output to a maximum of 50% of maintenance requirements. This is approximately 10 mL/kg of fluid per day. Fluid administration is subsequently adjusted according to the clinical status and serum sodium concentration.

Table 26.3 Prophylaxis regimens for contact of meningitis cases

Organism	Antibiotic	Those requiring prophylaxis
Haemophilus influenzae type b	Rifampicin 20 mg/kg (max 600 mg) p.o. daily for 4 days Infants <1 month of age: Rifampicin 10 mg/kg p.o. daily for 4 days Pregnancy/contraindication to rifampicin: Ceftriaxone 250 mg i.m. daily for 2 days	• Index case and all household contacts if household includes other children <4 years of age who are not fully immunised. • Index case and all household contacts in households with any infants <12 months of age, regardless of immunisation status. • Index case and all household contacts in households with a child 1–5 years of age who is inadequately immunised. • Index case and all room contacts, including staff, in a child care group if index case attends >18 h/week and any contacts <2 years of age who are inadequately immunised. • Children who are not up to date with Hib should be immunised.
Neisseria meningitidis	Rifampicin 10 mg/kg (max 600 mg) p.o. 12 hourly for 2 days Infants <1 month of age: Rifampicin 5 mg/kg p.o. 12 hourly for 2 days Pregnancy/contraindication to rifampicin: Ceftriaxone 250 mg i.m. as a single dose or Ciprofloxacin 500 mg p.o. as a single dose	• Index case (if treated only with penicillin) and all intimate household or day care contacts who have been exposed to index case within 10 days of onset. • Any person who gave mouth-to-mouth resuscitation to the index case.
Streptococcus pneumoniae	Nil	• No increased risk to contacts

Notes:
- It is important that Rifampicin is given early to both the index case and contacts, especially for *N. meningitidis* disease, because of the rapidity with which secondary cases may develop.
- As prophylaxis is not infallible, any febrile household contact should seek urgent medical attention.
- Nasopharyngeal carriage of Hib is not eradicated by a single injection of ceftriaxone.
- Rifampicin interferes with the metabolism of several medications, including the oral contraceptive pill (alternative contraception

The control of seizures is vital. Careful attention is paid to the child's respiratory rate, both before the selection and following the use of an anticonvulsant.

Early consultation with an intensive care unit is necessary for any child who is under 2 years of age or who is experiencing deterioration in his or her conscious state, haemodynamic instability or seizures.

Fever persisting for more than 7 days or a secondary fever commonly results from nosocomial infections (usually viral), subdural effusions, other suppurative lesions or immune-mediated disease (accompanied by arthritis, rash and haematuria). Uncommonly, fever may also arise from inadequately treated meningitis (see PRP, above), a parameningeal focus or drugs. Management, including a repeat LP, must be individualised.

Although widely practised, routine administration of dexamethasone is controversial and is not routinely recommended at RCH. Studies using dexamethasone have drawn criticism, and benefits have only been proven in Hib meningitis. Since the introduction of immunisation, Hib meningitis has become very uncommon.

All patients require a hearing assessment 6–8 weeks after discharge, or sooner if hearing loss is suspected.

More than one in four survivors have mild disabilities that adversely affect school performance and behaviour. Consequently, all children surviving bacterial meningitis should be regularly reviewed during their early school years.

Viral meningitis

The most common causes of viral meningitis or meningoencephalitis are enteroviruses (Coxsackie and echoviruses) and HHV-6 (see p. 380). Most cases are self-limiting and their importance lies in the fact that their clinical presentation can mimic bacterial meningitis. Enterovirus may be isolated from throat swabs and stools, and PCR of the CSF may be positive. Treatment is symptomatic except in the rare instance of infection in the immunocompromised where IVIG may be used.

TB meningitis

TB meningitis is uncommon in Australia. It often presents in an insidious manner and can be difficult to recognise. Large volumes of

CSF are required (at least 10 mL) for diagnosis by isolation and culture of mycobacteria and/or PCR. Treatment with multiple antituberculous antibiotics should be started early and requires specialist advice. Steroids may also play an important role in treatment.

Encephalitis

Encephalitis is most commonly caused by HSV-1 and 2, EBV, varicella zoster virus, enterovirus, adenovirus, influenza virus and *Mycoplasma pneumoniae*. Encephalitis usually presents with one or more of the following: fever, headache, vomiting, change of behaviour, drowsiness, convulsions, focal neurological deficits and signs of raised intracranial pressure. CSF findings are non-specific (see Table 26.2). CT or MRI of the brain and EEG may be more helpful.

The recognition of herpes encephalitis is critical because treatment with aciclovir is indicated. Focal seizures and neurological signs are more typical of herpes encephalitis but clinical presentation, especially early in the disease, is not specific to any aetiological agent. Therefore, any child with encephalitis of uncertain aetiology should be started on i.v. aciclovir (see Antimicrobial guidelines). If the patient does not regain consciousness over a short period of time, i.v. aciclovir should be continued until:

- An alternative diagnosis is reached; or
- Herpes encephalitis is excluded by:
  - Absence of typical clinical features
  - Normal serial CT or MRI scans
  - Normal serial EEG
  - Negative CSF PCR for HSV.

Brain abscess

Brain abscess classically presents with fever, headache and focal neurological deficit. Although rare, early recognition is important because most cases are readily treated and delayed diagnosis can be disastrous. Diagnosis is by brain CT or MRI. Empiric treatment to cover the major aetiological pathogens is flucloxacillin 50 mg/kg (max 2 g) i.v. 4 hourly, cefotaxime 50 mg/kg (max 2 g) i.v. 6 hourly *and* metronidazole 15 mg/kg (max 1 g) i.v. stat, then 7.5 mg/kg (max 500 mg) i.v. 8 hourly (see Antimicrobial guidelines). Aspiration for diagnosis and neurosurgical intervention are sometimes necessary.

GASTROENTEROLOGY

See also Gastrointestinal Conditions, chapter 23.

Infectious diarrhoea

- Infectious diarrhoea continues to cause significant morbidity in children in developed and developing countries.
- In Australia, approximately 20 000 children (15/1000) under 5 years of age are admitted to hospital each year with acute gastroenteritis.
- Rotavirus is the aetiological agent in up to two-thirds of children in whom a pathogen is identified.
- Other important pathogens in children hospitalised with diarrhoea include:
  - Enteric adenovirus (10%)
  - *Salmonella* spp. (10%)
  - *Campylobacter jejuni* (6%)
  - *Giardia lamblia* (<1%)
  - Astroviruses and caliciviruses (<1%)
  - *Cryptosporidium parvum* (<1%)
  - Enteropathogenic (and other) *Escherichia coli* (<1%)
  - *Shigella* spp. (<1%)
  - *Yersinia enterocolitica* (<1%)
- There are several other diarrhoeal pathogens that occur less frequently.
- Children under 5 years of age with rotavirus-positive gastro-enteritis are unlikely to have another pathogen isolated from their faeces.
- It is unusual to find a protozoal parasite in the setting of acute diarrhoea.
- Repeat stool investigations are not helpful except in patients with chronic diarrhoea, suspected *Salmonella* carriage or parasitic infection.
- The cause of infectious diarrhoea can often be identified by simple laboratory studies but rarely alters management.

- Most bacterial causes of diarrhoea are self-limiting and do not usually require antibiotic therapy. The primary aim of treatment, as with viral gastroenteritis, is to achieve and maintain adequate hydration.
- Nosocomial infection is common. The prevention of its spread by adequate infection control measures is an essential component of hospital management.

Specific pathogens

Rotavirus

- Major cause of severe diarrhoea in children.
- Causes over 50% of hospitalisations for acute gastroenteritis in children under 5 years of age.
- Annual peak of infection and illness occurs in the winter–spring period.
- Common cause of nosocomial infection.
- Illness usually begins 12 h to 4 days after exposure, and lasts up to 1 week.
- Presents with diarrhoea, vomiting (may precede diarrhoea) and fever. Respiratory symptoms are common.
- May be complicated by dehydration, electrolyte imbalance and acidosis.
- Most children shed the virus in stools for up to 10 days. However, about one-third with severe primary rotavirus infection may continue to excrete rotavirus for >21 days.
- Diagnosed by enzyme immunoassay and latex agglutination assay.
- Treatment is supportive with particular attention to hydration.
- An oral tetravalent rhesus-human reassortant vaccine has been shown to have protective efficacy in large-scale clinical trials. A possible association with intussusception recently resulted in the withdrawal of the vaccine in the United States.

Adenovirus

Similar presentation to rotavirus, but there is no seasonality. It is more common under 12 months of age. Diarrhoea and vomiting may last longer, and high fever is less common.

Salmonella (non typhi)

- Causes a broad spectrum of clinical syndromes, including asymptomatic carriage, gastroenteritis, bacteraemia, enteric (typhoid) fever and focal infections (e.g. bone and joint).
- Age-specific attack rates are highest in children under 5 years of age (it peaks at under 1 year of age) and the elderly.
- Invasive infections and mortality are more common in infants, the elderly and those with underlying diseases.
- Faecal excretion of *Salmonella* persists longer in younger children.
- Antibiotic treatment is not usually indicated for uncomplicated gastroenteritis, and may prolong excretion.
- Antibiotic treatment is indicated for: bacteraemia, systemic involvement, or infection in infants under 3 months of age; those with underlying disease (e.g. immunocompromise) and the elderly. The choice and duration of treatment depends on the clinical manifestation and antibiotic susceptibility.

Campylobacter jejuni

- More common over 5 years of age.
- Causes diarrhoea with visible or occult blood, abdominal pain, malaise and fever.
- Antibiotic treatment is not usually necessary, except in special circumstances where the elimination of the carrier state is important, such as infection in food handlers.

Giardia lamblia

- The most common parasite identified in stool specimens from children.
- Transmission is more common in children (and staff) in childcare centres and returned travellers.
- The major reservoir and means of spread is contaminated water and, to a lesser extent, food. Person-to-person spread also occurs.
- Asymptomatic carriage is common.
- There is a broad spectrum of clinical manifestations, but the most common are:

- — Diarrhoea (usually persistent)
- — Abdominal distension
- — Flatulence
- — Abdominal cramps
- — Weight loss/failure to thrive (FTT).
- Diagnosis is confirmed by microscopy of stool specimens. These do not usually contain blood, mucus or leucocytes. Repeat specimens may be necessary.
- Metronidazole 30 mg/kg (max 2 g) p.o. daily for 3 days *or* tinidazole 50 mg/kg (max 2 g) p.o. as a single dose are effective treatments for symptomatic giardiasis.

Dientamoeba fragilis

- This parasite is thought to be transmitted with the eggs of *Enterobius vermicularis* (pinworm).
- Symptoms include acute or chronic diarrhoea and abdominal pain, although many infected children are asymptomatic.
- May be associated with eosinophilia.
- May be treated with metronidazole (dose as above).

Escherichia coli

There are at least five categories of diarrhoea-producing *E. coli*:

- *Enterohaemorrhagic E. coli* (EHEC): haemolytic uraemic syndrome (HUS) haemorrhagic colitis.
- *Enteropathogenic E. coli* (EPEC): watery diarrhoea in children less than 2 years of age in developing countries.
- *Enterotoxigenic E. coli* (ETEC): the major cause of traveller's diarrhoea (usually self-limiting).
- *Enteroinvasive E. coli* (EIEC): usually watery diarrhoea, but may cause dysentery.
- *Enteroaggregative E. coli* (EAEC): chronic diarrhoea in infants and young children.

Antibiotic treatment is not usually indicated for diarrhoea caused by *E. coli*, and is associated with a worse outcome in HUS.

Clostridium difficile

- Acquired from the environment or by faecal–oral transmission from a colonised host.

- Up to 50% of healthy neonates and infants under 2 years of age are colonised, in contrast to 5% of those over 2 years of age.
- Pseudomembranous colitis usually occurs in patients on antibiotics (particularly penicillins, clindamycin and cephalosporins).
- *Clostridium difficile* organisms and toxins are often present in the stool of asymptomatic infants.
- Rare cause of diarrhoea in those under 12 months of age.
- Only clinically significant diarrhoea or colitis should be considered to be caused by *Clostridium difficile*.
- Management includes the cessation of antibiotics and the use of *oral* metronidazole 7.5 mg/kg (max 400 mg) p.o. 8 hourly; (vancomycin should be avoided to decrease the emergence of resistance).

Enterobius vermicularis (threadworm, pinworm)

- The most common worm infection in Australia. School-age children, followed by preschoolers, have the highest rates of infection. In some groups, nearly 50% of children are infected.
- Causes pruritus ani and vulvae.
- Infection often occurs in more than one family member.
- Incubation period is at least 1 to 2 months from the ingestion of eggs until the adult female migrates to the perianal region to deposit eggs.
- Eggs are infective within a few hours of being deposited on the perianal skin.
- Eggs survive up to 2 weeks on clothing, bedding or other objects.
- Eggs often remain under the fingernails. Reinfection by auto-infection is common.
- Diagnosis is by visualisation of worms in the perianal region (at night) or microscopy of eggs collected on sticky tape briefly applied to the perianal skin in the morning.
- Treat with mebendazole 50 mg (<10 kg), 100 mg (>10 kg) p.o. (not in pregnancy or in those under 6 months of age) or pyrantel 10 mg/kg (max 500 mg) p.o. as a single dose, followed by a second dose 2 weeks later. All family members should be treated.

Hepatitis

Hepatitis A (HAV)

This is the most common viral hepatitis; it is particularly prevalent in children.

Transmission	Faecal–oral route
Incubation period	Usually about 4 weeks (2–7 weeks)
Infectious period	Viral shedding lasts 1–3 weeks; the highest titres in stool occur 1–2 weeks before the onset of illness, corresponding to the highest risk of transmission; lowest risk after onset of jaundice.
Clinical features	Usually an acute self-limited illness; mild, non-specific symptoms without jaundice in infants and preschoolers; fever, malaise, jaundice, anorexia and nausea in older children and adults.
Complications	Relapse (unusual), fulminant hepatitis (rare)
Diagnosis	Serology for HAV-specific IgM and IgG
Treatment	Supportive.
Control of case	Cases should be excluded from child-care or school for 7 days from the onset of illness.
Prevention	Inactivated HAV vaccine (or immunoglobulin for short-term protection) should be considered for travellers to endemic areas, those with high-occupational risk, and those with chronic liver disease (e.g. hepatitis B infection) or haemophilia.

Hepatitis B (HBV)

HBV infection is endemic worldwide. The prevalence of HBV and carriage rates vary in different parts of the world. In Australia, the carriage rate in Caucasians is about 0.2%, while that in some Aboriginal populations is over 10%.

Transmission	Blood or body fluids that are HBsAg positive; vertical transmission occurs in infants born to HBsAg-positive mothers; there is a high risk of horizontal transmission in the first 5 years of life.
Incubation period	7 weeks to 6 months

Infectious period	From several weeks before the onset until the end of the period of acute illness.
Clinical features	Symptomatic acute hepatitis (jaundice, anorexia, malaise and nausea) in adults; usually asymptomatic in young children, particularly in those under 1 year of age.
Complications	Twenty-five per cent of chronic carriers die later in life of primary liver cancer or chronic liver disease. Those infected as infants or young children are more likely to become carriers and to develop fatal complications as adults: 70–90% of infants infected at birth become chronic HBV carriers (particularly if the mother is HBeAg positive), in contrast to only 5% of adults. The remainder eliminate the virus and have no long-term effects.
Diagnosis	Serology for detection of HBsAg, HBeAg (also anti-HBsAb, anti-HBcAb, anti-HBeAb).
Treatment	No specific therapy for HBV is available; alpha-interferon and nucleoside analogues may resolve chronic infection but are less effective if infection is acquired during childhood. HAV vaccination is recommended.
Prevention	In Australia, recombinant HBV vaccine is currently recommended for all pre-adolescents, as well as those at high risk; universal infant vaccination is likely to be introduced shortly; infants born to HBsAg-positive mothers and individuals exposed to HBsAg-positive blood or body fluids should be given HBV-specific immunoglobulin plus HBV vaccination. See needle stick injuries (p. 402).

Hepatitis C (HCV)

HCV causes at least 95% of cases of acute and chronic hepatitis that were previously classified as non-A, non-B. The carriage rate is about 0.3% in apparently healthy new blood donors in Australia. However, this probably underestimates the prevalence in the population, which may be around 1%.

Transmission	Parenteral exposure to HCV-infected blood and blood products; vertical transmission occurs from about 6% of HCV-positive mothers (higher if the mother is co-infected with HIV); breast-feeding is not believed to be a major route of transmission; sexual transmission is uncommon.
Incubation period	6–7 weeks (range 2 weeks to 6 months)
Clinical features	Mild, insidious hepatitis; usually asymptomatic in children.
Complications	Persistent infection in >85% (most children with chronic infection are asymptomatic); 65–70% develop chronic hepatitis, 20% develop cirrhosis. HCV appears to have a role in primary liver cancer.
Diagnosis	Detection of anti-HCV antibodies using ELISA and/or recombinant immunoblot assay, PCR for HCV RNA.
Treatment	Patients must be monitored regularly (examination and liver function tests) for carriage and development of chronic liver disease. Optimal treatment regimens using alpha-interferon, ribaviran and other antivirals are under investigation. HAV and HBV vaccination is recommended.

HIV INFECTION AND AIDS

Cause	Acquired immunodeficiency syndrome (AIDS) is caused by human immunodeficiency virus (HIV).
Transmission	Perinatal (vertical) transmission is the most common means of paediatric HIV infection.
Incubation period	It is important to distinguish between infection with HIV, which may be asymptomatic during a variable latent period, and the progressive immunological derangement which leads to AIDS. Perinatally infected infants may be asymptomatic for several months or years.

Risk groups
- Infants of mothers who are known to be HIV positive or who are members of a high-risk group (e.g. sex workers, intravenous drug users and those with bisexual partners).
- Intravenous drug users.
- Homosexual or bisexual males.
- Sexual contacts (including sexually abused children) of individuals with HIV.
- Transfusion recipients, particularly patients with congenital bleeding disorders who received blood products before 1985.
- Individuals from countries with a particularly high prevalence of HIV infection.

Clinical features
Clinical presentations of HIV infection include: prolonged fever; failure to thrive or weight loss; generalised lymphadenopathy; hepatosplenomegaly; parotitis; chronic or recurrent diarrhoea; recurrent otitis; chronic candidiasis; chronic eczematous rash.

The indicator diseases for the diagnosis of AIDS in children include candidiasis, lymphoid interstitial pneumonitis, recurrent episodes of serious bacterial infection, opportunistic infection (e.g. *Pneumocystis carinii* pneumonia and disseminated *Mycobacterium avium* complex disease), CMV retinitis, cerebral toxoplasmosis, progressive neurological disease and malignancy (e.g. primary brain lymphoma).

Diagnosis
Patients require counselling and informed consent before testing for HIV, which should be performed on a confidential basis. Specific antibody detection is a sensitive indicator of HIV infection in adults and children, but passively transferred maternal antibody may persist for up to 18 months in infants. The presence of free viral protein (p24 antigen), a positive viral culture or PCR assay of non-cord blood, help confirm the diagnosis of HIV infection. The disease is

monitored using a combination of CD4+ T-cell count and quantification of HIV RNA (viral load). Patients may also have lymphopenia, abnormal T-cell subsets and hypergammaglobulinaemia.

Management

A multidisciplinary approach by a specialised team is vital for the unique needs of these patients and their families. Medical management of HIV-positive patients includes:

- Antiretroviral drugs (highly active antiretroviral treatment, HAART)
- Prevention of opportunistic and other infections (immunisation and prophylactic antimicrobials)
- The early diagnosis and aggressive management of opportunistic infections.

Control

Antiretroviral therapy given to the HIV-infected woman during pregnancy and delivery, and to the newborn, together with other measures, can decrease the rate of transmission to the child from 25–35% to <2%. Recognition of HIV-infected pregnant women is therefore critical.

Antiviral therapy and other interventions (e.g. immunisation, PCP prophylaxis) can have a significant impact on disease progression.

HIV can be transmitted in breast milk: wherever artificial feeding can be undertaken safely it is advised that HIV-infected women should not breast-feed.

NEEDLE STICK INJURIES (NSI)

Standard precautions

- All sharp objects and body fluids should be considered as potentially contaminated.
- Avoid contact with blood and other body fluids by:
  — Using protective barriers (e.g. gloves) if contact is likely
  — Immediately cleaning up accidental spills.

Table 26.4 Evaluation of needle stick injury sources

High risk of HIV and HBV	High risk of HCV
• Unsafe sex, particularly with multiple (or homosexual) partners • Intravenous drug users (IVDU) (particularly if they share equipment) and their sexual partners • Family members of an infected person • Individuals from communities with high HIV prevalence	• Recipients of blood products prior to 1985 • IVDU (particularly if they share equipment) and their sexual partners

Managing NSI or exposure to blood/blood-stained body fluid

- Squeeze the puncture wound.
- Wash blood off the skin with soap and water.
- Rinse blood from the eyes and mouth with running water.
- Document the date and time of exposure, details of incident, names of the source and exposed individuals.
- Inform source individual of exposure.
- Assess the risk of HIV, HBV and HCV in the source individual.
- Obtain consent for serological testing for HIV-1 and 2, hepatitis B and hepatitis C antibodies in the source and exposed individuals.
- Give HBV-specific immunoglobulin +/– HBV vaccine if appropriate (see Table 26.4).
- Consider HIV post-exposure prophylaxis.
- Arrange follow up.

Assessing risk

A significant exposure is considered to have occurred if there has been:

- An injection of blood/body fluid (particularly if >1 mL).
- A skin penetrating injury with a sharp that is contaminated with blood/body fluid.
- A laceration from a contaminated instrument.
- A direct inoculation in the laboratory with contaminated material.
- A contaminated wound or skin lesion.
- Mucous membrane/conjunctival contact with blood/body fluid.

The estimated risk of virus transmission from a *significant* NSI at the Royal Children's Hospital is:

- HBV-positive source: ~30%
- HCV-positive source: ~3%
- HIV-positive source: ~0.3%.

Note: these figures are for NSI from a positive source. When the source is unknown, the actual risk of infection for the affected individual depends on the probability of infection in the source population.

Table 26.5 Management of needle stick injury

Exposure	Virus	Bloods to take from the affected individual	Bloods to take from the source individual	What to give the affected individual
High-risk	Hepatitis B	Anti-HBsAb (within 48 h)	HBsAg (within 48 h)	*HBV immune:* Nil *HBV non-immune:* • Source HBsAg positive/unknown ⇒ HBV immunoglobulin (*within 48 h*)* + HBV vaccine • Source HBsAg negative ⇒ HBV vaccine
	Hepatitis C	ALT + hold serum	Anti-HCV Ab	Nil
	HIV	Hold serum	Anti-HIV I & 2 Abs	HIV prophylaxis† if HIV positive and/or risk of transmission is significant
Low-risk	All viruses	Anti-HBsAb (if unsure of immunity) Hold serum	HBsAg	*HBV immune:* Nil *HBV non-immune:* HBV vaccine

* HBV immunoglobulin should be given as soon as possible, but can be deferred for 48 h, while awaiting results of serology to confirm affected individual's immunity (when checking whether a vaccinated individual has maintained immunity or whether the individual is immune from previous infection).

† Current HIV prophylaxis is zidovudine, lamivudine and indinavir (this may change with ongoing developments in antiviral drugs). The treatment should be started promptly, preferably within 1–2 h of the exposure.

CHAPTER 27

METABOLIC CONDITIONS

Avihu Boneh
Stephen G. Kahler

Metabolic diseases, although generally rare individually, in aggregate are an important cause of illness in Western society. Some newborns admitted with a clinical presentation of 'neonatal septicaemia' will eventually be found to have an inborn error of metabolism. *A high index of suspicion is the primary rule in the diagnostic approach to metabolic disorders.* The presenting symptoms of metabolic diseases are non-specific (see Table 27.1).

A careful history regarding the pregnancy, delivery, neonatal period, food refusal or craving, and motor and cognitive development should be recorded. A review of the systems, including a record of medications given to the child, may be very helpful and should be done for every patient.

The family history should be recorded. Consanguinity should be noted. Relatives with seemingly unrelated disorders (e.g. 'retardation') may, in fact, have the same disorder as the patient. The signs of maternal morbidity during pregnancy (e.g. severe chronic vomiting, liver disease and intercurrent infections) should be recorded. Miscarriages, unexplained deaths of newborns and Sudden Infant Death Syndrome (SIDS), as well as other children having similar clinical signs in the family, should be noted as they may contribute to a diagnosis.

PHYSICAL EXAMINATION

Some findings on physical examination may be suggestive of a metabolic disease. These are summarised in Table 27.2.

Table 27.1 Clinical signs suggestive of a metabolic disease

Age	Clinical signs	Possible diagnosis
Day 1 of life	Seizures	Persistent – hyperinsulinaemia Mitochondrial – cytopathy Disorders of purines and pyrimidines
Neonatal period(*)	Vomiting, feed refusal, changes in respiration, prolonged jaundice, lethargy or irritability, movement disorder, seizures, hypo/hypertonia, changes in the level of consciousness	Organic acidaemias, non-ketotic-hyperglycinaemia Urea cycle defects Fatty acid oxidation defects Tyrosinaemia Galactosaemia Mitochondrial – cytopathy Disorders of purines and pyrimidines
1st year of life	Same as above, motor/cognitive developmental delay or regression	Organic acidaemias Urea cycle defects Fatty acid oxidation defects Lysosomal storage diseases
Early childhood	Mental retardation, seizures, behavioural abnormalities, learning difficulties, autistic features	Organic acidaemias Urea cycle defects Fatty acid oxidation defects Amino-acidopathies Lysosomal storage diseases adrenoleukodystrophy
Any age group(**)	Acute decompensation: change in consciousness, seizures, movement disorder, change in respiration	Organic acidaemias Urea cycle defects Fatty acid oxidation defects Adrenal insufficiency

* Symptoms should be considered in relation to the child's age (in days), fasting, food intake (i.e. specific sugars, protein and fat) and changes in diet.
** May follow an intercurrent infection, prolonged fasting, a large meal with high protein content, and so on.

Table 27.2 Physical examination: signs of metabolic disease

General appearance	Growth parameters: height and weight
	Dysmorphism
Skin	Rash
	Odour
	Hyperkeratosis
	Signs of chronic scratching
Head and neck	Craniomegaly
	Dysmorphism
	Bulging fontanelle
	Signs of rickets
	Abnormal eye movement
Chest	Signs of lung disease
Heart	Cardiomegaly
	Signs of cardiac failure
Abdomen	Hepato ± splenomegaly
	Signs of liver disease
Genitalia	Ambiguous genitalia
Skeleton	Signs of rickets
	Bone or joint pain, contractures
	Abnormal spine posturing/vertebral disease
Muscles	Muscle mass, wasting
Neurological	Muscle strength, tone
	Sensation
	Reflexes (tendon and primitive)
	Movement disorders
	Ataxia

LABORATORY INVESTIGATIONS

Blood, urine and CSF samples collected at the time of presentation may be diagnostic and are invaluable. Always attempt to collect these samples *before* commencing treatment, but do not delay treatment in crisis situations.

There are four initial questions to be answered:
- Is there acidosis and is it of metabolic origin?
- Is there hypoglycaemia?
- Is there hyper- or hypo-ketonaemia?
- Is there hyperammonaemia?

The following tests (see Table 27.3) should be done to answer these questions.

Table 27.3 Investigation of suspected metabolic disease

	First-line tests	Second-line tests*
Blood	Acid–base (arterial or capillary) Electrolytes Glucose (in 'lactate tube'; see below) Ammonia Lactate (1 mL blood in yellow lactate tube, place on ice.) Acylcarnitines (blood spots on a Guthrie ('PKU') Card)	Complete blood count Plasma amino acids (place on ice) Pyruvate (place on ice) FA/Ketones (specify: beta-hydroxy butyrate *and* acetoacetate) (place on ice) Liver transaminases Urea, creatinine, calcium, phosphate Uric acid Cholesterol Freeze additional plasma for further testing
Urine	pH, glucose, ketones, protein Reducing substances Organic acids (keep frozen if not analysed immediately)	Freeze additional urine for further testing
CSF	Glucose, protein, lactate	Freeze additional CSF for further testing (amino acids, neurotransmitters, etc.)

* Check with the laboratory for the preferred sample.

See Table 27.4 for interpretation of laboratory results.

In addition to these tests, brain CT or MRI and abdominal ultrasonographic examination may be helpful in the diagnostic process.

TREATMENT

There are three basic guidelines in the treatment of metabolic conditions:
- Enhance the disposal of the accumulating toxic metabolites. Adequate fluid intake is important, particularly as many of the toxic metabolites are excreted by the kidney. Correct dehydration and replace ongoing losses (diarrhoea, fever, etc).

  Haemofiltration should be considered in severe cases or when there are indications of rapid accumulation of toxic metabolites

Table 27.4 Interpretation of laboratory results

Metabolic condition	pH	Glucose	Ketones	Ammonia
Urea cycle defects	Normal or ↑	Normal	Normal	↑↑
Organic acidaemias	↓	↑, Normal or ↓	Normal or ↑	↑
Ketolysis defects	Normal or ↓	Normal or ↑	↑↑	Normal
FA oxidation defects	Normal or ↓	Normal or ↓	Normal or ↓	Normal or ↑
Hyperinsulinaemia	Normal	↓↓	Normal	Normal or ↑

(rapid deterioration in the level of consciousness, increasing intracranial pressure, etc.).

- Avoid catabolism, which might lead to an ongoing accumulation of these metabolites.

  It is of the utmost importance to provide the patient with an adequate amount of calories for age and weight. Intravenous glucose infusion (10–20% solution) is usually a safe mode of treatment. Intravenous fat solutions (Intralipid, 10 or 20% solutions) may serve as a good source of calories in a small fluid volume. Do not use intravenous fat solutions if you suspect a fatty acid oxidation disorder. Intravenous amino acids can usually be given at a low dose (e.g. 0.5 gm/kg per day for a newborn) to enhance anabolism, unless there is hyperammonaemia.

- Enhance enzymatic activity, whenever possible.

  Treatment with some vitamins and co-factors may be indicated to enhance the disposal of toxic metabolites or to enhance residual enzymatic activity. These are listed in Table 27.5.

URGENT AUTOPSY FOR SUSPECTED METABOLIC DISEASE

Collect samples as soon as possible after death, preferably within 2 h. Note the time between death and freezing or the attainment of the samples. Tissue samples should be no larger than 1.0 cm cubes; heart, kidney and brain samples may also be collected.

Muscle samples are preferably from the quadriceps. If the parents object to the two incisions (the muscle and liver), suggest a right upper quadrant incision to take samples from the liver, rectus muscle and skin biopsy.

Skeletal muscle

(i) Two × 0.5 cm cubes – wrap in aluminium foil, place in a small screw-cap tube and completely cover with *dry ice. Store in a freezer at –70°C.*

(ii) One piece in a glutaraldehyde bottle for EM. Store in a refrigerator at 4°C. *Do not freeze this sample.*

Table 27.5 Vitamin treatments

Compound	Dose (mg/day)	Indication
Carnitine	100–400 mg/kg per day (oral)	Organic acidaemias
	15–60 mg/kg per day (i.v.)	Fatty acid oxidation disorders
Thiamine (B_1)	100 mg/kg per day (i.v. or oral)	MSUD, PDH deficiency MRC disorders
Riboflavin (B_2)	50–400 mg/day	Glutaric acidurias MRC disorders
Pyridoxine (B_6)	100–200 mg/day (i.v. or oral)	Homocystinuria Seizures
Cobalamin (B_{12})	1 mg/day as hydroxycobalamin (i.m.)	Homocystinuria and MMA, combined or separately
Biotin	10–20 mg/day (i.v. or oral)	Hyper-lactataemia Biotinidase deficiency Holocarboxylase synthetase deficiency
Vitamin C	500 mg/day or 100 mg/kg per day (oral)	MRC disorders Organic acidaemias
Vitamin K (menadione)	10 mg/kg per day (oral) or 1 mg/kg per day i.m.	MRC disorders
Coenzyme Q	50–200 mg/day	MRC disorders
Folic acid	5 mg/day	MRC disorders with anaemia Some amino-acidopathies
Glycine	200 mg/kg per day	May be given in some cases instead of carnitine

PDH, pyruvate dehydrogenase.
MRC, mitochondrial respiratory chain.
MMA, methylamlonic aciduria.
MSUD, maple syrup urine disease.

Liver

(i)   *Two cores* from a 14 French gauge cannula or, if open biopsy, 2 × 0.5 cm cubes – wrap in Alfoil, place in a small screw-cap tube and completely cover in *dry ice*. Store in a freezer at –70°C.

(ii) One piece in glutaraldehyde bottle for EM. Store in a refrigerator at 4°C. *Do not freeze this sample.*

Skin fibroblasts

One piece full thickness (2–3 mm surface diameter) in a tissue culture medium bottle, or a viral medium bottle or sterile normal saline without preservatives. Store in a refrigerator at 4°C.

Do not freeze this sample.

Blood (for DNA tests)

Ten millilitres of heparinised blood (no mixing beads or separating gel) can be sent at room temperature if they are expected in the laboratory within 24 h, or frozen.

In addition to these samples, obtain blood, urine, CSF and bile samples, if possible (see Table 27.3), for further metabolic analysis. A vitreous humor specimen should be obtained if urine is unavailable. Organ biopsies for light microscopy should be placed in aluminium foil or parafilm, frozen immediately (on dry ice) and put in screw-cap tubes. Note the time of sampling.

CHAPTER 28
NEONATAL PAEDIATRICS

Peter McDougall
Lex Doyle
Colin Morley
Barbara Burge

This chapter on the newborn infant describes routine care and the variations from normal, common minor and major problems, and uncommon, but life-threatening problems. Feeding and intravenous nutrition; surgical; cardiac; ophthalmological; and metabolic problems, procedures and emergencies are covered in other chapters of this handbook. No attempt is made to cover intensive care for the newborn. Sections on postnatal depression, mastitis and some of the problems of the ex-very low birthweight infant are included.

ROUTINE CARE

Most aspects of routine care vary with the age of the baby.

The first minutes

The baby must start breathing. The major stimuli for this are hypoxia, acidosis and sensory bombardment from touch and temperature. The foetal circulation (<10% of cardiac output going to the lungs) changes to the adult-type circulation (with 100% of cardiac output going to the lungs) following a reduction in pulmonary artery pressure with aeration of the lungs.

- *Establishing breathing.* The Apgar score has been used to describe the infant's condition at 1 and 5 min after birth. Breathing, heart rate, colour, tone and response to stimulation are assessed and each scored from a range of 0 to 2. An Apgar score between 7 and 10 indicates the infant is well. A score between 4 and 7 indicates the baby needs assistance. A score between 0 and 3 indicates severe cardiorespiratory depression. In practice it is best to describe exactly what was happening to the infant.

- *Resuscitation.* When assessing an apnoeic baby the heart rate is the most important parameter. If the heart rate is above 100 beats per min (b.p.m.) the baby will respond to stimulation and the inflating of the lungs with a bag and mask. If the heart rate is less than 100 b.p.m. and the baby does not quickly respond to stimulation or bag and mask ventilation, the baby should be intubated and ventilated with sufficient pressure to make the lungs expand. This should cause a rapid improvement in heart rate and colour. A baby who does not respond needs cardiac massage and may need infusions of bicarbonate or blood depending on the underlying problem to aid cardiac output. *Admission to a neonatal intensive care unit is mandatory if ventilation is not established by 5 min of age.*

- *Heat losses,* particularly evaporative, should be minimised by drying and wrapping the baby in warm towels. A well, term infant will be kept warm by being cuddled by the mother. The baby's rectal temperature should stabilise around 37°C by an hour of age.

- The *umbilical cord* is clamped and cut close to the skin. The cut end and the base of the cord must be kept clean and dry. Antiseptic solution, such as chlorhexidine in alcohol, may be applied daily until the cord stump drops off. Omphalitis can occur if these measures are not followed. The plastic clamp can be removed at 2 days of age.

- After the infant's temperature is stable, the infant can be washed with soap and water.

The first hours

- Record the heart rate, colour, respiratory rate and effort, at frequent intervals, depending on the infant's condition. All major causes of respiratory distress will present within the first hour of life.

- Often the baby will be very alert and breast feeds should be started at these times.

Vitamin K

- All infants, regardless of size, maturity, or ill-health, should receive 1 mg of i.m. vitamin K. This eradicates haemorrhagic disease. Do not administer vitamin K in the delivery ward as other drugs may be given inadvertantly. Claims regarding the association between i.m. vitamin K and childhood cancer have not been substantiated.

- An increased incidence of both early and late haemorrhagic disease of the newborn has been observed in breast-fed infants who have received either oral, i.v., inadequate i.m., or no prophylactic vitamin K.
- Parents who insist on their infant having oral vitamin K should be informed that it must be given for three doses at 2 weekly intervals.

The first day

After an initial period of alertness the infant will sleep for long periods and may not be too demanding with feeds. The infant should:

- Suck and swallow: if not, consider unrecognised prematurity, neurological or anatomical abnormality, or infection.
- Pass meconium: if not, consider low bowel obstruction.
- Pass urine: many babies pass urine at birth and this is missed. If no urine is passed by a boy he may have urethral valves.

The first examination

The purpose of this examination is to detect congenital abnormalities, reassure the parents and to discuss their concerns. Before disturbing the baby observe the posture, behaviour, general appearance, colour and wellbeing.

- *Head and neck.* Look for scalp abnormalities; fractures; haematomas; lacerations; eye size, anatomy and red reflex; neck cysts, lumps or fistulae; cleft palate; tongue size and shape; ear position, shape, size and tags or fistulae; and facial symmetry at rest.
- *The chest.* Recession and laboured breathing are the most important signs of respiratory difficulty, heart sounds, rate, pulse characteristics and presence. Normal babies breath so shallowly when they are sleeping that it can be difficult to see. In awake babies the rate and depth of each breath can be very variable.
- *The abdomen.* Feel for the masses (liver, spleen, kidneys, bladder and ovaries), distension and tenderness; and examine the genitalia, hernial areas and anus.
- *Limbs.* Examine for abnormal fingers, hands, toes and feet; posture of the hands and feet; and the flexibility of the joints.

- *The hips.* Carefully examine for congenital dislocation.
- Weight, length, and head circumference should be measured, and recorded on a percentile chart.

The first week

After an initial phase of waking frequently until lactation is established, the breast-fed baby should establish a regular cycle of waking for feeds, followed mostly by sleeping. However, some babies will stay awake after some feeds, even in the first week of life.

- Stools change over the first 4–5 days from black meconium, to dark-green, yellow-green, and finally loose yellow once full breast-feeding is established. The frequency of bowel actions can be very varied, but will usually be about once per feed after feeding is established.
- Urine production is usually low in the first few days, but increases after feeding has been established, with a urinary frequency of usually at least once per feed.
- More than half the babies will become jaundiced after the first 24 h of age (see later).
- On the third day, blood will be taken from a heel prick to screen for phenylketonuria (incidence 1 : 10 000), hypothyroidism (incidence 1 : 5000) and cystic fibrosis (incidence 1 : 2500 in Caucasians). Results are available approximately 1 week after sampling. Negative (normal) results are not notified, but the laboratory will contact the baby's doctor regarding the management of children with positive (abnormal) results, and advise on appropriate management. This usually involves an immediate referral to a tertiary paediatric hospital for further testing, and treatment, if appropriate.
- After an initial weight loss of up to 10% over the first few days, the baby's weight should stabilise and then increase towards the end of the first week.

The first month

- Weight gain for term babies varies from 150–250 g per week. For premature babies it is about 15 g/kg per day
- Problems usually relate to crying, not sleeping enough, not gaining weight, or poor feeding. These are discussed elsewhere in this handbook.

VARIATIONS FROM NORMAL

When the baby is fully examined, many normal variants or minor problems will be obvious. If they are obvious to the doctor, some will also be obvious to the parents. The amount of anxiety provoked in the parents by an abnormality is usually related to what is obvious to them, rather than to its medical importance. The management of most of these conditions is through competent and confident explanation.

Skin

- *Naevus flammeus* ('stork-bite'). Dilated capillaries, on the nape of the neck and on the bridge of the nose and adjacent forehead. They fade over 6–12 months.
- *Milia*. Small white blocked sebaceous glands on the nose. They disappear over the first month.
- *'Mongolian' pigmentation*. This condition results in areas of increased melanin deposition over the lower back and sacrum; however, it can be more extensive. Sometimes this condition is mistaken for bruising. It presents in babies born to parents with increased melanin in their skin, irrespective of race. It gradually lightens as the remaining skin increases its pigmentation.
- *Miliaria*. There are two types – 'crystallina' and 'rubra'. Miliaria crystallina are beads of sweat trapped under the epidermis and are most prominent on the forehead in babies who are overheated. Miliaria rubra, also called 'heat rash', usually appear after a few weeks of age, fluctuate over 2–3 weeks and disappear. They are related to an increasing activity of the sweat glands. They are prominent on the face and in babies who sweat.
- *Dry skin*. Babies who are more mature have a thicker epidermis and hence drier-looking skin after birth. This dry skin may occasionally crack and bleed around the ankles or wrists during the first few days. Usually it needs no treatment but emollients may help.
- *Puffy eyelids/scalp oedema*. The newborn infant has excess body fluid at birth. Fluid accumulates easily in the eyelids and, after lying on one side, the lower eye may be more swollen. Scalp oedema is common in the first few hours after a normal birth, but can persist for several days. If it persists or is generalised this needs investigating.

- *Bruising/petechiae/subconjunctival haemorrhages.* The presenting part is commonly bruised after birth. If the cord was wrapped tightly around the neck, the baby may have petechial haemorrhages on the face and head (traumatic cyanosis). Subconjunctival haemorrhages occur in up to 25% of babies delivered normally and do not adversely affect vision. Bruising is common after forceps deliveries, particularly over bony prominences, but disappears over the first week of life. Less commonly after forceps deliveries, firm nodules may be noted in the subcutaneous tissue at the same sites. This is subcutaneous fat necrosis. It resolves spontaneously over the first month of life.
- *Sucking blisters.* These are common on the lips, particularly the upper lip.
- *Breast hyperplasia.* A breast bud is palpable in most term babies regardless of their gender. In some they become enlarged during the first week as they respond to hormonal changes and breast milk may be observed. The breasts should be left alone and the hyperplasia will subside over several months. However, infected breast tissue that is swollen, hot, red and tender may need surgical drainage.
- *Erythema toxicum* ('toxic erythema' or 'urticaria of the newborn'). A harmless skin condition of unknown aetiology that peaks at 2–3 days of age, and is rarely present after the first week of life. New lesions have a broad erythematous base up to 2–3 cm diameter with a 1–2 mm papule. If the fluid in the pustule is examined it contains eosinophils and is sterile. Lesions can appear simultaneously anywhere on the body. They come and go over a few hours during the first few days. The diagnosis of erythema toxicum can be made with confidence on clinical appearance alone. The differential diagnosis is staphylococcal skin infection, which is persistent and purulent. An examination of the fluid reveals neutrophils and Gram-positive cocci in infection.

Behaviour

In the first days, babies tend to sleep deeply, breathe quietly and regularly and do not move much. The rest of the time they are in a restless type of sleep (rapid eye movement (REM) sleep), where they breathe erratically, make various noises (including crying, vocalising and yawning), have many body movements, and may seem to be waking up. Babies may switch from one type of sleep to the other every 5–10 min or so. This behaviour can be confusing to inexperienced parents.

Deformities

The skull changes shape (moulding) to enable the baby to be delivered. In addition there may be postural deformities of the face, skull and limbs that are related to the baby's position in the uterus. These gradually improve after birth, but sometimes they do not disappear completely – very few people are symmetrical, especially in their face.

COMMON MINOR PROBLEMS

- *Hiccups*. These occur frequently after a feed. They are not caused by inadequate burping and are harmless.
- *Snuffles*. These occur in about one-third of normal babies. Despite the noise, the baby is otherwise quite well and is able to feed normally. The problem diminishes with time as the baby's feeding becomes more efficient and the nasal passages enlarge. It is only important if it interferes with the baby's ability to suck.
- *Vomiting*. Small vomits are harmless. The serious signs are vomit that is bile stained (green), blood-stained, projectile, persistent, or associated with frequent choking or failure to thrive.
- *A bleeding umbilical cord*. Small amounts of bleeding rarely occur as the cord is separating and require no treatment. More profuse bleeding may indicate a bleeding disorder. It may also indicate infection.
- *Umbilical hernia*. This presents in approximately 25% of babies and resolves in almost all. They require surgery if persistent beyond 2 years of age.
- *Hymenal skin tag*. The vaginal skin commonly protrudes between the labia in newborn girls. It is benign and disappears as the labia become larger.
- *Vaginal discharge*. A small amount of vaginal mucus is universal. In some it can be blood-stained during the first week as the endometrium involutes.

- *Red urine.* A red–orange discoloration of the napkin when the urine is concentrated (the first few days of life) is mistaken for blood but it is usually due to urates.
- *Clicky hips.* Some ligamentous clicking is common in all large joints, including the hips. It can be considered normal in the absence of any abnormal movement of the femoral head, restriction of hip movement, strong family history, or breech presentation. However, if there is any doubt, hip ultrasound is indicated.

JAUNDICE

Jaundice is common in the newborn period and is almost always caused by unconjugated hyperbilirubinaemia. Its significance largely depends on the age of the infant at its onset.

The first 24 hours

- Jaundice in the first 24 h is abnormal.
- It is mostly caused by haemolysis, usually Rh or ABO incompatibility, between mother and foetus. The severe haemolysis leads to a rapid rise in serum bilirubin over a few hours.
- It may rarely be conjugated hyperbilirubinaemia, however; this needs investigation.
- Any baby with jaundice in the first 24 h should be admitted to hospital and the following need to be investigated and performed urgently: serum bilirubin (total and direct), the mother and baby's blood group, direct Coombs' test, full blood examination and red cell antibodies .
- Further investigations are indicated if there is no evidence of haemolysis or if conjugated hyperbilirubinaemia is present.
- Phototherapy should be commenced if the bilirubin level is >150 mmol/L in the first 24 h. An exchange transfusion is considered if the jaundice is due to rhesus incompatibility and the infant is anaemic. This primarily corrects the anaemia and removes antibodies. Further exchange transfusions may be required to control the jaundice.
- Frequent monitoring of bilirubin levels is essential as rapid changes may occur and clinical assessment of the severity of jaundice, particularly under phototherapy, is impossible.

Days 3 to 7

The jaundice is considered to be 'physiological' if the following criteria are satisfied:

- The jaundice appeared on day 3 or 4.
- The baby is not premature.
- The baby is well (afebrile, feeding well and alert).
- The baby is passing normal-coloured stools and urine.
- There are no other abnormalities.

It is not necessary to measure bilirubin levels if the above criteria apply. More than 50% of term babies become visibly jaundiced by 2–4 days of age. This usually occurs when the serum bilirubin rises above about 85–120 mmol/L. In 97% of cases it does not exceed 221 mmol/L.

If the criteria are not fulfilled a bilirubin level is indicated. If the unconjugated bilirubin is >221 mmol/L, further investigations are needed, particularly for infection.

Treatment

A well term infant with no haemolysis is at minimal risk of kernicterus. The following are some guidelines for treatment:

- If the serum bilirubin >285 mmol/L give phototherapy.
- If the serum bilirubin >360 mmol/L an exchange transfusion may be needed.

Ill-term infants, in particular those exposed to hypoxic insults, or infants with evidence of haemolysis, are at a higher risk of kernicterus and treatment needs to be started at lower bilirubin levels. Preterm infants may be at an increased risk of kernicterus.

Prolonged jaundice (>14 days)

Most prolonged neonatal jaundice in a well infant is due to breast-feeding and is benign. However, a serum bilirubin should be performed to check whether the hyperbilirubinaemia is conjugated or unconjugated.

Causes

- Unconjugated bilirubinaemia is mostly caused by breast-feeding, and benign but hypothyroidism, infection or red cell enzyme abnormalities should be considered.

- A sudden onset at this age is suggestive of haemolysis caused by a red blood cell enzyme abnormality, most frequently glucose-6-phosphate dehydrogenase (G-6-PD) deficiency that can cause rapid haemolysis. Urgent admission to hospital is indicated.
- Conjugated bilirubinaemia is uncommon and always pathological. Consider biliary atresia (the stools are white), neonatal hepatitis, a choledochal cyst obstructing the bile duct, galactosaemia or parenteral nutrition.

If the above are excluded – the baby is well and breast-feeding – the likely diagnosis is breast milk jaundice. This occurs in 2–4% of breast-feeding infants, is not associated with kernicterus and does not need any treatment. Reassurance that breast-feeding should continue is very important.

A prolongation of the jaundice from the first few days of life can initially be managed as an outpatient.

RESPIRATORY DISTRESS

This is recognised by a respiratory rate greater than 60 b.p.m. and is associated with subcostal and intercostal recession and cyanosis in air.

Aetiology
Common pulmonary diseases
Respiratory distress syndrome (RDS) or hyaline membrane disease (HMD)

- The incidence increases with decreasing gestation. It is primarily caused by lung immaturity. It is present in most babies born at less than 30 weeks' gestation. The lungs do not expand easily or evenly. This causes damage to the epithelium and protein exudes on to the surface forming the hyaline membranes.
- There is respiratory difficulty soon after birth, which increases in severity over the next few hours and may progress to respiratory failure.
- The diagnosis is confirmed by the chest X-ray that has a generalised fine reticulogranular ('ground glass') appearance with air bronchograms.

Transient tachypnoea of the newborn (TTN) or 'wet lung syndrome'

- This is caused by delayed clearance of foetal lung fluid and commonly occurs in term babies born by elective Caesarean section. It also contributes to RDS in premature infants.
- It presents as mild respiratory distress and lasts for 1 or 2 days.
- It is diagnosed from a chest X-ray that has coarse streaking of lung fields with fluid in the fissures.

Bacterial infections

- Group B β-haemolytic streptococcus is the commonest and most serious cause of pneumonia in the newborn and is associated with septicaemia. It is acquired at birth from the colonised mother.
- It presents with early onset severe progressive respiratory failure. If not treated early there is rapid progression to collapse and death.
- Later infections present with a combination of lethargy, temperature instability, poor feeding, respiratory difficulty, apnoea or poor perfusion.
- The chest X-ray of group B streptococcus (GBS) pneumonia is similar to that of severe RDS and is not diagnostic. Other pneumonias may show consolidation.

Meconium aspiration syndrome

- Hypoxia causes the infant to gasp *in utero* and inhale meconium. This causes respiratory difficulty that is often associated with pulmonary hypertension and right to left shunting.
- The chest X-ray shows hyperinflation and patchy consolidation (pneumothorax and pneumomediastinum may follow) or a diffuse hazy appearance may be evident.

Milk aspiration

Infants are unlikely to aspirate feeds unless they are sick, preterm, neurologically abnormal, or an anatomical abnormality is present.

Pneumothorax

Occurs spontaneously at birth or may be secondary to lung disease and ventilation. The diagnosis should be confirmed by X-ray. Transillumination can be useful. Needle aspiration should only be used when the situation is life-threatening.

Uncommon pulmonary diseases

- *Viral infections* (respiratory syncytial virus, rhinovirus, para-influenza) are acquired after birth, often at home, and may present with apnoea, difficulty feeding or recession.
- *Pulmonary haemorrhage* occurs in ventilated preterm infants.
- *Chronic lung disease* occurs in premature infants who have received mechanical ventilation. It is diagnosed by X-ray showing cystic and fibrotic areas with a need for oxygen treatment beyond 28 days of life.
- *Congenital diaphragmatic hernia* is usually left-sided with poor breath sounds and a mediastinal shift to the right. The abdomen is scaphoid. It is diagnosed by chest X-ray, and often by ultrasound antenatally.
- *Chylothorax* is often bilateral with reduced chest movement and breath sounds. A chest X-ray shows a general granular appearance with fluid in the pleural space. Diagnosis is done by aspirating (under ultrasound control) and analysing the fluid.
- *Pulmonary interstitial emphysema (PIE)* is where air in the lungs outside the airways occurs in ventilated premature infants.
- *Congenital lobar emphysema and congenital lung cysts* are diagnosed by chest X-ray.

Airways obstruction

- *Nasal.* May be due to an upper respiratory tract infection, choanal atresia or traumatic deviated nasal septum. It presents with difficulty in breathing or feeding.
- *Oral.* Macroglossia may be associated with Beckwith–Wiedemann syndrome or hypothyroidism. Micrognathia may result in a tongue that obstructs the pharynx.
- *Neck.* Goitre.
- *Larynx.* Vocal cord palsy, subglottic stenosis or laryngomalacia present with inspiratory stridor.
- *Trachea.* Tracheomalacia and vascular ring present with inspiratory and expiratory wheeze.

Non-pulmonary

- *Cardiac.* These conditions cause increased blood flow through the lungs. They comprise left to right shunts through a patent ductus arteriosus, a ventricular septal defect or left outflow obstruction.

- *Pulmonary hypertension.* This is usually secondary to hypoxia and acidosis during the perinatal period.

Management
Before birth

- Anticipate these high-risk babies, if possible, and transfer to a hospital with a level 3 nursery for delivery and neonatal care.
- Betamethasone given between 48 h and 7 days before preterm labour reduces the severity of HMD, and halves the mortality and incidence of brain haemorrhages.

After birth

- If particulate meconium-stained liquor is present use a laryngoscope to aid aspiration of the oropharynx, larynx and trachea. Intubate and aspirate the trachea if meconium is seen below the cords. If possible avoid positive pressure ventilation until the airway is clear.
- Assess the baby's cardiorespiratory status and resuscitate as needed. If the baby is known to have a diaphragmatic hernia, intubate and ventilate at birth as spontaneous breathing or bag and mask ventilation can cause the distension of the thoracic intestinal contents.
- Most extremely low birthweight infants will need intubating. Babies who have laboured breathing may benefit from early continuous positive airway pressure (CPAP).
- In cases of oesophageal atresia, frequent (10–15 min) oropharyngeal suction prior to operative repair is necessary.

General care

- Temperature control is essential – incubator care may be necessary.
- Avoid enteral feeds if the baby needs >40% oxygen – give intravenous fluids.
- Measure blood glucose, electrolytes and carry out a full blood count.
- A septic work-up should include blood culture as a minimum.
- Treat with benzylpenicillin and gentamicin until the blood cultures are known to be clear.

Respiratory care

- A *chest X-ray* is mandatory for all neonates who have respiratory difficulty. It provides the diagnosis in most cases.
- In premature babies *surfactant* should be administered down the endotracheal tube as early as possible because this improves survival and reduces the severity of RDS and its complications.
- *Monitor* cardiorespiratory and blood gas measurements.
- *Inspired oxygen* is initially set using the pulse oximeter. Aim for an oxygen saturation of between 92 and 95%. In babies who need >40% oxygen, or who have respiratory difficulty, the arterial blood gases should be used to determine the inspired oxygen concentration. Aim for a P_aO_2 level between 50 and 85 mmHg. Oxygen is toxic to the lungs, especially at levels >70%. If you are using these levels, increase the mean airway pressure by CPAP or ventilation. Oxygen can be delivered into the incubator, via a head box, nasal cannulae, nasal CPAP tube or intubation. The route depends on the severity of the baby's illness.
- *Continuous positive airway pressure (CPAP)* distends the lungs and upper airway. It is given via nasal tubes. It is effective during RDS or for treating apnoea of prematurity. CPAP should be used for any baby who is grunting and/or showing increased respiratory effort. It is better to use it earlier rather than later. The level of CPAP depends on the problem. First assess the X-ray. A baby with 'solid' lungs needs a pressure of at least 5 cmH_2O.
- The *indications for ventilating a baby* vary depending on his or her gestational age and condition. The decision to ventilate a baby is made on the following criteria:
  - Apnoea not responding to simple treatment.
  - There are unsatisfactory arterial blood gases. There are no absolute cut-offs because the decision to ventilate depends on the size of the baby, the diagnosis and how the baby is managing. Reasonable values to consider ventilation are pH <7.25 with a PcO_2 >55 mmHg, or the need for a high inspired oxygen or hypoxia resistant to other treatments. In a very small baby, ventilation should probably be started earlier.
  - There is increasing evidence that babies can be treated with early nasal CPAP and do not always need ventilating. If the

baby has RDS and is breathing adequately use nasal CPAP at 10 cmH_2O to prevent intubation.

- *Endotracheal tubes*: use at least a 3.0 mm tube unless the baby weighs <750 g when a 2.5 mm tube is most appropriate. Term babies need a 3.5 mm tube unless very large when a 4.0 mm tube would be better. Pass the tube so that the black area near the tip can still just be seen above the cords.

- *Arterial pH* should be maintained between about 7.35 and 7.45. A level of 7.25 or just under is acceptable, depending on the circumstances (often chronic lung disease). *Remember:* life is all about maintaining pH.

- *Arterial Pco_2* should be between 35 and 55 mmHg. A low P_aco_2 means over-ventilation. This is usually because the infant is ventilated and the pressures or rates, or both, are too high. A high P_aco_2 indicates under-ventilation. If the pH is also low then it is a respiratory acidosis. Respiratory support should either be commenced with CPAP or intermittent positive pressure ventilation (IPPV) or the rates/pressures increased.

- *Arterial Po_2.* A low P_ao_2 means that the baby is hypoxic. If the pH is also low the baby may have a metabolic acidosis. Oxygen or a higher inspired oxygen need to be used. If this does not have any effect suspect cyanotic heart disease as a cause (see Cardiovascular Conditions, chapter 16).

- *Arterial bicarbonate* should be between about 22 and 30 mmol/L. A low level is due to a metabolic acidosis. The pH will also be low unless the baby has compensated by blowing off CO_2. A high level is a metabolic alkalosis. This is commonly due to the kidneys compensating for a respiratory acidosis in broncho-pulmonary dysplasia (BPD).

- *The base excess* should be between +2.5 and –2.5. If it is low it indicates a metabolic acidosis. A level of –5 is usually tolerated in small babies before intervention.

HYPOGLYCAEMIA

This is a true blood glucose level of <2.5 mmol/L. 'Dextrostix' or 'BM stix' are useful for screening purposes. However, if these suggest hypoglycaemia a true blood glucose level should be measured before starting any intravenous therapy.

Blood glucose should be measured at 1 h of age for infants with the following conditions: infants of diabetic mothers, small for gestational age infants, premature infants, large for gestational age infants, asphyxiated infants, infants with seizures and infants receiving intravenous infusions.

Clinical features

There are no specific clinical features of hypoglycaemia. The infant may be asymptomatic or have apathy, hypotonia, poor feeding, temperature instability, jitteriness or convulsions.

Treatment

- For asymptomatic infants with a true blood sugar in the range of 1.5–2.5 mmol/L give early, increased and frequent enteral feeds. If there is no response within 2 h, intravenous dextrose must be given.
- Intravenous dextrose (10% or 15%) is indicated if the true blood glucose <1.5 mmol/L. A bolus of 25% dextrose 2 mL/kg should be followed by an infusion providing 5–10 mg/kg per min of glucose. The response to therapy should be monitored by frequent blood glucose measurements.
- For an infant with severe hypoglycaemia (<1 mmol/L), where it is difficult to insert an intravenous line, give 0.5 units/kg of glucagon i.m.
- Further investigation and treatment is necessary if the glucose requirement is 10 mg/kg per min.

NEONATAL INFECTION

Infection is one of the commonest preventable causes of neonatal mortality and morbidity. They may be acquired from the mother's genito-urinary tract before or at birth (early onset) or postnatally from the environment by droplet spread or handling (late onset).

The most frequently encountered bacteria are:
- Early onset: Group B β-haemolytic streptococcus, *Escherichia coli* and *Listeria monocytogenes.*
- At late onset: Coagulase-negative staphylococci, *Staphylococcus aureus*, Group B β-haemolytic streptococcus, *Klebsiella* spp. and *Pseudomonas* spp.

The most serious viral infection is herpes.

The early symptoms and signs may be minimal, but if ignored rapid progression to overwhelming sepsis may occur. The following are important warning signs: respiratory difficulty, poor feeding, vomiting, abdominal distension and tenderness, drowsiness, floppiness, pallor, apnoea, seizures, temperature instability, tender limb.

Investigations

If one or more of the warning signs are present it is important to investigate infection. This includes:

- Blood culture: arterial or venous – at least 2–4 mL.
- Urine: suprapubic aspiration (SPA). If one SPA fails try with the assistance of ultrasound imaging. A catheter specimen could be obtained with an aseptic technique. A bag specimen is of little value.
- Throat swab and rectal swab.
- Swab any obviously infected lesion.
- Lumbar puncture: exercise caution in a sick baby with a bulging fontanelle.
- Cultures or specific polymerase chain reaction (PCR) for viral infections.

Treatment

Any ill neonate should be investigated and treated in hospital. Start with i.v. benzylpenicillin and gentamicin. Add cefotaxime i.v. if meningitis is suspected and metronidazole i.v. if abdominal sepsis is suspected. If there is any possibility that the baby may have herpes (i.e. the mother has active genital herpes) give aciclovir. The antibiotics may need to be changed when cultures are available. (See antimicrobial guidelines.)

Careful attention to temperature stability, ventilation, fluid and electrolytes, blood pressure, blood glucose and haematology is essential.

NEONATAL SEIZURES

Clinical features

- Subtle: deviation of the eyes, staring, abnormal sucking or lip smacking, or cycling movements of the limbs.

- Tonic: limbs go stiff, frequently associated with apnoea and eye deviation.
- Clonic: movement of one or all limbs not stopped by holding the limb.

These can be distinguished from 'jitteriness' or tremulousness, which have no ocular phenomena, are stimulus sensitive, and can be stopped by gentle passive flexion of the limbs.

Benign sleep myoclonus occurs in a neurologically normal infant only during sleep. The electroencephalogram (EEG) is normal and no treatment is necessary.

Aetiology

The aetiology can usually be found for neonatal seizures.

(1) Hypoxic ischaemic encephalopathy: the seizures occur within 48 h of the hypoxic episode.
(2) Intracranial haemorrhage.
(3) Infection: bacterial (group B streptococcus, *E. coli* and *Listeria* spp.) or viral (herpes, and enteroviruses) meningitis.
(4) Metabolic:
    (i) Hypoglycaemia
    (ii) Hypocalcaemia/hypomagnesaemia
    (iii) Hypo- or hypernatraemia
    (iv) Alkalosis
    (v) Local anaesthetic intoxication
    (vi) Urea cycle disorders
    (vii) Non-ketotic hyperglycinaemia
    (viii) Fatty acid oxidation defects
    (ix) Amino acid/organic acid/hyperammonaemia
(5) Pyridoxine dependency.
(6) Kernicterus.
(7) Drug withdrawal.
(8) Developmental brain abnormalities.
(9) Autosomal dominant neonatal seizures.
(10) Idiopathic.

Investigations

- Blood glucose.
- Electrolytes, calcium and magnesium.

- Blood gases.
- Cranial ultrasound.
- Urine analysis including ketones and reducing substances.
- Lumbar puncture, blood cultures and viral investigations.
- Metabolic screen: blood ammonia, plasma lactate, urinary organic acids, plasma amino acids and plasma carnitine.
- Cranial CT scan: if focal seizures, birth trauma or uncertain aetiology.
- MRI scan: for suspected developmental brain abnormality.
- EEG: to detect seizure activity and to aid prognosis.

Treatment

Admission to a neonatal intensive care unit is mandatory for all neonates with seizures. Attention to optimal ventilation, blood pressure control, fluid and electrolyte balance and normoglycaemia are essential.

Anticonvulsants

- Phenobarbitone: 20 mg/kg i.v. over 30 min (beware it may cause apnoea in a non-ventilated baby). A further 10 mg/kg may be given for refractory seizures followed by 5 mg/kg per day.
- Phenytoin: 20 mg/kg, i.v. over 1 h.
- Clonazepam: up to 0.25 mg. This may cause apnoea. Careful monitoring and the availability of mechanical ventilation are essential.
- Pyridoxine: 50–100 mg i.v. or p.o. should be considered for intractable seizures.

Most infants can be weaned from anticonvulsant therapy within 2 weeks of their last seizure. Some infants who have residual seizures or abnormal neurological signs with an abnormal EEG should be treated for months.

POSTNATAL DEPRESSION IN THE MOTHER

Mild to moderate postnatal depression occurs in about one in six women – a much higher incidence than previously recognised. If severe it may be a risk to the life of both the mother and baby.

It can have profound effects on the family and on the development of the child. The diagnosis may not always be obvious, so a high level of awareness is needed.

Warning signs

The mother is:

- Highly anxious about small things
- Totally disorganised, does not want to go out and cries a lot
- Difficult to reassure or keeps presenting to health professionals
- Overly 'fussy'
- Inattentive to her crying baby
- Subject to panic attacks.

A crying baby can and often accompanies a mother who is depressed. Crying babies can cause women who are unsure and vulnerable to reach this state.

Management

- Recognise and acknowledge the problem.
- Give the appropriate support and counselling.
- Medication, as well as support is often necessary.
- Referral to a mother–baby unit or a psychiatric hospital facility may be needed and is often of benefit.

MATERNAL MASTITIS

Mastitis is common in breast-feeding women.

- It presents with aches and pains and fever. Patients often think they have the 'flu'.
- An examination reveals a tender engorged segment in one or both breasts.
- The organism is usually *Staphylococcus aureus*.

Management

- Prompt treatment is important to prevent abscess formation.
- Oral antibiotics – flucloxacillin 500 mg 6 hourly.
- Panadol and increased fluids.
- Breast-feeding should continue.
- Good emptying of the affected breast. The baby is more efficient at this than expression.

PROBLEMS OF THE EX-VERY LOW BIRTHWEIGHT INFANT (VLBW)

While it is not the intention of this chapter to discuss the problems of managing VLBW infants (birthweight <1500 g) it is important to be aware of some of the problems that occur after discharge from the neonatal unit.

Bronchopulmonary dysplasia (BPD)

This is a common chronic lung disease occurring in infants after mechanical ventilation. It is characterised by an abnormal chest X-ray and oxygen dependency for >28 days. The majority of VLBW infants with chronic lung disease can be weaned from oxygen treatment within 4 weeks of the expected date of delivery. A small number require oxygen therapy for months and some are managed at home in oxygen.

These babies are particularly susceptible to respiratory infections in the first 18 months of life and may deteriorate rapidly and need to be readmitted to hospital. If the baby is feeding poorly because of dyspnoea, has retractions of the lower sternum and ribs, or apnoeic episodes, urgent admission to hospital is indicated.

In the absence of these signs the infant may be managed at home, but the parents need to be informed of the warning signs and the child reviewed frequently.

Necrotising enterocolitis (NEC)

This is due to inflammation of the intestine in the early neonatal period. While many babies recover with conservative management (nil orally, intravenous alimentation and antibiotics), some develop necrosis that necessitates bowel resection. The risks to these babies after discharge from hospital are:

- *Stricture formation.* This can present weeks or months after the initial episode. The presenting features of obstruction include: bile-stained vomiting, distension, constipation and failure to thrive.
- *Gastroenteritis.* This can produce severe dehydration very rapidly in a baby who has had a bowel resection. Admission to hospital for intravenous fluids is mandatory.

Hearing deficits

Hearing deficits are common in these babies and hearing must be carefully assessed.

Visual defects

Visual defects are common and must be screened for.

Further common problems

- *Umbilical hernia*: does not require treatment.
- *Inguinal hernias*: these require surgical repair soon after they are diagnosed as they frequently strangulate.
- *Immunisation*: (see also Immunisation, Chapter 5) an infant should receive the three doses of DTP, Sabin polio and Hib at 2, 4 and 6 months from the date of birth irrespective of the degree of prematurity. Hepatitis B vaccination is also recommended. There are no grounds for delaying immunisation or reducing the vaccine dose based on size or prematurity.
- *Apnoea*: this is a common problem until about 34 weeks' gestation. However ex-VLBW infants are at risk of apnoea until the age of 3 months past their due date after general anaesthesia, or if they catch respiratory infections. Close monitoring is advised at these times.
- *Capillary haemangiomas* (strawberry naevus): these appear after birth as small raised, red, lobulated and compressible lesions that increase in size over a few months. Most involute during the first 2 years. Failure to involute or difficult locations may be indications for a referral to a dermatologist for laser or intralesional steroid therapy.

CHAPTER 29
NEUROLOGIC CONDITIONS

Lloyd Shield
Simon Harvey
Geoffrey Klug

FEBRILE CONVULSIONS

- Febrile convulsions (FC) are usually brief, generalised seizures associated with a febrile illness, in the absence of any central nervous system (CNS) infection or past history of afebrile seizures.
- They occur in 3–4% of children aged 6 months to 5 years, and are recurrent in 25–30%.
- In otherwise healthy children they are not accompanied by an increased risk of intellectual disability, cerebral palsy, other neurological disorders or death.

Management

- A continuing convulsion (>10 min duration) may be terminated by i.v. or rectal diazepam 0.2–0.4 mg/kg (max 10 mg) (see Fig. 1.2).
- General temperature-lowering measures such as removing clothing and administering paracetamol 15 mg/kg may be helpful.
- A careful search for the cause of fever is conducted. Most will be due to viral respiratory infections.
- A lumbar puncture need not be performed routinely following a simple FC, but meningitis should be considered in any unwell child, especially when there is a persistently depressed conscious state, and in children with multiple or prolonged convulsions. The younger the child the higher should be the index of suspicion of meningitis.

Recurrence of FC is more likely if the seizure occurs in early infancy and if there is a family history of FC. As FC are usually benign, and as anticonvulsants may have significant side effects and do not alter long-term prognosis, these drugs are not routinely recommended for children with recurrent FC. In some circumstances (e.g. children with a history of prolonged FC) parents may be taught to administer rectal diazepam.

Three per cent of children with FC subsequently develop afebrile seizures (i.e. epilepsy). Predictors include:

- Previous abnormal neurological development
- A history of epilepsy in first-degree relatives
- Prolonged (>10 min) FC
- Focal features present during, or after, the FC
- Multiple convulsions during a single febrile episode.

When counselling parents, one should remember that many will have felt that their child nearly died. The excellent long-term prognosis, a 30% risk of FC recurrence but low risk of epilepsy need to be emphasised. Advice on the management of future febrile illnesses and FC is given. A follow-up visit is recommended to review FC, and minimise the development of fever phobia in the parents. An electro-encephalogram (EEG) is of no value in single or recurrent, simple FC.

EPILEPSY

Primary generalised epilepsy

- This term describes the group of childhood epilepsies characterised by recurrent generalised tonic–clonic seizures, absence, or myoclonic seizures of unknown (presumed genetic) aetiology.
- The first seizure is usually between 4 and 16 years of age, in an otherwise normal child.
- The EEG invariably shows generalised spike wave patterns.
- The prognosis is generally good for seizure control and remission in later childhood or adulthood.

Partial (focal) seizures

Partial seizures arise from a localised area of cortex in one or both cerebral hemispheres, and may be idiopathic or due to underlying structural pathology. Metabolic disturbances (e.g. hypoglycaemia and hypocalcaemia) may also produce partial seizures.

Two common but distinct forms of partial epilepsy are temporal lobe epilepsy and the benign focal epilepsies of childhood.

Temporal lobe epilepsy

- Complex partial seizures are the main seizure type, and usually manifest by the arrest of activity, staring, autonomic features, mouthing movements, semi-purposeful motor activity and an altered conscious state, sometimes preceded by epigastric or olfactory auras. Seizures may secondarily generalise.
- Seizures typically occur in clusters, and are often difficult to treat.
- These children frequently have learning and behavioural problems.
- An EEG may show localised epileptic activity and structural pathology should be sought by imaging.

Benign focal (partial) epilepsies of childhood

- Onset is typically in mid-childhood (peak 7 years).
- Seizures are commonly nocturnal or early morning. They are usually focal motor or sensory phenomena related to the face, mouth or jaw. The occipital variety may have visual manifestations. Secondarily generalised tonic–clonic seizures may also occur.
- EEG spike discharges typically occur in the centrotemporal region or occipital region.
- The prognosis is excellent as the seizures are usually infrequent and readily controlled on carbamazepine if treatment is required. They usually remit before the teenage years.
- Imaging is normally only necessary if clinical features or EEG are atypical or if seizure control is difficult.

Breath-holding attacks

See Table 29.2.

Status epilepticus

See Medical emergencies, chapter 1.

Anticonvulsant therapy

Indications for commencing anticonvulsants

The decision to investigate and treat a child following a seizure depends on many factors. Consideration should be given to a routine EEG in any child with non-febrile, generalised or partial seizures. Brain imaging with CT or MRI is reserved for those in whom there is suspicion from history, examination or EEG that there may be an underlying cerebral lesion. Many children have only a single convulsion, and treatment would not normally be commenced unless there are clinical features to suggest an increased risk of recurrence. These include:

- The seizure was prolonged (>10 min).
- The seizure was partial (but not due to a benign epilepsy syndrome).
- There is evidence suggesting organic cerebral damage, such as intellectual disability, a history of birth injury, head injury or previous meningitis.
- The epilepsy syndrome is associated with a high rate of recurrence.

Anti-epileptic medication is generally indicated in children with recurrent epileptic seizures (see Table 29.1).

Principles of anticonvulsant therapy

- Most patients can be controlled well with one anticonvulsant; polypharmacy should be avoided if possible.
- Introduce or change one anticonvulsant at a time, except in emergency situations.
- Most anti-epileptic medications are commenced at a low dose and titrated up to the maintenance dose, to avoid side effects during their introduction ('start low and go slow').
- Individuals vary greatly in dosage requirements and tolerance. Young children and infants typically require relatively large doses.
- Give anticonvulsants an adequate trial before withdrawal.
- If seizure control is inadequate or non-compliance or clinical toxicity is suspected, anticonvulsant blood levels might be measured for drugs such as phenytoin, phenobarbitone, carbamazepine and valproate. 'Routine' monitoring of phenytoin,

Table 29.1 Guidelines for the use of common anticonvulsants

Drug	Status epilepticus	Generalized tonic–clonic seizures	Partial: simple, complex or 2° generalised	Typical absence (petit mal)	Myoclonic/ tonic/atypical absence	More common or severe side effects	Oral maintenance dosage
Carbamazepine (Tegretol)	–	++	+++	–	–	Drowsiness, irritability, GIT, rash	10–20 mg/kg per day
Clobazam (Frisium)	–	+	++	+	++	Drowsiness, irritability	5–30 mg/day
Clonazepam (Rivotril)	+++	+	++	+	+++	Irritability and behaviour disorder, increased secretions	0.1–0.2 mg/kg per day i.v. up to 0.5 mg per dose depending on age
Diazepam (Valium)	+++	–	–	–	+++ (i.v. only)	Drowsiness, respiratory depression	Intravenous PR
Ethosuximide (Zarontin)	–	–	–	+++	+	Gastrointestinal disturbance, thrombocytopenia	0.2–0.6 mg/kg slowly
Gabapentin (Neurontin)	–	–	++	–	–	Drowsiness, dizziness, ataxia, fatigue	20–40 mg/kg per day
Lamotrigine (Lamictal)	–	++	++	++	++	Skin rash in 3%; may be severe. Increased risk if rapid introduction or on sodium valproate	See Pharmacopoeia
Nitrazepam (Mogadon)	–	–	–	–	++	Drowsiness, increased bronchial secretions	Increase slowly from 1.25 mg/day

Table 29.1 Guidelines for the use of common anticonvulsants *Cont'd*

Drug	Status epilepticus	Generalized tonic–clonic seizures	Partial: simple, complex or 2° generalised	Typical absence (petit mal)	Myoclonic/ tonic/atypical absence	More common or severe side effects	Oral maintenance dosage
Phenobarbitone	++	++	+	–	–	Cognitive, irritability, overactivity or drowsiness	3–5 mg/kg per day
Phenytoin sodium (Dilantin, DPH)	++	++	++	–	–	Gum hyperplasia, ataxia, nystagmus, serum sickness-like illness, cognitive, rash	5–8 mg/kg per day
Sodium valproate (Epilim)		+++	++	++	+++	Nausea, anorexia vomiting. Rarely severe hepatotoxicity	20–50 mg/kg per day
Vigabatrin (Sabril)	–		++	–	++ (Infantile spasms)	Excitation, agitation, drowsiness, dizziness, headache, weight gain, mild GI upset, constriction of visual fields	See Pharmacopoeia

* This table shows the relative effectiveness of each drug against each of the major seizure types. It does not represent a comparison of one drug against another. Sodium valproate should be used with caution in children under 3 years, particularly if multiple anticonvulsants are being used and underlying cerebral pathology is present. Cognitive side effects may be seen with all anticonvulsants, particularly benzodiazepines, barbiturates and phenytoin.

The above represents suggestions only. The final decision re the most appropriate choice of anticonvulsant can only be made by a physician in possession of details such as age of patient, neurological status, comorbidities, epilepsy syndromes, EEG, patient and parent attitudes, and after discussion of potential side effects.

phenobarbitone or carbamazepine levels is indicated in young infants or developmentally impaired older children in whom even severe side effects may not be evident.

Depending on the type of epilepsy, several years of freedom from seizures are generally required before anticonvulsants are withdrawn. This is done gradually over several months.

WEAKNESS OF ACUTE ONSET (ACUTE FLACCID PARALYSIS)

The acute onset of symmetrical limb weakness usually has a peripheral neuromuscular or spinal cord origin. Toxins (e.g. snake or tick bite), metabolic disturbance, systemic illness and psychogenic causes need to be considered under appropriate circumstances. Oral polio vaccine is a rare cause of acute flaccid paralysis.

Two key questions require urgent consideration:
- Is there a treatable cause?
- Is there respiratory or pharyngeal dysfunction of sufficient degree to warrant management in an intensive care unit?

Myasthenia gravis
- This diagnosis should be considered in any child with relatively acute onset limb weakness, particularly if accompanied by ptosis, eye movement disorder, pharyngeal or respiratory insufficiency.
- A diagnostic/therapeutic trial of parenteral anticholinesterase is warranted if myasthenia is a possibility.

Guillain–Barré syndrome
- This condition is often not recognised in its early stages when there may only be an 'ataxic' gait.
- The child should be transferred to a tertiary referral centre at the time of diagnosis, as respiratory weakness may occur rapidly, and plasma exchange or gamma-globulin need to be commenced early if they are to be effective.

Infant botulism
Suspect in children 2–9 months of age with constipation and rapid onset of weakness, particularly with ophthalmoplegia and bulbar/

respiratory weakness. A child with suspected infant botulism should be transferred urgently to a centre capable of undertaking long-term ventilation.

Spinal cord compression

- Myelopathy should always be considered when there is paraparesis or quadriparesis without neurological dysfunction at higher levels.
- Brisk deep tendon reflexes or extensor plantar responses may not be prominent early, and a sensory level is often the most important clue to a myelopathy.
- The confirmation or exclusion of trauma, tumour, abscess, haematoma or skeletal anomaly is an urgent priority.
- Spinal imaging is required even when acute 'transverse' myelopathy is suspected.

CHRONIC AND RECURRENT HEADACHE

- Migraine is the most common identifiable cause of recurrent or chronic headache in childhood.
- In adolescence, muscle contraction (tension-type) headache is also important.
- Although rare, raised intracranial pressure and systemic illness must also be considered.
- A careful history, examination and follow up will usually yield the correct diagnosis.

History

- Determine the location of the headache, and its quality, duration, frequency and time of onset.
- Identify trigger factors, associated symptoms (e.g. nausea or vomiting, visual disturbance and hemisymptoms) and the disruption to normal activities.
- Inquire whether the symptoms are progressive and if there is a family history of migraine or cerebral tumours; recent head injury; development of visual, gait or coordination difficulties; or changes in personality or intellectual functioning.
- Take a detailed social history.

Distinguishing features

- Migraine without aura is usually a frontotemporal or bilateral headache and in older children it is frequently accompanied by nausea and vomiting, followed by lethargy or sleep. Marked pallor is common and there is commonly a positive family history.
- Migraine headaches with aura or prolonged neurological symptoms are uncommon.
- Migraine has a fluctuating temporal pattern, while tension-type headache tends to be persistent but usually does not interfere with sleep.
- Recurrent morning headaches; headaches that are intense, prolonged and incapacitating; or that show a progressive change in character over time suggest intracranial pathology. Such patients, or those with abnormal examination findings, the rarer variants of migraine or those who do not respond to simple treatment measures, require paediatric referral.

Examination

- Measure head circumference and blood pressure.
- Auscultate the skull for intracranial bruits; palpate over the sinuses, cervical spine and teeth.
- Perform a thorough neurological examination, including examination of the visual acuity and fields, eye movements, optic fundi, coordination and gait.
- Assess the child's growth and pubertal status; inspect the skin for neurocutaneous stigmata.

Management: if the diagnosis is migraine

- Reassuring the child and parents that migraine is not usually a serious condition is an important part of its management.
- In migraine, trigger avoidance, stress management and the early use of paracetamol 15 mg/kg per dose orally, 4 hourly (max 90 mg/kg per 24 h) during an acute attack is frequently all that is required. Non-steroidal anti-inflammatory medications (e.g. ibuprofen 2.5–10 mg/kg per dose (max 150–600 mg) orally, 6–8 hourly) can be useful in the acute attack, but the role of sumatriptan in childhood is not yet clear.

- Prophylactic therapy for those with severe or frequent attacks is best done in consultation with a paediatrician. Propranolol 0.2–0.5 mg/kg (max 10–25 mg/kg) twice daily or pizotifen 0.5 mg mane and 1.0 mg nocte are commonly used initially. Sodium valproate 5–15 mg/kg (max 1 g) 12 hourly is also effective in some children with recurrent or chronic migraine syndromes.
- Two-thirds of children cease having attacks but 50% of these have recurrences in adult life.

NON-EPILEPTIC PAROXYSMAL EVENTS

- Many children referred for assessment of epilepsy do not have epilepsy, but some other non-epileptic paroxysmal disorder.
- In differentiating epileptic from non-epileptic events the description of the event is important, but equally important is a description of the circumstances in which the event occurred and the details of what the child was doing immediately before the event.
- Many non-epileptic paroxysmal disorders can be diagnosed positively on history alone, although in some special circumstances more detailed investigations such as video–EEG monitoring may be required.
- The long Q–T syndrome should be considered in any episode of fainting or seizure that is not clearly due to typical breath-holding, vaso-vagal syncope or a definable epilepsy syndrome.

Table 29.2 lists some of these events and their salient features.

HEAD INJURIES

Assessment
History
It is essential to determine the nature of the injury, its severity, the time of occurrence and the clinical course prior to the consultation.

Table 29.2 Non-epileptic paroxysmal events

	Breath-holding attacks	Shuddering	Benign paroxysmal vertigo	Infantile self stimulation	'Day dreams'	Night terrors	Nightmares	Syncope
Age	Infancy	Infancy	Preschool	Preschool	School	Preschool/ school age	All ages	All ages
Circumstances	Always upset	Anytime/ anywhere	Anytime/ anywhere	Anytime/ anywhere	Commonly school, watching TV, times of inactivity	First third of sleep (non-REM)	Second half of sleep (REM)	Always triggering factor or situational
Frequency	Varies greatly	Sometimes many per day	1 month or less	Daily or less	Varies but not large numbers per day	Nightly or less. Rarely more than one per night	Nightly or less	Occasional
Onset	Sudden, with or without crying	Sudden	Sudden	Sudden	Vague	Sudden	Sudden	Gradual or sudden
Recovery	Slow if hypoxic seizure occurs	Rapid	Rapid	Rapid	Vague. May be 'snapped out'	Returns to sleep	Remains asleep	Gradual
Duration	Seconds to minutes	Seconds	1–5 min	Minutes to hours	Seconds to minutes	Minutes	Minutes	Seconds to minutes

Table 29.2 Non-epileptic paroxysmal events Cont'd

	Breath-holding attacks	Shuddering	Benign paroxysmal vertigo	Infantile self stimulation	'Day dreams'	Night terrors	Nightmares	Syncope
Impairment of consciousness	Usually	No	No	No	Apparent but not real	Apparently awake but does not respond	Asleep	Yes
Observations	Cyanotic or pale, limp, may develop opisthotonos/ seizure	Rapid shivering movements maximal in head, trunk and arms	Frightened, pale, holds onto objects to maintain balance or falls	Posturing with stiffening and while lying on side or supine, leaning against firm edge. Irregular breathing, flushing, sweating	Blank staring but no motor automatisms or blinking despite long episodes. Not precipitated by hyperventilation	Screaming, crying inconsolably, may get out of bed. Appears terrified	Nil	May describe light headedness, dizziness or loss of vision. Tonic or tonic/clonic seizure may occur at end
Post-event impairment	Mild unless hypoxic seizure occurs	No	No	No	No	No recollection of event	Good recall of events	Minimal
Main differential	Epilepsy	Epilepsy	Epilepsy	Seizures/ abdominal pain, movement disorder	Absence seizures	Frontal lobe epilepsy	Night terrors	Epilepsy/Cardiac

General and neurological examination

- These findings will provide a baseline for further assessment and must be carefully recorded.
- Assessment using the Glasgow coma chart is advisable.
- Cervical spine injury must also be diagnosed or excluded as it may occur in association with head injury.

Radiological examination

- A skull X-ray is not performed routinely in patients presenting with head injury, nor is it used to determine whether or not a child requires admission. If a child is assessed as being clinically unwell after a head injury, he or she should be transferred immediately to a centre with paediatric neurosurgical expertise; the transfer should not be delayed by the taking of a skull X-ray.
- If the child is unwell enough to warrant a skull X-ray, he or she should be in hospital under observation. There is no place for a skull X-ray 'just in case'. The only exception is the child with a large scalp haematoma who is otherwise perfectly well, where a depressed skull fracture cannot be excluded clinically.
- A cervical spine X-ray is necessary when there is a suggestion that the spine has been damaged, and as a routine in all patients with severe head injuries.
- A CT scan is indicated in all patients with significant head injury, particularly if there is the possibility of an intracranial haematoma, as suggested by severe headache and vomiting, a depressed conscious state or focal neurological signs.

Blunt head injury

This form of injury is due to an impact on a flat surface that produces an acceleration–deceleration type of injury.

Effects

- Scalp haematomas are common – in the infant or young child it may be responsible for a significant reduction in the circulating blood volume.
- Skull fracture – significant injuries may not necessarily have a skull fracture, but the majority do. Conversely, a skull fracture may not be associated with significant brain injury. The fracture is usually linear and it may extend to the skull base. The

involvement of the nasal, paranasal or middle ear spaces implies that the injury is compound, with the risk of infection. Check for CSF rhinorrhoea or otorrhoea.

- Concussion – the duration of unconsciousness is an indicator of the severity of the concussion.
- Localised brain damage – this is due to either local deformity at impact (which is not generally an important factor except for some injuries in infancy), or surface laceration of the brain due to brain movement within the skull.
- Intracranial haemorrhage – subarachnoid and subdural haemorrhages are usually due to a surface laceration of the brain. In extradural haemorrhage, a dural vessel is torn by distortion at or near the point of impact, especially if on the lateral aspect of the head.
- Intracerebral haemorrhage may result from local damage or a shearing injury within the brain.

Clinical course

Most patients rapidly recover from the effects of concussion in 12–24 h. A delay or reversal of recovery suggests haemorrhage, brain swelling, infection or an extracranial complication – most commonly an impairment of ventilation (hypercarbia→brain swelling).

Management
Mild

- A brief loss of consciousness (<5 min) suggests a mild injury, and these patients can be sent home after an initial 4 h observation in emergency.
- An adequate explanation must be given to the parents and they must be given written information regarding signs suggesting deterioration, and indications for re-presentation (see below).
- The patient should be reviewed the following day, either by the local medical officer (LMO) or in emergency.

Blows to the side of the head are potentially serious, and these patients should be admitted.

Serious

A more serious head injury is indicated by:

- A longer period of unconsciousness.
- Increasingly severe headache with or without vomiting.

- A deterioration in the conscious state, behaviour or vital signs.
- Neurological defects.
- Bleeding or CSF leak from the nose or ear.
- Severe bleeding from a scalp wound.
- A superficial haematoma on the side of the head may be associated with an extradural haematoma, even if no fracture is seen on the X-ray.

Children with these sings will require admission and must be observed carefully for at least 48 h.

Delayed presentation
These can be grouped into four categories:
- Symptoms and signs as described for potentially serious head injuries – admit.
- Patients with a wide linear fracture and a large scalp haematoma – admit.
- Patients presenting with a skull X-ray showing a narrow linear fracture, but who do not require admission on clinical grounds – discuss with a neurosurgeon.
- Apparently well patients – send home after appropriate advice, with instructions to return immediately if there is any deterioration.

Localised head injury
In these injuries the damage is predominantly confined to a focal area of the head. Injuries of this type are relatively more common in children than in adults.

Effects
- Simple or compound depressed fractures are common.
- Infection may occur with compound injuries.
- Focal contusion or laceration of the brain may be present to a varying size or depth, and may produce neurological signs or seizures.
- Concussion may be absent.

Management
- X-rays are always required, and should be performed as part of the admission including, where indicated, tangential views. CT is indicated in these focal injuries.

- Admission for neurosurgical assessment is required in most cases.
- To prevent wound infection all patients with external compound injuries with head wounds should be placed on antibiotics (such as flucloxacillin 15 mg/kg (max 500 mg) orally, 6 hourly for 24–48 h), and the wound covered by a head dressing. Prophylactic antibiotics are not indicated, however, for patients with internal compound fractures (base of skull) with CSF leaks. These patients should be observed closely and, if they develop a fever with no obvious focus, given empiric antibiotics (e.g. flucloxacillin 50 mg/kg (max 2 g) i.v. 4–6 hourly and cefotaxime 50 mg/kg (max 2 g) i.v. 6 hourly).

Care of the unconscious patient

- Maintain the airway.
- Observe for vital and basal neurological signs.
- Ensure temperature regulation.
- Fluid and electrolyte balance.
- Nasogastric aspiration to avoid the inhalation of gastric contents (orogastric if the base of the skull is fractured).

Anticipate complications

Early evaluation to assess the development of complications, such as compression and infection, is essential. Observing for complications associated with extracranial injury is also important. The patient who is not improving should be referred to the neurosurgeon.

Head injury instruction to parents

For the next 24 h keep a careful watch over the patient who should be roused at least every 2 h. The child must be brought back to the emergency department immediately if the parent notices any of the following:

- The child becomes unconscious or more difficult to rouse.
- The child becomes confused, irrational or delirious.
- There are convulsions or spasms of the face and limbs.
- The child complains of persistent headache or neck stiffness occurs.
- Vomiting occurs repeatedly.
- There is bleeding from the ear or recurrent watery discharge from the ear or nose.

CSF SHUNT PROBLEMS

Subacute shunt obstruction

Aetiology

- *Upper end block*. The tube is too long or blocked by the choroid plexus.
- *Lower end block*. The tube is too short or blocked by abdominal tissues.
- *Disconnection*.

Symptoms

- Headache.
- Drowsiness.
- Vomiting.
- Fits.
- The same as a previous episode.

Signs

- Fontanelle tension.
- Abnormal cranial percussion note.
- Focal neurological signs.
- A change in vital signs.
- A deterioration in the conscious state.
- A recent increase in head circumference in infants.

Specific signs

- *Upper end block*. The pump depresses but it does not refill.
- *Lower end block*. The pump is difficult to depress. An X-ray of the chest or abdomen will give an indication of the length of the tube.
- Disconnection. The signs depend on the site of the disconnection. Ventricular tube disconnection is unusual and has the same signs as upper end block. Pump disconnection produces local swelling. Disconnection along the course of the tubing may produce local swelling. X-rays may demonstrate a disconnection.

Assessment

The neurosurgeon will want to know:

- The symptoms and signs, including the state of the pump and shunt tubing.
- The findings on plain X-ray, CT head scan or ultrasound.
- The type of shunt: atrial or peritoneal.

Shunt infection

These infections are often indolent, and should be suspected in any child with a shunt who is constitutionally unwell with fevers. There may be associated obstruction, with symptoms and signs as above.

CHAPTER 30
ORTHOPAEDIC CONDITIONS

Kerr Graham
Peter Barnett

NEONATAL ORTHOPAEDIC CONDITIONS

Developmental dysplasia of the hip

This condition was previously known as congenital dislocation of the hip; however, not all cases are present at birth, and the hips are not necessarily dislocated. Risk factors are breech delivery, caesarean section, family history, congenital foot abnormality, other congenital anomalies, being the first born and being female.

Diagnosis
General screening

All neonates should have a clinical examination for hip joint instability: the Ortolani and Barlow tests. The baby should be relaxed. With the knee flexed, the thumb is placed over the lesser trochanter and the middle finger over the greater trochanter. The pelvis is steadied with the other hand and the flexed thigh is abducted and adducted. Any clunk or jerk where a dislocation reduces, allowing the hip to abduct fully is Ortolani's sign. The demonstration of acetabular dislocation by levering the femoral head in and out of the acetabulum is Barlow's sign (see Fig. 30.1).

Selective screening

Infants in high-risk groups and those with an abnormal routine clinical screening examination should have an ultrasound examination of their hips.

- As clinical diagnosis can be difficult and ultrasound has diagnostic limitations, the repeated examination of children during the first year of life is important.
- X-rays are helpful after 3 months.

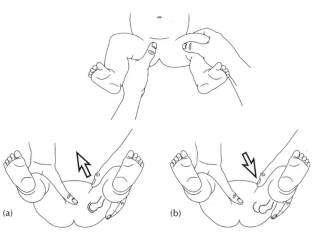

Fig. 30.1 Screening for developmental dysplasia of the hip. (a) Ortolani's sign, (b) Barlow's sign.

Management

The earlier the diagnosis the easier the management.

- Most neonates can be successfully treated by abduction bracing with a Pavlik harness.
- Operative treatments, including open reduction, may be required with later diagnosis.

Club foot (congenital talipes equinovarus)

Most infants with abnormal-looking feet are said to have 'talipes'. However, the majority have postural problems such as talipes calcaneovalgus (excessive dorsiflexion and eversion), metatarsus varus (adduction of the forefoot) or postural talipes equinovarus (see Fig. 30.2). These deformities are usually mild and mobile; i.e. they correct easily and fully with the pressure of one finger. They resolve spontaneously with no treatment.

The true club foot deformity is more severe and is often stiff. The foot is in equinus, with the hind foot in varus, and the forefoot supinated.

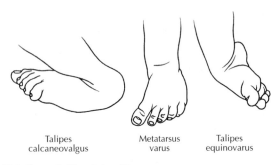

| Talipes calcaneovalgus | Metatarsus varus | Talipes equinovarus |

Fig. 30.2 Congenital foot deformities

Management

- All require manipulation and casting.
- Soft tissue surgery is required for many.
- Bone surgery is required for a few.

TORSIONAL AND ANGULAR DEFORMITIES IN CHILDREN

Many children are seen with normal angular or torsional variants. It can be difficult to distinguish physiological variation from pathological conditions. The range of 'normality' is very wide, but what parents accept is much narrower. The physiological variations in normal children can result in as much anxiety as the pathological disorders.

Intoeing

Intoeing in childhood can be due to metatarsus varus, internal tibial torsion or medial femoral torsion.

See Table 30.1 and Figures 30.3 and 30.4.

Out-toeing

Infants and toddlers have restricted internal rotation at the hip because of an external rotation contracture, not retroversion of the femur.

Infants

- Present with a 'Charlie Chaplin' posture between 3 and 12 months.

Table 30.1 Intoeing in childhood

	Metatarsus varus	*Internal tibial torsion*	*Medial femoral torsion*
Synonyms	Metatarsus adductus		Inset hips
Age at presentation	Birth	Toddler	Child
Site of problem	Foot	Tibia	Femur
Examination	Sole of foot bean shaped	Thigh–foot angle is inwards	Arc of hip rotation favours internal rotation
Management	Observe or cast	Observe and reassure	Observe, rarely surgery
When to refer if not resolved	3 months after presentation	6 months after presentation	8 years after presentation

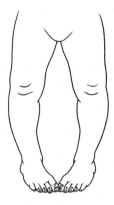

Fig. 30.3 Internal tibial torsion

- The child weight bears and walks normally.
- Resolution occurs with no treatment.

Children

- May be due to neurologic disorder.
- Surgery may be necessary.

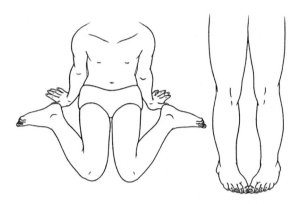

Fig. 30.4 Medial femoral torsion

Bow legs (genu varum)

The vast majority are physiological. Rare causes include skeletal dysplasias, rickets and Blount's disease (tibia vara).

Presentation

- Toddlers are usually bowed until 3 years of age.
- Physiological bowing is symmetrical, not excessive and improves with time.

Management

Monitor intercondylar separation (ICS; see Fig. 30.5). Refer when ICS is greater than 6 cm, is not improving or when it is asymmetric.

Knock knees (genu valgum)

Again, the vast majority are physiological. Rare causes are rickets and trauma.

Presentation

- Children are usually knock-kneed from 3 to 8 years.
- Physiological knock-knee is symmetrical, not excessive and improves with time.

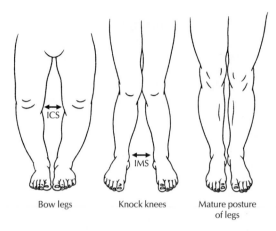

Fig. 30.5 Postural variants in the lower limbs

Bow legs   Knock knees   Mature posture of legs

Management

- Monitor the intermalleolar separation (IMS; see Fig. 30.5).
- Refer if IMS greater than 8 cm.

Note: Most children with bow legs or knock knees are normal with <1% having an underlying problem.

Flat feet (pes plano valgus)

This condition is painless and asymptomatic. Note: If painful or stiff, referral is needed.

Causes

- Physiological (in the vast majority): all newborns have flat feet due to fat that fills the medial longitudinal arch; 80% of children develop a medial arch by their sixth birthday.
- Tarsal coalition (in older children and adolescents only).

Management

- No treatment is required unless the condition is painful or stiff.
- The condition is unaffected by orthotics or exercises.
- The majority of cases resolve spontaneously.

TRAUMA

The management of fractures and dislocations is an integral part of the overall management of the traumatised patient. Common fractures in children involve the wrist, elbow, clavicle, distal tibia, and fibula and femur. Each has distinct management strategies but common themes run through.

Assessment

Patients presenting with a suspected fracture or dislocation require a full evaluation of the fracture, and damage to other structures needs to be excluded.

An accurate history of the mechanism of injury will determine which structures may potentially be damaged.

Examination

- A closed or open fracture (the latter will require operative intervention).
- Deformity or swelling (*note*: acute swelling in children usually indicates a fracture).
- Neurological status distal to the injury.
- Peripheral pulses – if the blood flow to the limb is compromised, emergency orthopaedic consultation is necessary.

Management

- The affected limb should be splinted by a board or plaster slab prior to an X-ray.
- Analgesia (usually parenteral) is required (e.g. pethidine 0.5– 2 mg/kg (max 25–100 mg) or 0.5–1.0 mg/kg (max 25–50 mg) i.v.).
- An X-ray should be obtained to examine the joint above and below the suspected fracture site. An anteroposterior and lateral view should be obtained.
- If the angle between the shaft of the bone and the fractured fragment is greater than 15–20°, manipulation of the fracture needs to occur prior to the placement of a plaster. Forearm fractures in children 6 years or older can usually be manipulated using a local anaesthetic block (e.g. Bier's Block).

- If the fracture involves both cortices of the bone, a plaster involving the joint above and below should be placed (e.g. above the elbow for a forearm fracture).
- A simple undisplaced greenstick or buckle fracture can be treated in a short cast.

Home treatment after a full plaster

- Elevate the limb above the heart level for the next 24–48 h.
- A sling should only be worn after this period and the hand should not be below the elbow while in the sling.
- Crutches should only be used by children over 6–7 years of age.
- Written plaster instructions should be explained and given to parents.

Follow up

For patients who have had a manipulation of fracture or a fracture involving both cortices of the bone, a repeat X-ray should be obtained in 1 week to ensure the correct position is maintained. Plaster should remain in place for 3–6 weeks, depending on the degree of injury. Following the removal of the cast, the bone is still at risk of re-fracture for the next 8–12 weeks; therefore, contact sports are not recommended during this period.

SPECIFIC MANAGEMENT OF SOME COMMON FRACTURES

Clavicle

- Sling for 2–3 weeks.
- Inform the parents of the lump that will develop at the fracture site and that may be visible for up to 1 year.
- No contact sports for 6 weeks.
- No follow-up X-ray is necessary in children, but proximal ephiphysis is required in adolescents.

Humerus
Surgical neck

- *Undisplaced* – sling for 3 weeks.
- *Displaced* – frequently treated with a collar and cuff – refer for an orthopaedic opinion.

Shaft

- Check the integrity of the radial nerve.
- *Undisplaced* – collar and cuff. A U-shaped plaster slab may be applied to the humerus to reduce movement and minimise knocks.
- *Transverse/displaced/comminuted* – refer for an immediate orthopaedic consultation.

Supracondylar

- Check the integrity of the radial artery, radial nerve, median nerve and ulnar nerve.
- If there is vascular compromise, extend the elbow until perfusion returns.
- *Undisplaced* – collar and cuff with the elbow flexed for 3–4 weeks.
- *Angulated, displaced or comminuted* – refer for an immediate orthopaedic consultation.

Epiphyseal and intra-articular

- Refer for an immediate orthopaedic consultation.

Radius and ulna

Shaft

- *Undisplaced* – above elbow plaster, follow up with an orthopaedic opinion.
- *Displaced* – refer for an immediate orthopaedic consultation.

Distal end

- *Undisplaced* and non-deformed clinically:
  - if a single cortex is only involved, use a short arm cast for 3–4 weeks
  - if both cortices are involved, plaster above the elbow – refer for an orthopaedic opinion within a week.
- *Displaced and clinically deformed* – use LAMP (local anaesthesia manipulation plaster) in the emergency department.
- *Totally displaced* with fracture ends not touching – use GAMP (general anaesthesia manipulation plaster) in theatre.

Metacarpals

- Check carefully for rotation at the fracture site.
- *Undisplaced* – volar slab; follow up with an orthopaedic opinion.
- *Displaced* – refer for an immediate orthopaedic consultation.

Phalanges (hand)

- Check carefully for rotation at the fracture site.
- Intra-articular fractures require anatomical reduction.
- *Undisplaced* – strap to the adjacent finger.
- *Displaced* – refer for an immediate orthopaedic or plastic surgical consultation; some may be reduced under regional nerve block.

Femur

- Isolated femur fractures in young children rarely cause hypotension; however, in adolescents and patients with multi-trauma an intravenous line should be inserted.
- Ensure adequate analgesia with entonox, opioids and a femoral nerve block.
- Apply simple skin traction, refer for an immediate orthopaedic consultation.

Tibia

Undisplaced:

- *Proximal* – above-knee plaster, follow up with an orthopaedic opinion within 1 week (there is a risk of valgus deformity).
- *Distal* – below-knee plaster, follow up with an orthopaedic opinion.
- *Displaced* – will need manipulation, refer for an immediate orthopaedic consultation.

Toddlers' fracture

- This is a clinical diagnosis in a young child where a fractured tibia is suspected on clinical grounds (i.e. non-weight bearing after a fall or tender tibia/fibula on palpation), but no abnormality is detected on the X-ray.
- Exclude septic arthritis/osteomyelitis.

- Apply an above-knee plaster for pain relief, or allow weight bearing as the child desires if the pain is minimal.
- Limping will continue for 6 weeks.

Ankle

- *Undisplaced* – below-knee plaster, follow up with an orthopaedic opinion.
- *Displaced* – will need manipulation, refer for an immediate orthopaedic consultation.

Metatarsals

- *Undisplaced* – lower leg plaster slab, followed by elevation, follow up with an orthopaedic opinion within 1 week.

Note: Consider child abuse in infants with fractures.

ANKLE INJURY

True sprains or soft tissue injuries are more common in adolescents. Younger children with open growth plates are more likely to sustain a growth plate injury or fracture and should be treated in a plaster cast.

Clinical assessment

- Mechanism of injury – it is usually caused by an inversion injury to the ankle.
- Was the patient able to bear weight immediately after the injury?
- Where is the swelling most prominent?
- What is the point of maximal tenderness?

Investigation

X-rays are required if:

- Deformity is present
- Maximal tenderness occurs over the tibia or fibula
- The patient is unable to weight bear.

Note: If the patient is tender over the growth plate of the tibia or fibula and the X-rays are normal, the patient has a Salter-Harris 1 epiphyseal injury and it should be treated in a below-knee plaster. However, if there is a large amount of swelling use a plaster slab.

If none of the above conditions apply the treatment will depend on the severity of symptoms.

Management: mild–moderate sprain

Remember the RICE acronym:

- *R*est – non-weight bearing should occur for a few days to a period of 2–3 weeks.
- *I*ce – should be applied every 2–3 h for 15 min during the first 48 h; then heat can be applied.
- *C*ompression – should be accomplished either with a firm bandage or a plaster slab.
- *E*levation – the limb should be elevated on a few pillows whenever possible to allow the swelling to subside.

Management: severe sprain

Treat like a fracture:

- Use below-knee plaster (or if the swelling is severe, a plaster slab followed by a full plaster) for 2–4 weeks.
- Non-weight bearing for the first week.
- Gradual rehabilitation should occur after several days of rest. This includes gentle weight bearing and ankle exercises to strengthen the damaged ankle ligaments (initially plantar- and dorsiflexion exercises as soon as possible; later toe raises and inversion/eversion exercises when the pain has subsided).

PULLED ELBOW

Clinical features

- This injury tends to occur usually at the age of 1–3 years.
- The cause of injury is usually another person pulling the child's arm forcefully. There may be a crack or popping sound at the time. Occasionally, it may occur after a fall.
- The arm is held pronated and slightly flexed (i.e. limp by their side as if they are ignoring it).
- The child is not distressed and is not using the apparently lifeless limb.
- Palpation from the clavicle to the wrist does not demonstrate any swelling or tenderness.
- Supination of the arm causes pain.

Investigations

If the symptoms are typical of a pulled elbow, no investigations are necessary.

Management

- Hold the child's hand as if to shake it and with your other hand encircle the elbow with the thumb over the annular ligament of the radius.
- Gently apply traction and supinate the hand. Flex the forearm at the elbow all the way to the shoulder. You should feel a pop as the radial head is relocated.
- The child should be moving the arm normally within 10–15 min.

Note: If the history is not typical or there is swelling or your attempts fail, an X-ray of the elbow should be obtained to exclude a radial head fracture.

LIMP IN CHILDHOOD

Limp is a common presenting complaint in childhood (see Table 30.2).

Clinical assessment

- Is the limp acute, subacute or chronic?
- Is there associated pain or fever or both?
- Are there other constitutional symptoms?
- Have there been previous episodes of pain or limp?
- What position is the leg held in (e.g. flexed and externally rotated)?

Table 30.2 Differential diagnosis of limp in childhood

Acute	Subacute	Chronic
Fracture	Juvenile rheumatoid arthritis	Cerebral palsy
Irritable hip	Tumour/leukaemia	Developmental dysplasia of the hips
Septic arthritis	Acute on chronic SCFE	Perthes' disease
Osteomyelitis		Chronic SCFE

SCFE, slipped capital femoral epiphysis.

- Does joint movement or bony pressure cause pain?
- Is there limitation of movement?

Investigations
- Full blood examination (FBE), differential, erythrocyte sedimentation rate (ESR); and C-reactive protein.
- Take a plain X-ray of the joint or affected limb.
- Ultrasound of hip if it is painful (looking for fluid in the joint).
- Arrange a bone scan (after orthopaedic consultation).

Management
This will depend on the underlying problem:
- Slipped capital femoral epiphysis (SCFE), tumours, Perthes' disease or developmental dysplasia of the hip should be referred immediately to an orthopaedic surgeon.
- Toddlers' fractures may be occult and not seen on an X-ray. If the child is afebrile then observation is appropriate.
- A bone scan should be arranged for worsening or changing symptoms.

Irritable hip (transient synovitis)
This is a common condition. A child who is constitutionally well presents with a painful hip and difficulty walking. This condition needs to be distinguished from the others listed in Table 30.2. Although it is the commonest reason for limp in the preschooler, irritable hip is a diagnosis of exclusion.

Clinical features
- This usually occurs in 3–8 year olds.
- There is a history of a recent viral illness (which lasts 1–2 weeks).
- There is an absence of trauma.
- Children are usually able to walk, but with pain.
- The severity of the symptoms may vary with time.
- The child is afebrile and appears well.
- There is a mild to moderate decrease in the range of motion due to pain, particularly internal rotation.

Note: The less movement in the joint, the more likely the cause is infective.

Investigations

- This is the same as for limp (see above; ultrasound usually demonstrates an effusion).
- X-rays and FBE are normal with an ESR of <20.

Note: The history, symptoms and signs of an irritable hip overlap with septic arthritis, which is a serious condition requiring urgent treatment. *If there is any suspicion of bone or joint sepsis, paediatric orthopaedic consultation is required and admission to hospital should be arranged.*

Management

Rest in bed and simple analgesics are the treatment of choice. The more the child can rest the quicker the recovery. Patients may have a relapse if they increase their activity too quickly. Occasionally, these patients need to be admitted to hospital for bed rest and traction.

Acute bone and joint sepsis (septic arthritis (SA) and osteomyelitis (OM))

This can affect any joint or bone, but most commonly involves the lower limbs. *SA is an orthopaedic emergency with drainage and antibiotics essential to prevent long-term morbidity.*

Clinical features

- There is an acute onset of limp/non-weight bearing/non-movement of the limb (may be delayed in OM).
- The pain is localised to the joint or the metaphysis of the bone.
- There is irritability and poor feeding in infants.
- The temperature is usually >38.5°C.
- The joint is held in a mid position.
- There is pain on all movements with a decreased range of movement (severe in SA).

Investigations

(As for limp (see above).)

- The ESR is usually >20–30.
- The white cell count (WCC) is raised in SA and is usually raised in OM.
- A bone scan may be indicated if the diagnosis is not clear.

Management

- Admit to hospital; keep nil orally.
- Intravenous antibiotics (covering *Staphylococcus aureus, Haemophilus influenzae* and Gram-negative organisms in neonates). See Antibiotic guidelines.
- Urgent paediatric orthopaedic consultation is required, and possibly surgery.

Perthes' disease

This is a specific hip disease of childhood. Affected children have a generalised disorder of growth with a tendency to low birthweight and delayed bone age. The pathology is avascular necrosis of the capital femoral epiphysis followed by a sequence of changes including resorption of necrotic bone, reossification and remodelling. This sequence of events is seen radiologically as density of the capital epiphysis, patchy osteolysis, new bone formation and remodelling with a variable degree of femoral head deformity.

Clinical features

- Age range: 2–12 years, but the majority present between 4 and 8 years.
- Sex ratio: five males to one female, 20% bilateral.
- Symptoms: pain and limp, usually for at least 1 week.
- Signs: restriction of hip motion.

Investigations

- X-ray.
- A bone scan is useful in the early stages before the signs are clear on an X-ray.

Management principles

- Resting the hip in the early irritable phase.
- Regaining motion if the hip is stiff.
- Containing the hip by bracing or surgery in selected patients.

Slipped capital femoral epiphysis (SCFE)

Can occur acutely or chronically. Its early detection will prevent later morbidity.

Clinical features

- Age: this occurs in late childhood to early adolescence. Maximum incidence in girls aged 10–12 years and boys 12–14 years.
- Patient weight is usually >90th percentile.
- There is pain in the hip or knee.
- There is a limp.
- The hip appears externally rotated and shortened.
- There is decreased hip movement, particularly internal rotation.

Note: The condition can be bilateral.

Investigation

Take an X-ray of the pelvis and a *frog leg lateral* of the affected hip.

Management

- The patient should not weight bear if the diagnosis is entertained.
- Urgent orthopaedic referral and surgery to prevent further slipping is required.

SCOLIOSIS

Definitions

- Scoliosis is a curvature in the spine when viewed from the frontal (coronal) plane.
- A structural scoliosis occurs when the curvature has an element of rotation and may progress with growth.
- A non-structural scoliosis may be secondary to a problem outside the spine, such as unequal leg lengths.

Detection

The most common type of scoliosis is adolescent scoliosis, affecting girls in 90% of cases. Because abnormal spinal curvatures start small and may progress with time and growth, efforts have been made to detect the condition at an early stage by school screening programs. This is usually done by the forward bend test, in which the examiner observes the spine from behind as the subject bends forwards. Flexion of the spine usually demonstrates the deformity much more clearly because of the asymmetry of the ribs and chest wall. Very small curves are relatively common and it can be difficult to decide when an X-ray is required, which curves are likely to progress and which require brace treatment or surgery. The risk of curve progression is related to the age at presentation and the size and cause of the curve.

Ten per cent of normal teenagers have a curve of 5° or more, but only 2% have curves of >10°.

Management

All children with scoliosis should be referred to a paediatric orthopaedic surgeon.

- If the curvature <20° – observe.
- If the curvature is 20–40° – a brace is recommended.
- If the curvature is >40° – surgery is required.

CHAPTER 31
RENAL CONDITIONS AND ENURESIS

Colin Jones
Harley Powell
Rowan Walker
Annie Moulden

Significant renal disease in childhood usually presents in one of the following ways:

- Antenatal ultrasound abnormality of the urinary tract
- Urinary tract infection (UTI)
- Functional voiding disorder
- Proteinuria (including nephrotic syndrome)
- Haematuria
- Hypertension
- Acute renal failure
- Chronic renal failure.

ANTENATAL ABNORMALITIES

See Fig. 31.1.

URINARY TRACT INFECTIONS

All children with a first UTI need investigation.

Diagnosis
Urine infections are diagnosed by bacterial growth on midstream urine (MSU), catheter (CSU) or suprapubic aspirate (SPA) specimens of urine.

Bag urine specimen collection
- A bag urine specimen that has no growth excludes a UTI; however, a UTI cannot be diagnosed from a bag specimen.

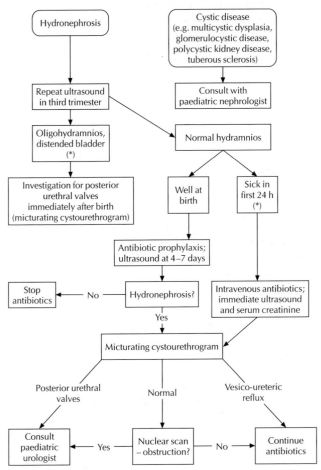

* Consult a paediatric nephrologist or urologist early in all cases

Fig. 31.1 Antenatal abnormalities

- In sick infants or those where the suspicion of UTI is high (e.g. renal tract anomaly or previous UTI), a bag specimen should not be taken, as it only delays the diagnosis. An SPA (preferred) or CSU sample should be obtained.

Urine 'ward test' strips

The ward test strips for leucocytes or nitrites are negative in up to 15% of UTI in infants.

Midstream urine specimen collection

This can be obtained from children who are able to void on request (usually by 3–4 years of age). The child's genitalia are first washed with warm water. In girls the labia should be separated. The child is asked to void. After discarding the first few millilitres, a specimen is collected. A pure growth of >10^5 colony-forming units per litre (c.f.u./L) can be used as evidence of infection; up to 50% of urine specimens from patients with symptomatic UTI have no pyuria or nitrituria or both. Confirmatory testing may be needed in selected patients.

Suprapubic aspirate collection

Aspirated urine should be sterile, hence any growth of bacteria indicates infection (see Procedures, chapter 3 for collection technique).

Catheter specimen collection

These are useful in infants after a failed SPA, or in older children who are unable to void on request. A pure growth of >10^5 c.f.u./L indicates infection (see Procedures, chapter 3 for collection technique).

Management

- Most infants who are <6 months of age with a UTI and older children with acute pyelonephritis (fever, vomiting and loin/abdominal pain) require i.v. benzylpenicillin 50 mg/kg (max 3 g) 6 hourly and gentamicin 7.5 mg/kg (max 240 mg) daily.
- In older children without pyelonephritis, a 5-day course of oral antibiotics is usually sufficient (see Antibiotic guidelines). Antibiotic sensitivity should be checked when available (usually at 48 h).
- Prophylactic antibiotics should be commenced immediately after the treatment antibiotic course has finished.

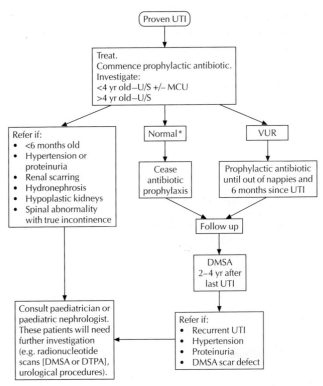

U/S   ultrasound
MCU   micturating cystourethrogram
VUR   vesico-ureteric reflux
* A normal U/S does not exclude scarring

Fig. 31.2 An outline of the management of a proven urinary
tract infection (UTI)

- Prophylactic antibiotics should be continued until the minimal
  initial investigations have been performed, and a decision is
  then made on the basis of the anatomy of the urinary tract
  (see Fig. 31.2). See Antimicrobial guidelines.
- For neonates <1 month old or preterm infants, discuss with a
  paediatrician.

Minimal initial investigations

Forty per cent of children with UTI have renal tract abnormalities, including vesico-ureteric reflux (VUR, 35%), reflux nephropathy (renal scarring, 12%), pelviureteric junction (PUJ) or vesico-ureteric junction (VUJ) obstruction (together 4–6%), and other congenital abnormalities. The following can be utilised:

- Renal ultrasound (U/S).
- A DMSA scan performed 2–4 years after the last UTI to indicate whether the renal injury requires further follow up.
- Micturating cystourethrogram (MCU), which is mandatory in children <12 months of age. It is currently recommended for children <4 years of age.

Figure 31.2 outlines further management.

Investigation of siblings of a child with VUR

- Fifty per cent of siblings of a child with VUR will have or have had it.
- If the sibling <1 year or a newborn – MCU and U/S.
- If sibling >1 year – U/S alone.

PROTEINURIA

Isolated proteinuria

See Fig. 31.3.

Nephrotic syndrome

Diagnosis

The diagnosis of nephrotic syndrome is made on the basis of proteinuria (>40 mg/m² per h on a recumbent urine, usually >3 g/1.73 m²/day; usually 3+ to 4+ on dipstick testing), generalised oedema, hypo-albuminaemia (<25 g/L) and hypercholesterolaemia (>4.5 mmol/L).

Management

Exclude life-threatening complications:

- Sepsis (e.g. peritonitis).
- Symptomatic hypovolaemia (e.g. cool extremities and postural hypotension).

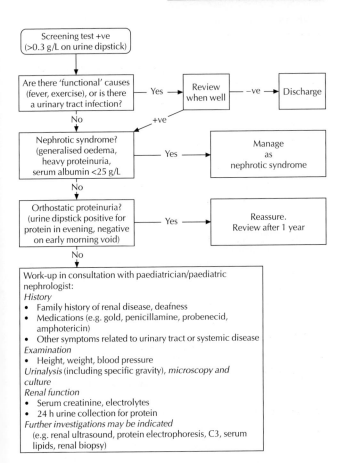

Fig. 31.3 Isolated proteinuria

- Symptomatic thromboembolism (e.g. venous sinus thrombosis: convulsions and a reduced conscious state; deep venous thrombosis, and pulmonary embolism).
- Symptomatic oedema (e.g. marked ascites, respiratory distress with pleural effusions, and skin breakdown).

Admit to hospital: for initial assessment, as well as patient and family education.

Treatment

(*Note:* Minor variations in protocol may exist between different centres.)

- Prednisolone: administer according to the following dosage schedule:
    - 60 mg/m^2 per day as a single dose up to a maximum of 80 mg/day until there is a remission of proteinuria (to trace or negative on urinalysis) for 4 days
    - 45 mg/m^2 per day for 8 days
    - 60 mg/m^2 per alternate day for 8 days (four doses)
    - 45 mg/m^2 per alternate day for 8 days
    - 30 mg/m^2 per alternate day for 8 days
    - reduce by 5 mg every 8 days until finished.
- Phenoxymethylpenicillin: 12.5 mg/kg (max 1 g) oral twice daily to prevent pneumococcal sepsis while oedematous.
- Aspirin: 10 mg/kg per alternate day to reduce the incidence of arterial thromboses.

Note: The long-term prognosis of nephrotic syndrome is dependent on the response to predisolone.

Treatment of complications

- Symptomatic oedema – concentrated albumin (i.e. 20%) 1 g/kg (5 mL/kg), i.v. over 4 h with frusemide 1 mg/kg at 2 and 4 h after the start of the infusion.
- Circulatory insufficiency – concentrated albumin 1 g/kg, i.v. over 4 h. (Administer frusemide only if the circulation is markedly improved at the end of the infusion – it is dangerous in hypovolaemic patients.)
- Thrombo-embolism – systemic anticoagulation with heparin, followed by warfarin for 3–6 months.
- Sepsis – high-dose antibiotic therapy to cover *Streptococcus pneumoniae*, *Haemophilus influenzae* and *Escherichia coli* (e.g. cefotaxime 50 mg/kg (max 2 g) i.v., 6 hourly). In suspected primary peritonitis:

- Use a peritoneal tap to establish diagnosis.
- If early diagnosis and minimal symptoms, antibiotic therapy alone may be sufficient.
- It usually requires laparotomy for a peritoneal lavage.

Additional treatments

If the patient does not respond to steroids, refer to a paediatric nephrologist for consideration of cyclophosphamide or cyclosporin A treatment.

Indications for renal biopsy

- Age: less than 1 year of age.
- Failure to respond to prednisolone within 3–4 weeks of treatment using 60 mg/m^2 per day, either at diagnosis or with relapse.
- Nephritic/nephrotic syndrome (increased blood pressure, moderate haematuria, and renal impairment without evidence of peripheral circulatory insufficiency).
- Low complement (C3).

Relapse

Most (75%) patients relapse.

- This is usually precipitated by a febrile illness or an allergic reaction.
- Four days of heavy proteinuria (>100 mg/dL; i.e. 3+ to 4+ on urine dipstick) distinguishes relapse from transient proteinuria associated with a febrile illness.
- Treat as for the initial diagnosis, with the use of penicillin and aspirin if the patient becomes oedematous.

Indications for referral

Refer to a paediatric nephrologist in cases of:

- Nephritic/nephrotic syndrome
- Complications
- Failure to respond to steroids in 2–3 weeks
- Frequent relapsing nephrotic syndrome or steroid dependence.

HAEMATURIA

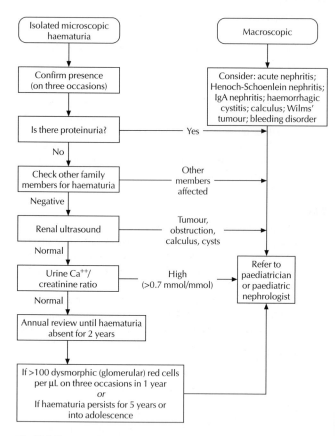

Fig. 31.4 Haematuria assessment

HYPERTENSION

Measurement
- Use a cuff with a bladder that covers at least 75% of the arm's length.
- Take in the right arm, with the patient sitting; if initially increased, retake after resting quietly.

Definition
The 95th percentiles for blood pressure (BP) at different ages in childhood are as follows:
- Newborn: 95/70
- 0–6 years: 115/75
- 6–13 years: 120/80
- 13–16 years: 135/85
- 16–18 years: 140/90.

Cautions
- As in adults, treatment of the asymptomatic child should not be based on a single BP measurement. BP should be repeated on three occasions to confirm sustained elevation. Twenty-four hour ambulatory blood pressure monitoring is suitable for most children >5 years of age.
- BP 'tracks' poorly (i.e. only 20–40% of children with BP higher than the 80th percentile still remain in that group 10 years later). Children placed on medication for essential hypertension should undergo a trial of no treatment after their BP has been controlled for 9 months.
- There are no proven advantages of lowering asymptomatic blood pressure in terms of modifying adult cardiovascular risk in normal children.
- BP reduction slows the progression of renal impairment in people with renal disease. Children with renal impairment should have their BP target range set at less than the mean BP for their age.
- Hypertensive children should be referred to a paediatrician or paediatric nephrologist for investigation for causes outlined in Tables 31.1 and 31.2.
- In asymptomatic hypertension the BP should be lowered slowly.

Table 31.1 Causes of secondary hypertension in childhood

Secondary causes	
Renal (75%)	Post-infectious glomerulonephritis
	Chronic glomerulonephritis
	Obstructive uropathy
	Polycystic kidney disease
	Autosomal recessive
	Autosomal dominant
	Reflux nephropathy
	Renovascular
	Haemolytic uraemic syndrome
Cardiovascular (15%)	Coarctation of the aorta
Endocrine (5%)	Phaeochromocytoma
	Hyperthyroidism
	Congenital adrenal hyperplasia
	Primary hyperaldosteronism
	Cushing's syndrome
Other (5%)	Neuroblastoma
	Neurofibromatosis
	Glucocorticoids
	Increased intracranial pressure

Table 31.2 Initial investigation of established hypertension

Urine	m.s.u., careful urinalysis (dipstick)
	Microscopy
	Urinary catecholamines
Blood	Creatinine
	Potassium
	Bicarbonate
Imaging	Renal ultrasound
	DMSA scan

- Angiotensin-converting enzyme inhibitors are the usual drug of choice for chronic treatment, and should be started in low doses and increased with monitoring of potassium and creatinine.

Management
Asymptomatic hypertension
Refer to paediatric nephrologist.

Symptomatic hypertension

This requires immediate treatment:

- In a conscious child, not vomiting, a nifedipine tablet crushed and given by nasogastric tube or swallowed with water. The dose is 5 mg for those <2 years of age; 10 mg for those >2 years of age. Repeat 20 minutely titrating to BP control.
- In a child with impaired consciousness or vomiting either:
  - labetalol 0.2 mg/kg i.v. push over 2 min. If no response in 5–10 min, increase to 0.4 mg/kg (max 60 mg) *or*
  - nitroprusside 0.3–8.0 µg/kg per min constant infusion (need ICU monitoring), *or*
  - diazoxide 1 mg/kg i.v. push repeated 5–10 minutely to 5 mg/kg.
- Catecholamine production: phentolamine 0.1 mg/kg i.v. bolus (to 5 mg).
- Head trauma/increased intracranial pressure: labetalol or nitroprusside. (*Note*: Nifedipine/diazoxide contraindicated.)

ACUTE RENAL FAILURE

Definition

Acute renal failure is the change in glomerular filtration such that the renal solute load (electrolytes, other ions and nitrogenous wastes) cannot be excreted. There are two main forms:

- Oliguric – acute reduction in urine output to <0.5 mL/kg per h. This form is more complex to manage (see Fig. 31.5).
- Polyuric – often subacute and clinically unapparent, until the fluid intake is reduced and the patient becomes dehydrated due to an inappropriately high urine output.

Causes

Pre-renal

- Dehydration (e.g. gastroenteritis).
- Shock.
- Sepsis.
- Nephrotic syndrome.

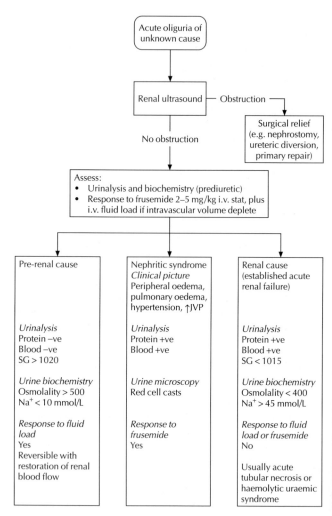

Fig. 31.5 Differentiation of types of oliguria

Renal

- Crescentic glomerulonephritis: acute post-infectious glomerulo-nephritis; membrano-proliferative glomerulonephritis; Henoch–Schoenlein purpura; and antineutrophil cytoplasmic antibody-associated haemolytic uraemic syndrome.
- Acute tubular necrosis.
- Crush injury (myoglobinuria).
- UTI with septicaemia.
- Nephrotoxin (e.g. gentamicin).

Post-renal

Obstruction, especially to a single kidney. The cause is usually apparent from the clinical context of the illness.

Management

Water

Limit to insensible losses (300 mL/m^2) plus urine output.

Sodium

Principle: intake = urine sodium + other sodium losses.

- Oliguric: minimal Na$^+$ intake.
- Polyuric: measure the urine [Na]$^+$ and volume of urine. Generally, about 75 mmol/L is required.

Potassium

There should be no intravenous or oral intake until losses of K$^+$ are established.

For hyperkalaemia:

- Repeat venous or arterial serum K$^+$ urgently. Arrange haemo-filtration or dialysis with the patient who has renal failure.
- ECG – peaked T waves, wide QRS, increased PR interval, de-creased P and R waves, ST segment depression and a prolonged QT interval.
- If K$^+$ >7 mmol/L with ECG changes:
  — 10% calcium gluconate 0.5 mL/kg i.v. over 3–5 min (do not mix with bicarbonate). Works in seconds.
  — Insulin plus concurrent glucose infusion: 0.1 U/kg rapid-acting insulin and 2 mL/kg 50% dextrose. Works in minutes.
  — Arrange a dialysis urgently.

- If K+ >7 mmol/L, no ECG changes:
  - NaHCO$_3$ 1–3 mmol/kg (shifts K+ intracellularly); however, there is the risk of hypocalcaemic tetany with decreased pH. Works within the hour.
  - Dextrose 0.5 g/kg per h (10% dextrose at 5 mL/kg per h) until blood glucose reaches 14 mmol/L (shifts K+ intracellularly). Works within the hour.
  - Arrange dialysis urgently.
- If K+ >6 mmol/L:
  - Na+ – K+ exchange resin; e.g. Resonium A, 1 g/kg p.o. (action within 6–12 h) or p.r. (action within 30 min; may repeat in 1–2 h).
  - Arrange dialysis.

Acidosis

Correct with bicarbonate (mmol = base deficit × weight × 1/3) over 4 h as long as:

- The patient is not severely hypocalcaemic (HCO$_3$ may lower Ca and cause convulsions).
- The accompanying Na load does not cause fluid overload (e.g. hypertension and pulmonary oedema).

Hypocalcaemia

This is usually due to increased serum phosphate.

- A low phosphate diet.
- Calcium carbonate (phosphate binder).
- Symptomatic hypocalcaemia may require i.v. calcium gluconate.
- There is a danger of metastatic calcification if the $Ca^{2+} \times PO_4^{3-}$ product is >5–6.
- If there is increased phosphate, consider dialysis.

Uraemia

- The acute rise in serum urea to more than 30 mmol/L may cause CNS symptoms.
- Protein restriction and high-quality protein food are required.
- A high carbohydrate diet.

Indications for dialysis/haemofiltration
- Fluid overload (hypertension or pulmonary oedema) not responding to frusemide.
- Hyperkalaemia.
- Severe metabolic acidosis.
- Progressive uraemia.
- Dialysable nephrotoxin.
- Hyperammonaemia.
- The reduction of intravascular volume to facilitate total parenteral nutrition or blood transfusion.

CHRONIC RENAL FAILURE

Presentation
- Known renal disease.
- Growth failure.
- Rickets.
- Anaemia: normochromic, normocytic.
- Laboratory test: increased serum creatinine, increased urea, increased phosphate and metabolic acidosis.
- Radiological studies: small kidney, with other renal disease; e.g. obstruction uropathy.
- Proteinuria.
- UTI.

Management
The investigation of the cause and treatment of chronic renal failure should be performed in conjunction with a paediatric nephrologist.

MONOSYMPTOMATIC NOCTURNAL ENURESIS

Nocturnal enuresis is defined as bed-wetting in a child of 5 years of age or older. It is the second commonest paediatric condition affecting 20% of 5 year olds, 5% of 10 year olds and up to 1% of adults.

Cause

Despite the widely held belief that enuresis is a behavioural or psychological problem, it is now well documented that enuresis is due to a genetically based arousal disorder that may also be associated with nocturnal antidiuretic hormone (ADH) insufficiency.

Nocturnal enuresis is usually inherited in an autosomal dominant manner with variable penetrance. It is essential to discuss family history as enuretics are often very relieved to know other family members were affected.

Enuresis occurs if the bladder becomes full and the child is unresponsive during sleep to the sensation of bladder fullness. Hence, all children with enuresis have an arousal disorder that interferes with their ability to wake to bladder distension. The bladder may become full as a result of a small functional bladder capacity or nocturnal polyuria due to ADH insufficiency. Normally, increased ADH secretion overnight reduces urine output during sleep. About 60% of children with nocturnal enuresis have failed to develop the normal circadian rhythm of ADH secretion.

There is no association between isolated bed-wetting and structural urological pathology or urinary tract infection, hence there is no need for investigation. Psychological issues are often present but are usually due to the enuresis, not the cause of it, and improve with resolution of the wetting.

Management

Many families, knowing that the wetting will eventually resolve spontaneously, choose to do nothing. As the spontaneous remission rate is only 15% per year, all children 6 years and over for whom wetting has become a problem should be offered treatment. Initial measures should include cessation of fluid restriction, treatment of constipation if present and the keeping of charts to document progress.

First-line treatment is an alarm, either a bed alarm or a personal alarm. The alarm rings as the child begins to wet, and by a combination of conditioning and other factors this treatment will cure about 60% of children. Alarm treatment is most effective when all involved are motivated and regular practitioner support is provided during the treatment period of 6–8 weeks. Alarms can be hired through the Royal Children's Hospital or privately from pharmacies or continence services in the community. The correct technique is important and it is vital that it is the child who turns off the alarm, even if he or she needs to be woken by a parent to achieve this. See Fig. 31.6.

Relapse rates after discontinuing the alarm vary from 10–25% but can be minimised using a fluid load (overlearning) for a week at the end of the treatment period (300 mL + at bed time to ensure a full bladder during the night).

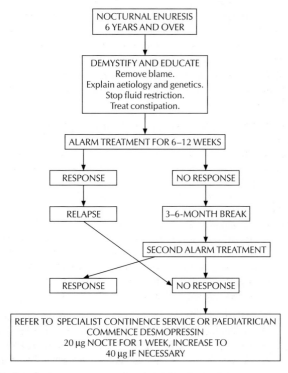

Fig. 31.6 Management of nocturnal enuresis

If a child fails to respond to an alarm on two occasions (with a 3-month break between treatments), a trial of desmopressin (Minirin), 20 µg, intranasal at night is indicated. The remission rate to Minirin is about 60% and it is palliative rather than curative. It can be used for long periods and is safe provided an excessive fluid load is not ingested after a dose is given.

The alarm should be retried each year as the response improves with increasing age. There is no indication for the use of imipramine (Tofranil) now that desmopressin is available as a safer palliative alternative. Fluid restriction, star charts, hypnosis, chiropractic treatments and other remedies have not been shown to be effective.

DAY-WETTING (FUNCTIONAL VOIDING DISORDER)

Daytime wetting is a distressing and embarrassing symptom with a significant impact on self-esteem. It affects about 5% of Australian children between 5 and 12 years of age, girls more often than boys. It is difficult to treat and should be managed in consultation with an experienced paediatrician.

There are a number of different causes of day-wetting. The following classification is useful in determining appropriate investigations and management.

Urge incontinence

- Symptoms are urgency, frequency, posturing (squatting) and wetting.
- The condition is caused by detrusor (bladder) instability; i.e. dysfunctional overactivity in the detrusor muscle during bladder filling.
- More girls are affected than boys.
- There is an association with recurrent UTIs, vulvovaginitis and constipation.
- The condition often coexists with vesico-ureteric reflux and reflux nephropathy.
- Management includes treating any coexistent UTIs and constipation, regular voiding, bladder training with the aim of increasing bladder capacity and anticholinergic medication to reduce detrusor spasm.

Dysfunctional voiding
- There is a lack of coordination between detrusor and bladder neck activity with poor relaxation of the external sphincter during voiding.
- The condition is associated with increased intravesical pressure, high residual urine volumes and at times upper tract dilatation.
- Management relies on teaching sphincter relaxation (i.e. pelvic floor relaxation) and ensuring optimal voiding techniques.

Diurnal enuresis
- This condition is characterised by complete bladder emptying of reasonably large volumes of urine in children who appear to be unaware of the need to void, especially when distracted by other activities (typically when watching TV or on the computer).
- It is likely to be due to a combination of developmental and personality factors with some of these children being inattentive and unaware of their bodily needs.
- Management is dependent on increasing the child's awareness of bladder sensation; it involves engaging the child in treatment, behaviour modification and rewarding progress.

Neurological and urological pathology
- Exclude ectopic ureter, urethral obstruction, fistulae and neurogenic bladder by compiling a history of constant dribbling and examining the external genitalia and direct visualisation of the urethra.
- Examining the back and assessing the lower limb neurological function should highlight spinal cord anomalies, especially a tethered cord.

Investigation
- All children with day-wetting should have a urine microscopy and culture, and renal and bladder ultrasound, including an assessment of residual urine volume.
- Ultrasound should be repeated 2 yearly in children refractory to treatment.

CHAPTER 32
RESPIRATORY CONDITIONS

Anthony Olinsky
Michael Marks

UPPER RESPIRATORY TRACT INFECTIONS (URTIs)

The average child has between four and 12 upper respiratory tract infections a year, the peak incidence being between 1 and 6 years.

Aetiology

Viruses are responsible for at least 90% of upper respiratory tract infections. The only common important bacterial pathogen is Group B haemolytic streptococcus. See Table 32.1.

Beware of the child with signs of a mild upper respiratory tract infection who has severe constitutional symptoms. Look for another diagnosis such as meningitis.

Table 32.1 Clinical features of upper respiratory tract infections

	Viral	Streptococcal
Age	Any age	4–15 years
Nasal symptoms	Usually	Infrequent
Cough	Frequent	Rare
Vomiting	Sometimes	Frequent
Level of fever	37–40°C	Usually >38.5°C
Tender, enlarged tonsillar lymph nodes	Not present	Usually present
Exudate on tonsils and pharynx	Sometimes	Frequent

Management
Viral

- Symptomatic if necessary. Give paracetamol if the child is distressed.
- Ephedrine nose drops for nasal obstruction interfering with feeding or sleeping (max duration of therapy is 48 h).

Probable streptococcus

- Penicillin – a total course for 10 days is given as phenoxymethyl-penicillin orally, 30 mg/kg (max 1 g) 12 hourly.
- If the child is very sick the initial therapy may be by injection.
- In remote communities, or in situations where compliance may not be reliable, procaine penicillin 50 mg/kg (max 1.2–2.4 g) is an acceptable alternative. *Note:* This is a very painful injection.
- Give paracetamol if the child is distressed.

WHOOPING COUGH (PERTUSSIS)

Whooping cough continues to be widespread in many communities mainly because of a poor uptake of childhood immunisation. However, the current vaccines give protection only for 5–10 years, and adolescents and adults can acquire the infection and pass it on to younger children who are inadequately protected.

Clinical features

- A cough that endures for some weeks, occurs in paroxysms and may be associated with facial suffusion and vomiting. In some children the paroxysm is terminated by an inspiratory whoop.
- Between the paroxysms the child appears normal.

Diagnosis

- The diagnosis is dependent on taking a careful history.
- Early in the illness, the diagnosis can be confirmed by identifying *Bordetella pertussis* in a nasopharyngeal aspirate.

Management

- No pharmacological agents favourably alter the course of whooping cough. Erythromycin estolate 15 mg/kg (max 500 mg) orally, 8 hourly for 14 days, may reduce the period of infectivity and should be used in children who may pass on the infection to infants under the age of 12 months (who are most at risk from complications). Household and other close contacts should be similarly treated.

- Almost all infants under the age of 6 months (and some between 6 and 12 months) with whooping cough require admission to hospital.
- In hospital, careful observation, including the use of a monitor, is essential. If paroxysms occur frequently and are associated with marked cyanosis, nursing in oxygen may be of some help.

PHARYNGITIS/TONSILLITIS AND ACUTE OTITIS MEDIA

See Ear, Nose and Throat Conditions, chapter 21.

LARYNGOTRACHEOBRONCHITIS (CROUP)

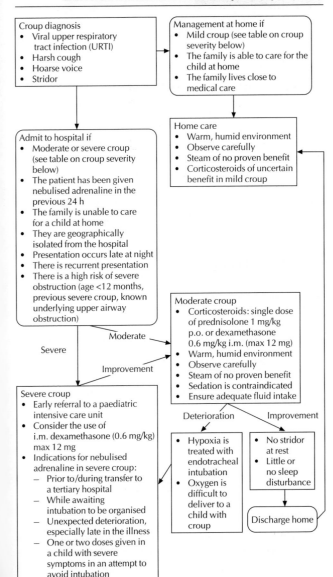

Croup diagnosis
- Viral upper respiratory tract infection (URTI)
- Harsh cough
- Hoarse voice
- Stridor

Management at home if
- Mild croup (see table on croup severity below)
- The family is able to care for the child at home
- The family lives close to medical care

Admit to hospital if
- Moderate or severe croup (see table on croup severity below)
- The patient has been given nebulised adrenaline in the previous 24 h
- The family is unable to care for a child at home
- They are geographically isolated from the hospital
- Presentation occurs late at night
- There is recurrent presentation
- There is a high risk of severe obstruction (age <12 months, previous severe croup, known underlying upper airway obstruction)

Home care
- Warm, humid environment
- Observe carefully
- Steam of no proven benefit
- Corticosteroids of uncertain benefit in mild croup

Moderate croup
- Corticosteroids: single dose of prednisolone 1 mg/kg p.o. or dexamethasone 0.6 mg/kg i.m. (max 12 mg)
- Warm, humid environment
- Observe carefully
- Steam of no proven benefit
- Sedation is contraindicated
- Ensure adequate fluid intake

Moderate

Severe

Improvement

Severe croup
- Early referral to a paediatric intensive care unit
- Consider the use of i.m. dexamethasone (0.6 mg/kg) max 12 mg
- Indications for nebulised adrenaline in severe croup:
  - Prior to/during transfer to a tertiary hospital
  - While awaiting intubation to be organised
  - Unexpected deterioration, especially late in the illness
  - One or two doses given in a child with severe symptoms in an attempt to avoid intubation

Deterioration

Improvement

- Hypoxia is treated with endotracheal intubation
- Oxygen is difficult to deliver to a child with croup

- No stridor at rest
- Little or no sleep disturbance

Discharge home

Fig. 32.1 Assessment and management of laryngotracheobronchitis (croup)

Fig. 32.1 Assessment and management of laryngotracheobronchitis (croup) *Cont'd*

CROUP SEVERITY

Sign/symptom	Mild	Moderate–severe
Stridor*	None or only with agitation	Stridor at rest
Respiratory rate	Usually normal	May be ↓
Retractions	None	+ to +++
Air entry	Normal	Normal to ↓↓
Colour	Normal/flushed	May be pallor
Cyanosis	None	Late sign only
Conscious state	Normal	May be restless or in a ↓ conscious state

* The loudness of the stridor does not necessarily correlate with the severity of obstruction

Notes on drugs used in croup
Prednisolone 1 mg/kg (max) per dose. In hospitalised children this may be repeated for persistent symptoms.
Dexamethasone 0.6 mg/kg (max 12 mg) i.m.
Adrenaline (nebulised) 0.05 mL/kg of 1:100 (1%), or 0.5 mL/kg of 1:1000 (0.1%) solution per dose (diluted to 2.5 mL) by inhalation.
Repeated doses of nebulised adrenaline may occasionally be given in a child in whom it is desirable to avoid intubation (e.g. established subglottic stenosis). It should not be used as a definitive treatment, and after its use the child must be observed very closely, as rebound obstruction frequently occurs.
Antibiotics have no role in management unless an associated bacterial infection is present.
Oxygen should not be used routinely in children with croup as it may mask cyanosis, which is an important sign of increasing obstruction.

EPIGLOTTITIS

See Medical Emergencies, chapter 1.

The incidence of acute epiglottitis has fallen markedly in countries where immunisation against *Haemophilus influenzae* type b is widespread. However, it continues to occur and, if the diagnosis is not made promptly, the child with it is likely to die.

Clinical features

This differs from laryngotracheobronchitis in the following ways:

- Most children appear sick because of associated sepsis.
- The onset is with fever and lethargy, and symptoms of respiratory obstruction develop after 2–6 h. There may be a history of a preceding upper respiratory tract infection.
- The stridor is soft, and the expiratory element is often dominant with a snoring or gurgling quality. *Cough is not a prominent feature.*
- Difficulty in swallowing and excess salivation with drooling are common.

Management

All children with suspected epiglottitis require urgent admission to a hospital with facilities to intubate children with acute upper airways obstruction. After intubation, most children should be transferred to a paediatric intensive care unit, preferably by a paediatric emergency transport service. All medical practitioners should know what facilities are available within their community for dealing with such emergencies.

- Do not lie the patient flat. Do not examine the larynx unless an anaesthetist is present and able to intubate.
- Ceftriaxone – an initial dose of 100 mg/kg (max 2 g) i.v., with a second dose of 50 mg/kg after 24 h.
- Rifampicin prophylaxis 20 mg/kg (max 600 mg) p.o. daily for 4 days, for contacts.
- Provide adequate fluids. If the patient has an intravenous line, fluids can be given intravenously. Do not give more than 40–60% of maintenance requirements.

ACUTE VIRAL BRONCHIOLITIS

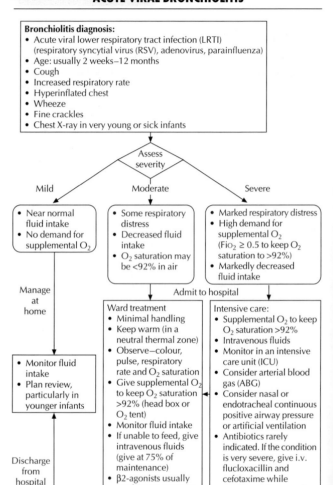

Bronchiolitis diagnosis:
- Acute viral lower respiratory tract infection (LRTI) (respiratory syncytial virus (RSV), adenovirus, parainfluenza)
- Age: usually 2 weeks–12 months
- Cough
- Increased respiratory rate
- Hyperinflated chest
- Wheeze
- Fine crackles
- Chest X-ray in very young or sick infants

Assess severity

Mild · Moderate · Severe

Mild
- Near normal fluid intake
- No demand for supplemental O_2

Manage at home

Moderate
- Some respiratory distress
- Decreased fluid intake
- O_2 saturation may be <92% in air

Severe
- Marked respiratory distress
- High demand for supplemental O_2 ($Fio_2 \geq 0.5$ to keep O_2 saturation to >92%)
- Markedly decreased fluid intake

Admit to hospital

- Monitor fluid intake
- Plan review, particularly in younger infants

Discharge from hospital

Ward treatment
- Minimal handling
- Keep warm (in a neutral thermal zone)
- Observe—colour, pulse, respiratory rate and O_2 saturation
- Give supplemental O_2 to keep O_2 saturation >92% (head box or O_2 tent)
- Monitor fluid intake
- If unable to feed, give intravenous fluids (give at 75% of maintenance)
- β2-agonists usually produce no response

Intensive care:
- Supplemental O_2 to keep O_2 saturation >92%
- Intravenous fluids
- Monitor in an intensive care unit (ICU)
- Consider arterial blood gas (ABG)
- Consider nasal or endotracheal continuous positive airway pressure or artificial ventilation
- Antibiotics rarely indicated. If the condition is very severe, give i.v. flucloxacillin and cefotaxime while awaiting culture results

Improve — Deteriorate

- Feeding adequately
- Improved respiratory status
- No requirement for supplemental O_2

Note:
Some infants can have recurrent episodes of bronchiolitis in the first 2 years. Most infants with recurrent wheeze will not develop asthma.

Fig. 32.2 Assessment and management of bronchiolitis

PNEUMONIA

Clinical features

- The child with pneumonia usually has tachypnoea (see Table 32.2), and there is often subcostal indrawing in young children.
- Focal signs in the chest may be difficult to detect.
- A diagnosis of pneumonia, especially in younger children, can usually only be made with radiological confirmation.

Table 32.2 Normal respiratory rates in childhood

Age	Respiratory rate
Birth–6 months	45
6 months–3 years	30
4 years–7 years	25
>8 years	20

Aetiology

- Viruses, especially respiratory syncytial virus and *parainfluenzae* type 3, are the most common cause of pneumonia in young infants in developed countries. There is generally only mild to moderate constitutional disturbance. There may be chest hyperinflation and scattered inspiratory crackles.
- *Mycoplasma pneumoniae* is the commonest pathogen in children over 5 years old, but it also causes pneumonia in younger children. Typically, symptoms develop over several days. Cough is prominent and crackles may be focal or widespread.
- *Streptococcus pneumoniae* is the commonest bacterial pathogen in all age groups. The next is *Haemophilus influenzae* (both non-typable and all serotypes) followed by *Staphylococcus aureus*. Children are usually unwell and focal signs are present in the chest. Many older children can be satisfactorily managed at home, but most under the age of 24 months should be admitted to hospital.

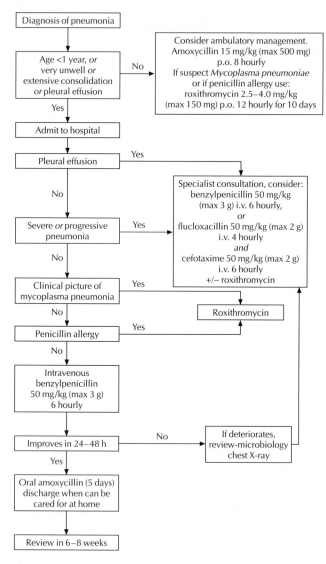

Fig. 32.3 Management of pneumonia

Management

- Chest X-ray is necessary to confirm the diagnosis.
- Blood culture, nasopharyngeal aspirate for viruses and Myco-plasma serology where indicated. Throat swabs and sputum are of no value for bacterial culture.
- Because of the inability to make a precise aetiological diagnosis, antibiotics are recommended, at least initially, unless symptoms are mild and a viral aetiology is highly probable.
- Management is determined by age and the severity of illness, and should follow the algorithm in Fig. 32.3.

General measures

- Minimal handling; careful observation of colour, pulse and respirations; pulse oximetry; keep warm (in neutral thermal zone).
- Increased inspired oxygen concentration.
- An adequate, but not excessive fluid intake. If fluids are given intravenously the rate should be at 40% maintenance, once any dehydration is corrected.

ASTHMA

The aims in the management of asthma are:

- To achieve a rapid resolution of acute episodes.
- To use prophylactic drugs when the morbidity from asthma is sufficient to justify their use in view of potential side effects.
- To prevent exercise-induced asthma.

Critical to these issues is the proper assessment of the severity of acute episodes and the degree of morbidity in the long term, based on the frequency of acute episodes and whether there are interval symptoms between the acute episodes (see Table 32.3).

Delivery devices

It is important to use delivery devices that are appropriate to the patient's age. Inhalations are given with a spacer mask firmly applied to the face (in younger children) and with the lips around a mouth-piece for older children.

Table 32.3 Managing acute episodes of asthma

Type of episode	Treatment
Mild acute episode Not cyanosed Audible wheeze No use of accessory muscles of respiration Respiratory rate not increased Active More than five to seven words between breaths	One to two doses of inhaled β_2-sympathomimetic with metered dose inhaler, via spacer. May need to continue β_2-sympathomimetic 4–6 hourly for a further 24–36 h
Moderate acute episode Not cyanosed Audible wheeze Use of accessory muscles of respiration Lower rib recession especially in younger children Three to five words between breaths Normal breath sounds Patient wants to sit or lie quietly	Three doses of inhaled β_2-sympathomimetic with metered dose inhaler and spacer over 60 min. Observe for a further 30–60 min. Possible outcomes: • Complete clearing of audible wheeze and respiratory distress: continue β_2-sympathomimetic 3–4 hourly for 24–36 h. If further treatment is required, consider a course of oral steroids (e.g. prednisolone 1 mg/kg (max 50 mg) daily for up to 3 days) • Improvement but not complete clearing: short course of oral prednisolone (1 mg/kg (max 50 mg) daily for up to 3 days*), continue β_2-sympathomimetic 3–4 hourly • No improvement after three doses of β_2-sympathomimetic: admit to hospital and treat as severe

Table 32.3 Managing acute episodes of asthma *Cont'd*

Type of episode	Treatment
Severe acute episode Cyanosed in air Obvious respiratory distress with increased respiratory rate marked use of accessory muscles of respiration lower rib recession Audible wheeze – may be soft One to three words between breaths Wants to lie or sit still Reduced breath sounds	Admit to hospital and administer oxygen. Very frequent or continuous inhaled β$_2$-sympathomimetic either by metered dose inhaler and spacer or with nebuliser driven by oxygen (e.g. 1 mL salbutamol in 3 mL saline). Inhaled ipratropium bromide – 0.25 or 0.5 mg/dose three doses given with β$_2$-sympathomimetic 20 min apart in first hour Corticosteroids – oral, or i.v. if patient is very distressed. Methylprednisolone 1 mg/kg per 6 hourly (max 50 mg/dose for 24 h), then 1 mg/kg per 12 h – for a further 24 h if necessary Then oral steroids 1 mg/kg per 24 h (max 50 mg) for 3 days* If not settling, transfer to ICU and consider: i.v. salbutamol: dose-load 5 µg/kg over 10 min then infusion 1–5 µg/kg per min i.v. aminophylline: dose-load 10 mg/kg (max 500 mg) over 1 h then infusion: 1.1 mg/kg per h <9 years, or 0.7 mg/kg per h ≥9 years. intermittent positive-pressure ventilation (IPPV)

* The period of therapy with oral corticosteroids for an acute episode in a patient on moderate to high dose inhaled corticosteroids may need to be longer than the standard 3 days and particularly with high doses, it may be wise to tail off the drug over a further 3–5 days. This certainly should always be the case in patients on maintenance oral corticosteroids.

The only role for β$_2$-sympathomimetics via a nebuliser is in the management of severe acute episodes. A metered dose inhaler plus spacer is as effective as a nebuliser in all other circumstances.

If nebulised β$_2$ drugs are used more frequently than hourly, the patient must be reviewed frequently. Early referral to an ICU is recommended for patients who fail to respond to standard treatment.

- Load with one puff at a time (and repeat).
- Shake the puffer initially and then after every three puffs.
- If the child uses tidal breathing, allow five to six breaths. If the child is able to take larger breaths (this is best), wait until they take one to two breaths.
- Frequency – in hospital, doses may be given frequently as indicated by severity and response. The use of oxygen between treatments does *not* preclude using a spacer.

After washing in ionic detergent, the spacers should be air-dried to decrease the deposition of aerosol particles (spacers should not be rinsed, rubbed or towel dried).

Acute episode

See also Medical Emergencies, chapter 1 and Table 32.3.

The efficacy of β_2-sympathomimetics delivered by a metered dose aerosol and spacer is at least equivalent to that delivered by a nebuliser (including moderate to severe acute asthma).

Aerosol dosage for children with a moderate or severe episode of asthma:
- Salbutamol (100 µg/puff)
    (i)   under 6 years – six puffs via a metered dose inhaler (MDI) and a small volume spacer and face mask
    (ii) 6 years and over – 12 puffs via MDI and a large volume spacer.
- Ipratropium (40 µg/puff) – may be added in severe asthma:
    (i)   under 6 years – two puffs via MDI and a small volume spacer and face mask
    (ii) 6 years and over – four puffs via MDI and a large volume spacer.

Patients should continue on the above doses until the current attack of asthma has resolved. More minor episodes can be treated with two puffs of salbutamol.

Long-term management

The aim of long-term management is to control symptoms that interfere with the enjoyment of a normal lifestyle (see Table 32.4). There is no evidence that the use of prophylactic drugs favourably alters the long-term course of asthma.

Table 32.4 Long-term management of asthma

Pattern of asthma	Prophylactic and acute therapy
Infrequent episodic (75% of asthmatic population) Significant episodes < every 4–6 weeks Minor wheeze after prolonged exercise No other interval symptoms Normal lung function between episodes	No prophylactic therapy Treat acute episodes as in Table 32.3
Frequent episodic (20% of asthmatic population) Significant episodes more frequently than every 4–6 weeks Wheeze with moderate exercise but usually prevented by prior use of β_2-sympathomimetic Occasional (less than weekly), interval symptoms Normal or near normal lung function between episodes	*Sodium cromoglycate* – as Intal Forte two puffs three times daily If there is no benefit after 2–3 months: • Simply treat acute episodes *or* • Use inhaled corticosteroids (see below) Treat acute episodes as in Table 32.3
Persistent asthma (5% of asthmatic population) Significant acute episodes generally more frequently than 4–6 weeks Wheezing or chest tightness with minor exercise not totally prevented by a β_2-sympathomimetic Other interval symptoms requiring a β_2-sympathomimetic more often than two to three times a week (e.g. waking at night, chest tightness on awakening in morning) Evidence of airways obstruction between episodes or diurnal variation in peak flow rates >20% (patients over 7 years)	• If mild symptoms, trial sodium cromoglycate • If it fails, or if symptoms are more troublesome, use *inhaled corticosteroids* (beclomethasone, budesonide). Initial dose: 400–800 µg daily depending on symptoms Once controlled, reduce dose to minimum necessary to have good quality of life and normal to near normal lung function Review dose every 3–6 months If control of symptoms is not adequate on seemingly appropriate prescribed therapy, consider inhalation technique and compliance prior to increasing dose

Continued overleaf

Table 32.4 Long-term management of asthma *Cont'd*

Pattern of asthma	Prophylactic and acute therapy
Persistent asthma Contd.	<ul><li>If persistent nocturnal symptoms and/or >1000 µg is needed to control symptoms, add *salmeterol*, twice daily</li><li>If >1200–1500 µg is needed, change to *fluticasone*</li><li>If >1000 µg fluticasone is needed, add maintenance *oral steroids*</li></ul>Acute episode: as above except may need a longer course of oral corticosteroids If β_2-sympathomimetic is needed more often than 3–4 hourly, give course of oral steroids If β_2-sympathomimetic is needed more frequently than every 2–3 hourly, admit to hospital

In this section, significant episodes of acute asthma are considered to be those that require the use of a β2-sympathomimetic 4–6 hourly for at least 24–36 h.

Lung function

- Children with presumed infrequent and frequent episodic asthma should have spirometry performed between acute episodes on at least one occasion to check that there is no unrecognised airways obstruction.
- Children with persistent asthma should have spirometry performed when seen for a consultant review.
- Children under the age of 6 or 7 years cannot perform lung function tests reliably.
- Peak flow measures are unreliable during acute episodes in many children and early adolescents.
- It is only patients with persistent asthma who should have a peak flowmeter at home. It should be used regularly only to confirm the diagnosis of persistent asthma, when it is being stabilised and when drug doses are being reduced.

Crisis management

- Action plans based on peak flow measurements are of much less value in children than they may be in adults.
- Every patient with asthma should know what to do if they get a sudden severe acute episode. See Appendix 3 for an example of an asthma management plan. The appropriate action is to take very frequent or continuous β_2-sympathomimetic and to summon an ambulance.

Other measures

- The prior use of an inhaled β_2-sympathomimetic can prevent exercise-induced bronchoconstriction.
- Non-pharmacologic measures have never been shown to be effective in the management of asthma in children and adolescents.
- Identify and avoid potential allergens that may contribute to asthma (see Allergy and Immunology, chapter 14).
- Avoid tobacco smoke.

COUGH IN CHILDREN

Cough is a common symptom in children. The degree to which a family becomes concerned about the frequency and severity of a child's cough seems to be extremely variable. There is often a poor correlation between a parental report of cough and objective measures.

Cough is best thought of in the following diagnostic groups:

Recurrent cough

These are episodes of cough lasting a few days to a few weeks with completely asymptomatic periods between. There are two causes: viral respiratory tract infection and asthma.

Viral respiratory tract infection

Cough with a viral respiratory infection, although typically lasting 7–10 days, may persist for 4 or 8 weeks or even longer. Initially it may be loose but later in the course it may become dry. It may be perceived by the family to be worse at night.

Asthma

While cough can be a troublesome symptom of asthma, it rarely occurs without some evidence of airways obstruction (e.g. wheeze). There is considerable doubt as to whether the entity of 'cough variant asthma', in which cough is the only symptom of asthma, exists in children. Be very reluctant to diagnose asthma in the absence of evidence of airways obstruction. The management of asthma is based on the severity and duration of the airways obstruction, not on the cough.

Subacute cough

There are a number of entities in addition to post-viral infection in which cough can last some weeks to 2 or 3 months. They include:

- Whooping cough
- An inhaled foreign body
- *Mycoplasma pneumoniae* infection
- Segmental or lobar collapse following an acute respiratory infection
- Tuberculosis
- Psychogenic.

Whooping cough and psychogenic cough should be diagnosed on the pattern of the cough. The others will usually be diagnosable by a chest radiograph, which is indicated in children with a first episode of cough lasting more than 3–4 weeks, particularly if it has not been triggered by a viral respiratory infection.

Persistent cough

This is a cough of many months or even years. There may be a temporary clearance of the cough with a course of antibiotics, but it rapidly recurs once they are ceased. The likely causes are:

- Cystic fibrosis.
- Other causes of bronchiectasis – immotile cilia syndrome, agammaglobulinaemia and other immune-deficient states.
- Insidious onset bronchiectasis without an apparent cause.
- Smoker's cough in adolescents.

Bronchiectasis probably commences with suppurative bronchitis. If this has been present for <6–12 months, it may be completely reversible without permanent lung damage, following a prolonged course of antibiotics (weeks to months) and physiotherapy.

Cough management

- The single most important aspect of management is to make a diagnosis and explain its nature to the parents. The effects of passive smoking should be reiterated.
- Almost all cough mixtures are ineffective. The possible exception is an opiate cough suppressant, which would rarely be used in a child.
- Specific therapy is indicated for asthma, *Mycoplasma* infection, tuberculosis and segmental or lobar collapse. A foreign body must be removed bronchoscopically.
- It is often much more difficult to control the cough of asthma than the wheeze.

FOREIGN BODY IN THE BRONCHIAL TREE

Clinical features
Symptoms

- Coughing or choking episodes while eating nuts or other solid foods, or while sucking a small plastic toy or similar object. This story should never be dismissed.
- Persistent coughing and wheezing. Remember 'all that wheezes is not asthma'.
- Beware of the sudden onset of a first wheezing episode in a toddler in whom there is no history of allergy, especially if it follows a choking episode.
- Parents may not volunteer the history of possible inhalation. One of every eight episodes of foreign body inhalation is not witnessed.

Signs

- Diminished breath sounds over the whole or part of one lung.
- Wheeze.

Investigations
A chest X-ray is taken in full inspiration and full expiration to exclude obstructive hyperinflation or an area of collapse. Normal X-rays do not exclude a foreign body.

Management
Admission is indicated for all patients with a suspected inhaled foreign body. If there is any doubt, consult a paediatric thoracic physician.

Bronchoscopy

- As the radiological examination may be normal, bronchoscopy is necessary in almost every child in whom there is a story that strongly points to an inhaled foreign body.
- Bronchoscopy in children is difficult and it requires an expert paediatric endoscopist teamed with an experienced paediatric anaesthetist. It should only be done in a major children's hospital.
- Once a foreign body has passed through the larynx it is very rare for there to be an immediate threat to life, and referral to the nearest children's hospital is usually quite safe.

CHAPTER 33
RHEUMATOLOGIC CONDITIONS
Roger Allen

Musculoskeletal signs and symptoms are common in children and adolescents, and a broad spectrum of conditions needs to be considered. As the clinical features and laboratory findings may be relatively non-specific, it is important to look for disease patterns when evaluating the presenting complaint and conducting a systems review.

This chapter contains two parts: (i) an approach to diagnosis by history, examination and investigation; and (ii) a brief outline of some of the more common rheumatologic conditions.

EVALUATION OF ARTHRITIS/ARTHRALGIA

History

- Check the nature of onset – is it acute or insidious? Acute onset monoarticular arthritis associated with fever is septic until proven otherwise.
- Check the timing of symptoms during the day – as a general guide early morning stiffness = inflammatory; post-activity pain = mechanical.
- Are there any intercurrent infections – respiratory, enteric or skin? Postviral infections are probably the commonest cause of transient arthritis.
- What does the child, or parent, consider to be the most symptomatic site – is it in the joint, muscle, adjacent bone or a more diffuse area?
- Check extra-articular symptoms – ensure a thorough systems review and keep the three 'major sleepers' in mind: (i) systemic lupus erythematosus; (ii) acute lymphoblastic leukaemia; and (iii) inflammatory bowel disease.
- See to what extent the normal physical activities/interests have been interrupted.

- Assess the functional milieu of the patient (e.g. school progress, family and peer relationships, and potential stress experiences).
- Check the family history for other inflammatory types of arthritis, particularly the spondyloarthropathies, autoimmune disorders and pain syndromes (e.g. fibromyalgia or other potential pain models).

Examination

- Examine all joints (not only the site of the presenting complaint).
- Aim to localise the site of maximal discomfort (e.g. is it the joint capsule, adjacent bone or muscle belly, tendon or ligament attachments?).
- Examine for signs of systemic diseases with an articular component or extra-articular features of juvenile chronic arthritis (JCA) or both.

A musculoskeletal assessment should include:

- Joint – signs of inflammation, the range of movement and deformity.
- Entheses – bone attachment sites of ligaments/tendons (e.g. the Achilles tendon).
- The tendon sheaths of fingers and toes (e.g. dactylitis in psoriasis).
- Gait – antalgic (pain) or limp, Trendelenburg's sign.
- Weakness (e.g. inability to toe or crouch walk).
- Patellar tracking pattern – does the patella move vertically on walking?
- Shoe sole and heel-wearing pattern.
- Leg length measurement.
- Spinal flexion, including Schober test (the measurement of the lumbosacral range should increase by at least 6 cm on maximal flexion; the starting range is between the lumbosacral junction and a point 10 cm above).

Investigations
Often useful

- Full blood examination, erythrocyte sedimentation rate (ESR) or C-reactive protein.
- Synovial fluid culture – only if sepsis is considered.

- Antinuclear antibody (ANA) – beware of over-interpretation as up to 20% of normal children may have a low positive ANA.

Occasionally useful

- Specific bacterial/viral studies (e.g. ASOT, antiDNase B, Yersinia and parvovirus serology) if the clinical picture is suggestive.
- Rheumatoid factor – in polyarticular patients, older children or if the pattern of disease appears unusual.
- Human leucocyte antigen (HLA) B27 – in an apparent spondylo-arthropathy (remember almost 9% of the Caucasian population are positive).
- Imaging – plain X-ray, bone scan and ultrasound. Early in an arthritis, plain films give no more information than a careful examination. They may be useful in difficult sites such as the hip, or if there is a long history of arthritis.
- Diagnostic aspirate – worthwhile if sepsis or haemarthrosis is considered, but will not necessarily differentiate between other inflammatory arthritides.

Not useful

Serum uric acid.

CAUSES OF ARTHRITIS/ARTHRALGIA IN CHILDHOOD

Juvenile chronic (rheumatoid) arthritis (JCA)
Assessment

- Age at onset – <16 years of age.
- Minimum duration of arthritis – 6 weeks (some criteria suggest 3 months).

Note: Most acute non-septic arthritis is not JCA.

Disease subtypes

- Pauciarticular – affects four or fewer joints:
  — Young, often ANA-positive female
  — Older, often B27-positive male.
- Polyarticular – affects five or more joints; sero (rheumatoid factor) positive or negative.
- Systemic – e.g. joints plus fever, rash and lymphadenopathy.

It is useful to look for: enthesitis (suggestive of a spondyloarthropathy); nail pits/scalp rash (indicative of psoriasis); Still's rash (faint urticarial-like erythema) – mostly when febrile; uveitis (especially pauci-JCA patient) by slit-lamp.

Management

Management depends on the clinical picture of disease severity and subtype.

Medication

See Table 33.1.

Physical therapy

Physical therapy is essential to maintain joint range and function. Splinting should be considered where appropriate.

Table 33.1 Medication therapy for juvenile chronic arthritis

Common drugs used	Dosage (mg/kg per day)
Non-steroidal anti-inflammatory drugs (NSAID)	
Indomethacin	1.5–3.0
Naproxen	10–15
Diclofenac	2–3
Ibuprofen	30–40
Aspirin	60–100
Slow-acting antirheumatic drugs (SAARD)	
Sulphasalazine	30–40
Hydroxychloroquine	5–6
Methotrexate	10–15 mg/m² per week*
Penicillamine	10–15
Gold (i.m.)	1 mg/kg per week
Corticosteroids	
Oral: may initially require 0.5 – 1.0 mg/kg per day, but if long term aim for alternate day <0.5 mg/kg or if necessary daily 0.1–0.2 mg/kg	
Intra-articular: triamcinolone acetonide – dose relates to joint size (e.g. knee 20–40 mg, ankle 7.5–10 mg)	

Henoch–Schoenlein purpura (HSP)
Clinical features
- Evolving crops of palpable purpura – predominantly buttocks and legs.
- Abdominal pain (occasionally melaena).
- Large joint migratory arthritis (of variable duration and severity).
- Nephritis.
- Other (e.g. oedema dorsum of the feet and hands, acute scrotal swelling and 'bruising').

Investigations
- Full blood examination (mainly to exclude thrombocytopenia).
- Urinalysis – haematuria/proteinuria.
- Renal function – urea/creatinine and urinary protein estimation.

Management
- Supportive – bed rest and analgesia.
- Corticosteroids – may reduce the duration of abdominal pain, but it is uncertain if it significantly affects other features.
- Other – it is rare that a more severe renal impairment may warrant immunosuppression or plasmapheresis and antihypertensive therapy (requiring supervision by a renal physician, see Renal Conditions and Enuresis, chapter 31); surgical intervention if appendicitis or intussusception (see Common Surgical Conditions, chapter 34).

Irritable hip (transient synovitis)
See Orthopaedic Conditions, chapter 30.

Septic arthritis
See Orthopaedic Conditions, chapter 30.

Kawasaki Disease
See Infectious Diseases, chapter 26.

POSTINFECTIOUS ARTHRITIS

Acute rheumatic fever
See Cardiovascular Conditions, chapter 16.

Post-streptococcal reactive arthritis

- Symmetrical non-migratory poly- or pauciarticular arthritis.
- Carditis may occur and may form part of a spectrum with acute rheumatic fever.
- Arthritis responds slowly to anti-inflammatories.
- Consider penicillin prophylaxis if carditis is present.

Postenteric reactive arthritis (Reiter's syndrome)

- Mainly *Salmonella*, *Shigella* and *Yersinia* (also reported with *Campylobacter* and *Giardia*).
- It is clinically similar to the spondyloarthropathies; therefore: predominantly lower limb, including sacro-iliitis, enthesitis common and a positive family history (especially if HLA B27 positive).
- Associated features – acute anterior uveitis and sterile pyuria.
- Treatment – non-steroidal anti-inflammatory drugs (NSAIDs): indomethacin 0.5–1.0 mg/kg (max 75 mg) p.o. 8 hourly is often the most effective.

Postviral arthritis

- Many viral illnesses are associated with arthritis.
- It is uncertain in most situations whether it is the primary (infective) or secondary (reactive) event; e.g. Epstein–Barr virus, rubella, adenovirus, varicella (beware septic arthritis secondary to infected skin lesion), parvovirus B19 and hepatitis B.
- A transient arthritis often follows a non-specific 'viral' illness, the confirmation of which may be difficult and unnecessary.
- Treatment – NSAID probably shortens the duration.

NON-INFLAMMATORY CAUSES OF JOINT PAIN

Benign nocturnal limb pain ('growing pains')

- Recurrent pain mainly involving the knee, calf and shin.
- No signs or symptoms of inflammation either on examination or history.
- Investigations (if carried out) are normal.
- Management involves analgesia (usually paracetamol) and reassurance; rubbing often helps.

Benign hypermobility

- Typical sites – hyperextension of the fingers parallel to the forearm; apposition of the thumb to the anterior forearm; hyper-extension of the elbows, knees or both more than 10°; excessive dorsiflexion of the ankles; and hip flexion allowing the palms to be placed flat on ground.
- Pain occurs typically in the afternoon or after exercise.
- The child may have features of patellofemoral dysfunction.
- The child may have transient joint effusions.

Reflex sympathetic dystrophy (Complex Regional Pain Syndrome Type I)

This condition is more common in paediatrics than is generally realised.

Clinical features

- Diffuse pain exacerbated by touch (hyperaesthesia).
- Diffuse swelling beyond the region of the joint.
- Ruddy or suffused colour change.
- Cool to touch.
- May follow relatively trivial trauma.

Investigation

- Bone scan often abnormal – increased or decreased uptake.
- Plain X-ray – osteopenia in prolonged cases.
- Acute phase markers normal.

Management

- Requires skilful physical therapy and pain management.
- Avoid immobilisation.
- Consider psychiatric assessment.
- Possible sympathetic nerve blocks.

CHAPTER 34
COMMON SURGICAL CONDITIONS

John Hutson

INGUINOSCROTAL CONDITIONS

The underlying pathological basis of an inguinal hernia, an encysted hydrocele of the cord and a scrotal hydrocele is persistence of the patent processus vaginalis after the completion of testicular descent.

Inguinal hernia

The opening of the processus vaginalis is large enough to allow the protrusion of the bowel through the inguinal canal and sometimes down to the scrotum. The younger the child, the greater is the danger that the bowel will become strangulated. Inguinal hernias always need surgery because of the ever-present danger of bowel strangulation and compression of the testicular vessels. The operation is short and children beyond the neonatal period are managed as day patients.

Reducible inguinal hernia ('6–2' rule)

- Birth to 6 weeks – surgical consultation on the day of diagnosis and surgery on the next convenient list (preferably within 2 days).
- Six weeks to 6 months – urgent surgical assessment with surgery within 2 weeks.
- Over 6 months – surgical assessment should be within 2 weeks and surgery within 2 months. This is normally done as a day case.

Irreducible inguinal hernia

These should be referred to a surgeon as soon as the diagnosis is made (see Fig. 34.1a). Normally, the surgeon is able to reduce the hernia manually and surgery is performed the following day. The child is admitted overnight and discharged the day after surgery.

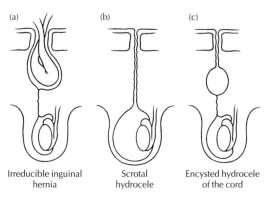

(a)   (b)   (c)

Irreducible inguinal hernia   Scrotal hydrocele   Encysted hydrocele of the cord

Fig. 34.1 Inguinoscrotal conditions

Scrotal hydrocele, encysted hydrocele of the cord

In both these conditions, the opening of the processus vaginalis is narrow and may close of its own accord in children up to 18 months to 2 years of age (see Fig. 34.1b, c). The important clinical signs to note are:

- A brilliantly transilluminable swelling.
- A narrow cord above the swelling.
- The swelling does not empty on squeezing.

If any of these features are absent, the swelling may be an irreducible hernia.

If the hydroceles persist beyond 2 years, surgery is recommended and inguinal herniotomy (i.e. a division of the patent processus vaginalis) is performed at a convenient time, usually as a day case.

Undescended testes

When the testis cannot be brought to the bottom of the scrotum, it is 'undescended'. An assessment of the undescended testis is easiest made between 3 and 6 months of life (avoiding confusion with retractile testis) and early referral to a surgeon is important. Experienced surgeons will perform an orchidopexy at about 6 months to 1 year as a day case.

Some children present later in childhood (4–10 years) with undescended testes: this is probably an acquired condition secondary to the failure of normal elongation of the spermatic cord with age. Surgery is recommended if the testis does not remain in the scrotum.

The acute scrotum

A child with a painful, tender and often red scrotum should be seen by a surgeon as a matter of urgency. It is usually impossible to differentiate the two common causes without surgical exploration:

- Torsion of the testicular appendage.
- Torsion of the testis.

A testis lying horizontally in the scrotum indicates an anatomical predisposition to torsion. In a boy with recurrent brief episodes of testicular pain, consider the possibility of intermittent testicular torsion. Epididymo-orchitis is a rare disease in prepubertal boys who do not have urinary tract infections. Mumps orchitis is not seen before puberty.

THE PENIS

The foreskin/prepuce

The foreskin is normally adherent to the glans at birth and remains so for a variable amount of time. Usually it is fully retractable by 4 years of age, but partial adherence is still normal up to 10 years. There is no need to retract foreskins in preschool children.

Smegma deposits

These present as yellow/white firm masses beneath the prepuce in young boys with non-retractable foreskins (see Fig. 34.2a). It is a normal variant and requires no treatment.

Balanitis

This is an infection under the foreskin with redness, inflammation, swelling and sometimes a white exudate (see Fig. 34.2b). Immediate treatment with local penile toilet (i.e. soak in an antiseptic solution), local antiseptic ointment (e.g. neomycin eye ointment) beneath the foreskin and oral antibiotics (e.g. cotrimoxazole (4/20 mg/kg (max 160/800 mg) 12 hourly) is usually sufficient. If the whole penis is red and swollen to the pubis, hospital admission and intravenous

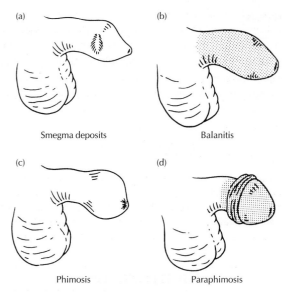

Fig. 34.2 Conditions of the penis

antibiotics (e.g. benzylpenicillin 50 mg/kg (max 3 g) 6 hourly and gentamicin 7.5 mg/kg (max 240 mg) daily) may be required.

Phimosis

This is a scarring of the preputial opening that causes:

- Urinary obstruction.
- A ballooning of the foreskin on micturition.

It is often the end result of recurrent episodes of balanitis (see Fig. 34.2c). It usually requires circumcision if severe, although mild cases respond to topical 0.05% betamethasone valerate cream applied three to four times daily for 10 days.

Paraphimosis

In this acutely painful condition, the retracted foreskin is trapped behind the glans and forms an oedematous ring of foreskin proximal to the exposed and swollen glans penis (see Fig. 34.2d). A surgeon should be consulted immediately if it cannot be reduced manually.

Circumcision

The indications for circumcision are phimosis and recurrent balanitis. Hypospadias is an absolute contraindication. It is important to stress to parents that circumcision is not required for cleanliness and that these days <10% of Australian male children are circumcised. It is an unnecessary operation with definite complications of surgery and anaesthesia.

UMBILICAL HERNIA

Umbilical hernia – the protrusion of the umbilicus – is a common finding in newborn children. In most it will resolve spontaneously and not require surgery. If it persists beyond 2 years of age, day surgical repair is recommended because the risk of strangulation increases with age.

ACUTE ABDOMINAL PAIN

Abdominal pain is a common symptom in children. Appendicitis needs to be distinguished from the other common causes: viral infection, urinary tract infection and constipation.

Appendicitis

Appendicitis may be straightforward if there is local peritonitis with guarding in the right iliac fossa. However, retrocaecal appendicitis may have no local peritonitis and merely vague fullness in the right side (retrocaecal abscess). In pelvic appendicitis there are no abdominal symptoms but vague suprapubic tenderness. Rectal examination is essential in this case.

Urinary tract infection should be excluded by urine testing. Viral infections often produce a local ileus but no peritonitis, which can be distinguished on physical examination as a 'squelchiness' or succussion splash (air and fluid in the ileum).

In the younger child, and especially in those <4 years of age, the diagnosis can be difficult. It is important to refer a child who complains of persistent abdominal pain, even if this is associated with vomiting or diarrhoea (i.e. do not assume it is gastroenteritis). If the child will not allow abdominal examination, one should suspect peritonitis.

Intussusception

In a 3-month to 2-year-old infant who presents with intermittent pallor, lethargy, vomiting and abdominal colic, the diagnosis of intussusception should be considered. These are the early symptoms and should be acted on, rather than awaiting the 'classical' red currant jelly stool, which is a feature of advanced disease. The abdominal mass is central beneath rectus abdominus and is often difficult to feel.

A child with suspected intussusception requires urgent surgical assessment and a contrast enema for diagnosis, treatment or both. If a hydrostatic pressure 80–100 mmHg fails to reduce the intussusception, emergency surgery is indicated. Contrast enema should not be performed in the presence of peritonitis, significant dehydration or established bowel obstruction. Early diagnosis is the key to easy and successful treatment.

VOMITING IN INFANCY

Malrotation and volvulus

It is important to determine whether the vomiting is bile stained or not. *Green vomiting is an indication for urgent surgical consultation to exclude the anatomical variant of intestinal malrotation and its associated lethal complication of midgut volvulus.* Initially, there may be no other symptoms or signs of abdominal disease. Abdominal distension is not present and should not be waited for. The twisted intestine may become gangrenous within 6 h after the onset of bile-stained vomiting.

Pyloric stenosis

In infants with non-bile-stained vomiting, pyloric stenosis needs to be distinguished from feeding problems, gastro-oesophageal reflux and infection (e.g. urinary tract infection and meningitis).

Pyloric stenosis should be suspected if the vomiting is projectile, persists despite the correction of feeding difficulties and/or the use of anti-gastro-oesophageal reflux measures, or is associated with a failure to thrive.

Examination

- Look for gastric peristalsis during test-feeding, and feel for the pyloric tumour, either during test-feeding or after vomiting.
- The passage of a nasogastric tube and drainage of the stomach is sometimes required to aid palpation of the tumour.
- The child should be referred to a paediatric surgeon on the basis of the symptoms, as the demonstration of signs can be difficult.

Investigations

Biochemistry

Metabolic alkalosis; chloride (usually <100 mmol/L) and sodium (usually <130 mmol/L) (cf. gastro-oesophageal reflux – electrolytes usually normal). Serum potassium may be normal despite significant losses.

Ultrasound

Required only if the diagnosis is unclear.

RECTAL BLEEDING

See Gastrointestinal Conditions, chapter 23.

NECK LUMPS

The enlargement of the cervical lymph nodes is common with upper respiratory infections, and there is no surgical problem if there is acute enlargement, tenderness and resolution. Bacterial infection with abscess formation should be considered in infants with large (2–4 cm), tender masses, even if there is no redness (the node is beneath the deep fascia).

Mycobacterial infection is seen in 1–3 year olds with indolent, but enlarging nodes over 4–6 weeks. Purple discoloration in the overlying skin indicates a collar–stud abscess that needs immediate surgical referral for excision. Nodes larger than 3–4 cm need a biopsy to exclude malignancy.

SURGICAL CONDITIONS OF THE NEONATE

Important warning signs

- *Excessive drooling of frothy secretions from the mouth may suggest oesophageal atresia.*
- *Bile-stained (green) vomiting is always abnormal.*
- *Malrotation may be present with minimal bile-stained vomiting at any age.* Admission to a paediatric hospital is essential.
- *Delayed passage of meconium* (beyond 24 h) *is abnormal* and may indicate Hirschsprung's disease or intestinal neuronal dysplasia.
- *Inguinal hernias need urgent attention to avoid strangulation.*

'Rare, dangerous or serious' conditions

Ambiguous genitalia

Genitalia that are frankly ambiguous need urgent consultation with an experienced paediatric endocrinologist or surgeon on the first day of life (see Endocrine Conditions, chapter 20).

An enlarged clitoris in an apparent female is also abnormal and needs immediate referral.

Hypospadias may overlap with ambiguous genitalia; this needs a careful initial assessment as someone already has assumed the gender should be male. If one or both testes are undescended, or the scrotum is bifid, or both, the baby should be treated as having ambiguous genitalia until proven otherwise by immediate referral for further investigation.

Oesophageal atresia

Excessive drooling or frothy, mucousy secretions from the mouth suggests an inability to swallow in a newborn. Test for oesophageal atresia by passing a 10-gauge catheter (which will not curl up) gently through the mouth: in atresia the catheter stops at about 10 cm from the gums, while in a normal baby it will pass to 20–25 cm and return acid on litmus testing. Proven oesophageal atresia needs urgent referral and transfer to a neonatal surgical unit. First aid includes nil orally, intravenous fluids and frequent (every 10–15 min) oropharyngeal suction to keep the airways clear (thereby preventing contamination of the lungs).

Diaphragmatic hernia

Respiratory distress in a newborn with a scaphoid abdomen suggests diaphragmatic hernia. Cardiac displacement and an X-ray of the chest and abdomen showing bowel loops in the chest (left more commonly) confirms the diagnosis. Urgent referral and transfer by the neonatal emergency transport service is needed. First aid includes intravenous fluids, nil orally, a nasogastric tube to prevent gaseous distension and respiratory support with oxygen. If a baby with suspected or diagnosed diaphragmatic hernia needs mechanical ventilation, then intubate the trachea. Bag and mask ventilation may exacerbate the respiratory distress by distending the bowel.

Exomphalos/gastroschisis

These anterior abdominal wall defects put the child at a great risk of heat and water loss from the exposed surface of the sac (exomphalos) or bowel (gastroschisis). First aid is needed urgently prior to the transfer: intravenous fluids, nil orally, nasogastric tube (to prevent gaseous distension) and wrapping the sac or exposed bowel in plastic kitchen wrap or aluminium foil to prevent evaporative cooling. The baby should be kept in an incubator while awaiting the neonatal transport service. Babies of excessive size and bodyweight (>4 kg) who have exomphalos should be suspected of having Beckwith–Wiedemann syndrome, with an excessive production of insulin. Blood glucose testing and i.v. 10% dextrose can avoid fitting, mental retardation or death caused by unrecognised neonatal hypoglycaemia.

Sacrococcygeal teratoma

Any lump over the coccyx of the baby should be assumed to be a teratoma until proven otherwise, and needs immediate referral at birth.

Malrotation with volvulus

Volvulus or twisting of the bowel is a potentially fatal complication of congenital malrotation, where the gut is abnormally positioned and inadequately fixed in the abdominal cavity. A well baby (or older child) may suddenly vomit bile-stained fluid without other symptoms (as would be seen with sepsis). Immediate referral for a barium meal to exclude midgut volvulus is required, as the twisted bowel will become infarcted in 6–12 h.

Table A1 Blood, serum and plasma

Test	Age	Reference range(s)	Comments
Acid/base (P)	Arterial or venous specimens: volume required (mL) 0.5		Arterial or capillary samples only are suitable for pH, Pco_2
pH	1 d	7.30–7.46	
	2 d–1 m	7.23–7.46	
	>1 m	7.34–7.43	
Pco_2		32–45 mmHg	Higher values seen in newborn
Base excess		−4 − +3 mmol/L	Lower values seen in newborn
Actual bicarbonate		18–25 mmol/L	
Alkaline phosphatase-ALP (S,P)	0–2 y	100–350 U/L	Higher values may be seen during periods of rapid growth
	2–10 y	100–300 U/L	
	10–16 y	100–350 U/L	
	Adult	30–120 U/L	
Aspartate aminotransferase – AST (S,P)	<1 y	20–80 U/L	Formerly SGOT. Upper limit of reference range, particularly in infancy, not well defined
	1–3 y	15–60 U/L	
	3–16 y	10–45 U/L	
	>16 y	0–40 U/L	

Table A1 Blood, serum and plasma Cont'd

Test	Arterial or venous specimens: volume required (mL)	Age	Reference range(s)	Comments
Bilirubin – unconjugated (S,P)	0.5	Full term 0–24 h	<65 μmol/L	Higher values in newborn due to increase in indirect (unconjugated) fraction. Even higher values in premature infants
		24–48 h	<115 μmol/L	
		3–5 d	<155 μmol/L	
		1 m	<10 μmol/L	
Bilirubin – conjugated (S,P)	<1 m	<10 μmol/L		Positive interference by sulphasalazine, nitrofurantoin
	>1 m			
Calcium – ionised (P)	0.5	Adult	1.19–1.29 mmol/L	Whole blood specimen needed. Must be collected anaerobically, in special syringe. Consult laboratory for details
Calcium – total (S,P)	0.5	<2 w	1.90–2.70 mmol/L	Lower limit of normal range in neonates not well defined
		2 w–1 y	2.10–2.70 mmol/L	
		>1 y	2.10–2.60 mmol/L	
Chloride			98–110 mmol/L	
Cholesterol – total (S,P)	0.5	6 m	2.3–4.9 mmol/L	Reference ranges based on USA data. Australian National Heart Foundation recommends adult cholesterol levels <5.5 mmol/L and children cholesterol levels <4.5 mmol/L
		1 y	2.5–4.9 mmol/L	
		2–14 y	3.1–5.4 mmol/L	

Test		Age	Value	Notes
Creatine kinase – CK (S,P)	0.5		40–240 units/L	Higher values in newborn. Specimens on three separate occasions recommended when testing for carriers of Duchenne muscular dystrophy
Creatinine (S,P)	0.5	1 m–1 y	0.01–0.03 mmol/L	Reference range related to muscle mass. Higher values seen in newborns
		1–4 y	0.01–0.05 mmol/L	
		4–10 y	0.02–0.06 mmol/L	
		10–16 y	0.03–0.08 mmol/L	
		>16 y	0.05–0.11 mmol/L	
Glucose f (S,P)	0.5	2 d–1 m	2.2–5.0 mmol/L	Lower values may be seen on day 1 and in premature infants. Therapy for hypoglycaemia should aim to keep the glucose level >3 mmol/L. Whole blood glucose approximately 10% lower than plasma
		>1 m	3.6–5.4 mmol/L	
γ-Glutamyltransferase – GGT (S,P)	0.5	0–1 m	<225 U/L	Newborns have very high levels of GGT that rapidly decrease to adult levels by about 3 months. Higher levels of GGT may be seen if on anticonvulsants or alcohol
		>3 m	<40 U/L	
Iron (S,P)	0.5		9–27 μmol/L	
Magnesium (S,P)	0.5		0.7–1.0 mmol/L	
Osmolality (S,P)	1		265–295 mmol/kg	
Phosphorus – inorganic (S,P)	0.5	<2 w	1.7–3.0 mmol/L	
		2 w–2 y	1.3–2.3 mmol/L	
		2–16 y	1.1–1.8 mmol/L	
Po_2 (P)	0.5	<2 w	55–100 mmHg	
	Arterial only	>2 w	80–100 mmHg	

Table A1 Blood, serum and plasma Cont'd

Test	Arterial or venous specimens: volume required (mL)	Age	Reference range(s)	Comments
Potassium		2 d–2 w	3.7–6.0 mmol/L	Ranges quoted are based on arterial/venous specimens. Capillary samples have higher potassium concentrations (up to 0.6 mmol/L higher)
		2 w–3 m	3.7–5.7 mmol/L	
		3 m–1 y	3.5–5.1 mmol/L	
		1–16 y	3.5–5.0 mmol/L	
		>16 y	3.5–5.0 mmol/L	
Proteins (s)	0.5			
Total protein		<1 m	45–70 g/L	
		1 m–1 y	50–71 g/L	
		1–4 y	55–74 g/L	
		4–16 y	57–80 g/L	
		>16 y	60–80 g/L	
Albumin		<1 m	23–43 g/L	
		1 m–1 y	29–45 g/L	
		1–16 y	33–47 g/L	
		>16 y	35–50 g/L	
Total globulins		<1 m	10–31 g/L	Consult with immunology laboratory regarding specific globulin fractions
		1 m–1 y	12–27 g/L	
		1–4 y	14–37 g/L	
		4–16 y	17–38 g/L	
Sodium			135–145 mmol/L	

Thyroxine				
total (TT4)		1–3 d	130–270 nmol/L	
		1–2 w	125–215 nmol/L	
		2–4 w	105–215 nmol/L	
		1–4 m	90–190 nmol/L	
		4 m–1 y	70–175 nmol/L	
		>1 y	70–155 nmol/L	
		Adult	9–26 pmol/L	Higher values in infants
free (FT4)				
T3 Resin uptake	<1 m	70–115%		
(T3 RU)	1–4 m	70–110%		
	4 m–1 y	70–110%		
	>1 y	75–115%		
	Adult	80–210%		
Free thyroxine index	<1 m	70–180%		
(FTI)	1–4 m	60–160%		
	4 m–1 y	60–155%		
	>1 y			
Triiodothyronine (T3)	Adult	1.0–2.7 nmol/L	Higher values in infants and children
Thyroxine binding	Adult	12–28 mg/L	Higher values in infants
globulin (TBG)				
Thyroid-stimulating	1–3 d	<40 mU/L		
hormone (TSH)	3–7 d	<25 mU/L		
	7–14 d	<10 mU/L		
	>14 d	<5 mU/L		
Triglycerides f (P)	0.5	Adult	0.9–2.0 mmol/L	Note: fasting is essential
Urea (S,P)	0.5	<1 m	1.3–5.7 mmol/L	Related to protein intake. Lower values in
		1 m–4 y	1.3–6.6 mmol/L	breast-fed infants and newborns
		>4 y	2.1–6.5 mmol/L	
Uric acid (S,P)	0.5	Prepubertal	0.13–0.39 mmol/L	Higher values may be seen in the first
		Adult male	0.18–0.48 mmol/L	2 years and following the onset of puberty
		Adult female	0.11–0.42 mmol/L	
Zinc (S,P)	2		11–22 µmol/L	

h, hour; d, day; w, week; m, month; y, year; f, fasting; P, plasma; S, serum; U, urine.

Table A2 Urine

Test	Specimens: Volume required (mL)	Age	Reference range(s)	Comments
Calcium	24 h		<0.12 mmol/kg per day	Include weight of patient on request card. Specimen must be collected into special bottle containing acid
Calcium/creatinine ratio	Random		<0.7 mmol/day	
Creatinine clearance	24 h	>2 y	1.4–2.4 mL/s per 1.73 m^2	Plasma sample for creatinine required during urine collection period. Height and weight must be recorded on request card. See special note in general instructions
Drug screen	Random (20 mL)			
Potassium	Random		Variable (mmol/L)	Many factors determine excretion rates; e.g. intake, renal function, hormonal influences and drug therapy
Protein	Timed collection overnight		mg/h per m^2 <4	The height and weight of the patient must be recorded on request card
Protein/creatinine ratio	Random (early morning)		mg/mmol <30	Consult the laboratory
Sodium	Random		Variable (mmol/L)	Many factors influence urinary sodium concentration. This test is of value in differentiating causes of hyponatraemia

h, hour; y, year.

Table A3 Sweat

Test	Specimens: volume required (mL)	Age	Reference range(s)	Comments
Sodium chloride	–	Prepubertal	<40 mmol/L <40 mmol/L	Contact gastroenterology department. At least 100 mg of sweat must be collected. If sodium is >50 mmol/L and chloride is >60 mmol/L, the result is definitely abnormal. All other results outside the reference ranges are doubtful. Higher values may be seen in normal adolescents and adults

Table A4 Serum drug levels

Test	Arterial or venous specimens: volume required (mL)	Reference range(s)	Comments
Carbamazepine (S,P)	1	20–50 µmol/L (therapeutic)	
Chloramphenicol (S,P)	0.5	Peak 20–30 mg/L (therapeutic)	Therapeutic range not well defined
Clonazepam	1	60–150 nmol/L (therapeutic)	Collect sample in EDTA. Consult laboratory regarding therapeutic range
Cyclosporin (B)	1	µg/L	
Digoxin (S,P)	1	Low <0.6 nmol/L Borderline low 0.6–1.0 nmol/L Therapeutic 1.0–2.5 nmol/L Borderline high 2.5–3.0 nmol/L High >3.0 nmol/L	
Ethosuximide (S,P)	1	0.30–0.70 mmol/L (therapeutic)	Therapeutic range not well defined
Gentamicin (S,P)	0.5	Peak 5–10 mg/L Trough <2 mg/L (therapeutic)	For thrice daily dosing only
Nitrazepam (S,P)	1		Consult with laboratory regarding therapeutic range
Paracetamol (S,P)	0.5		Only measured in suspected overdose – consult laboratory
Phenobarbitone (S,P)	1	80–120 µmol/L (therapeutic)	
Phenytoin (S,P)	1	40–80 µmol/L (therapeutic)	Only the phenobarbitone metabolite is measured as this usually gives sufficient information for therapeutic monitoring
Primidone (S,P)	1		

Salicylate (S,P)	0.5	0.7–2.00 mmol/L (therapeutic)	
Theophylline (S,P)	0.5	Neonatal apnoea 40–80 µmol/L (therapeutic) Asthma 55–110 µmol/L (therapeutic-peak)	
Thiopentone (S,P)	0.5	150–200 µmol/L (for anaesthesia)	
Tobramycin (S,P)	0.5	Peak 5–10 mg/L Trough <2 mg/L (therapeutic)	For thrice daily dosing only
Valproate (S,P)	0.5	0.30–0.70 mmol/L (therapeutic)	
Vancomycin (S,P)	0.5	Peak 25–40 mg/L Trough <10 mg/L (therapeutic)	

B, blood (whole); P, plasma; S, serum.

Table A5 Haematology reference ranges

	Haemoglobin (g/L)	Haematocrit (L/L)	Reticulocytes $\times 10^9$ /L (%)
Birth	110–170	0/30–0/40	
28 weeks' gestation	120–180	0.35–0.50	
34 weeks' gestation	140–200	0.40–0.55	
38 weeks' gestation	135–195	0.42–0.60	200–300 (2.6)
40 weeks' gestation			
1 week	135–205	0.42–0.62	<5 (0)
2 weeks	125–205	0.40–0.62	<5 (0)
1 month	100–180	0.31–0.55	
2 months	90–135	0.27–0.40	
3 months	95–140	0.29–0.41	5–250
6–24 months	105–140	0.33–0.42	10–100 (0.5–1.5)
2–5 years	115–140	0.35–0.42	10–100 (0.5–1.5)
6–11 years	115–155	0.35–0.48	10–100 (0.5–1.5)
12–18 years (male)	130–160	0.37–0.48	10–100 (0.5–1.5)
12–18 years (female)	120–160	0.36–0.48	10–100 (0.5–1.5)

Table A6 Red cell indices

	MCV (fL)	MCH (pg)	MCHC (g/L)
Birth			
28–37 weeks' gestation	120		320–360
38–40 weeks' gestation	110		320–360
1 week	110		320–360
1 month	90	24–34	320–360
2 months	80	24–34	320–360
3–12 months	70	24–31	320–360
Older	84–94	24–34	320–360

Table A7 Normal white cell levels

Age	Total (×10⁹/L)	Neutrophils (×10⁹/L) (%)	Lymphocytes (×10⁹/L) (%)	Monocytes (×10⁹/L) (%)	Platelets (×10⁹/L)
Birth	9.0–30	6.0–26 (60)	2.0–11.0 (30)	1.1 (7)	150–400
1 week	5–21	1.5–10 (45)	2.0–17.0 (40)	1.1 (9)	150–400
6 months	6–17.5	1.0–8.5 (30)	4.0–13.5 (60)	0.6 (5)	150–400
2 years	6–17.5	1.5–8.5 (33)	3.0–9.5 (60)	0.5 (5)	150–400
6 years	6–14.5	1.5–8.0 (50)	1.5–7.0 (42)	0.4 (5)	150–400
10 years	4.5–13.5	1.8–8.0 (54)	1.5–6.5 (38)	0.4 (4)	150–400
16 years	4.5–13.5	1.8–8.0 (60)	1.0–4.8 (33)	0.3 (4)	150–400

ESR0–6 mm in 1 h (micro Westergren)

Table A8 Haemoglobin electrophoresis

Age	Percentage
Hb F Birth (40 weeks' gestation)	60–90
2 months	30–55
3 months	15–30
4 months	5–15
6 months	2–5.0
1 year	0.2–2.0
Hb A$_2$ > 1 year	1.5–3.5

Table A9 Erythropoietic factors

Test	Reference range
Serum iron	9–27 µmol/L
Total iron binding capacity	45–72 µmol/L
Percentage saturation	16–33%
Serum ferritin	
<1 year	10–300 µg/L
>1 year	16–300 µg/L
Folate	
Serum	>4 µmol/L
Red cell	>270 µmol/L
Whole blood	>110 µmol/L
Vitamin B$_{12}$	150–590 pmol/L

Table A10 Coagulation

Test	Reference range
Bleeding time	1.6–7.0 min
Prothrombin time (International Normalised Ratio)	0.8–1.3 s
Activated partial thromboplastin time	22.0–39.0 s
D–Dimers	<0.25 µg/mL
Fibrinogen <6 months	1.5–4.0 g/L
>6 months	1.9–5.0 g/L

Table A11 Immunoglobulin: normal ranges (g/dL)

Age in years	IgG (g/L)			IgA (g/L)			IgM (g/L)		
	5th	50th	95th	5th	50th	95th	5th	50th	95th
Cord	5.34	10.52	16.94	ND	ND	ND	<0.10	<0.10	0.18
0.1	2.78	6.35	13.38	<0.09	0.14	0.34	0.10	0.37	0.62
0.2–0.4	1.39	4.65	10.83	<0.09	0.24	0.54	0.20	0.51	0.84
0.4–0.6	1.39	4.48	8.04	0.14	0.30	0.69	0.20	0.67	1.30
0.6–0.8	1.94	5.57	11.15	0.13	0.33	0.91	0.24	0.70	1.25
0.8–1.0	2.02	6.42	11.76	0.16	0.37	1.17	0.30	0.75	1.40
1 year	2.71	7.28	13.78	0.17	0.43	1.34	0.35	0.74	1.35
2 years	3.17	7.58	13.38	0.21	0.54	1.42	0.26	0.67	1.30
3 years	4.10	8.75	16.01	0.26	0.69	1.93	0.29	0.69	1.40
4–6 years	4.72	8.90	16.94	0.26	0.80	2.18	0.30	0.76	1.43
6–9 years	4.95	9.59	16.56	0.30	0.86	2.35	0.32	0.70	1.40
>9 years	5.18	9.59	17.80	0.33	1.08	2.67	0.32	0.76	1.35

Table A12 Immunoglobulin multiplication factors

Conversion of immunoglobulin values	IU/mL to g/L	g/L to IU/mL
IgG	0.0774	12.93
IgA	0.0141	71.13
IgM	0.008	123.84
IgE	IU = 2.4 ng	

APPENDIX 2
GROWTH CHARTS AND PUBERTAL STAGING

GIRLS IN UTERO 24–42 WKS
POST NATAL 0–3 YEARS

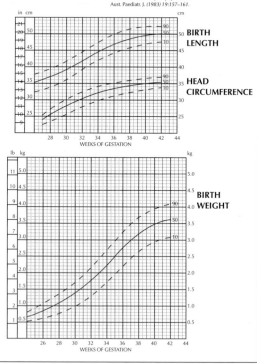

INTRAUTERINE GROWTH CURVES (COMPOSITE MALE/FEMALE)

Measuring techniques: (as for ages 0–36 months—see over page)

Additional Notes: Gestational ages are recorded in completed weeks from the first day of the mother's last menstrual period. Foetal growth is influenced by many factors including age, body weight, height, parity, ethnic origin of the mother and sex of the foetus. Corrections for some of these factors are found in the quoted reference.

Data Source: W.H. Kitchen et al Revised intrauterine growth curves for an Australian hospital population. Aust. Paediatr. J. (1983) 19:157–161.

Designed by the Department of Endocrinology, The Adelaide Children's Hospital, 1989.

GIRLS 0–3 YEARS
LENGTH PERCENTILE CHART

Reproduced with permission of
the Pharmacia Growth Service

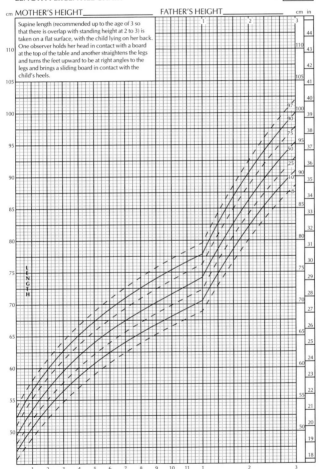

cm MOTHER'S HEIGHT_____   FATHER'S HEIGHT_____ cm in

Supine length (recommended up to the age of 3 so
that there is overlap with standing height at 2 to 3) is
taken on a flat surface, with the child lying on her back.
One observer holds her head in contact with a board
at the top of the table and another straightens the legs
and turns the feet upward to be at right angles to the
legs and brings a sliding board in contact with the
child's heels.

Data Source: Hamill P.V.V.: NCHS growth curves for children. DHEW publication (PHS) 78–1650

GIRLS 0–3 YEARS
WEIGHT PERCENTILE CHART

Weight should be taken in the nude, or as near thereto as possible. If a surgical gown or minimum underclothing (vest and pants) is worn, then its estimated weight (about 0.1 kg) must be subtracted before weight is recorded. Weights are conveniently recorded to the last completed 0.1 kg above the age of six months. The bladder should be empty.

DATE	AGE	LENGTH	WEIGHT	HEAD CIRCUM.

SIMPLIFIED CALCULATION OF BODY SURFACE AREA (BSA)

$$BSA (m^2) = \sqrt{\frac{Ht (cm) \times Wt (kg)}{3600}}$$

Ref: Mosteller R.D.
Simplified calculation of body surface area
N.Engl. J.Med. 1987; 317:1098.

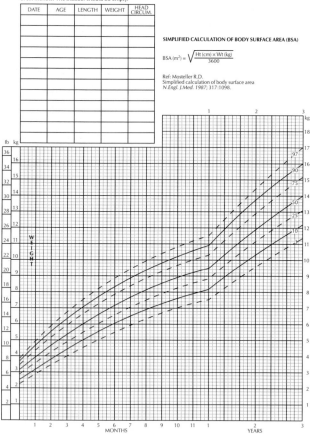

HEAD CIRCUMFERENCE
GIRLS
In utero 28–40 weeks, 0–12 months

Reproduced with permission of
the Pharmacia Growth Service

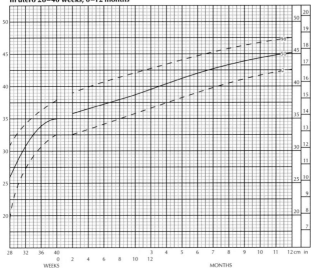

1–3 years

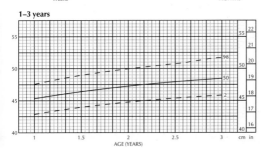

MEASURING TECHNIQUE
HEAD CIRCUMFERENCE

The tape should be placed over the eyebrows, above the ears and over the most prominent part of the occiput taking a direct route. A paper tape is preferable to plastic which stretches unacceptably. Record to nearest 0.1 cm.

SOURCES
Head circumference 0–3 years from NSW Health Commission Publication (Jones DL and Hemphill W, 1974).
Head circumference 28–40 weeks gestation from Kitchen WH Aust. Paediatr. J. (1983) 19:157–161.

BOYS   IN UTERO 24–42 WKS
POST NATAL 0–3 YEARS

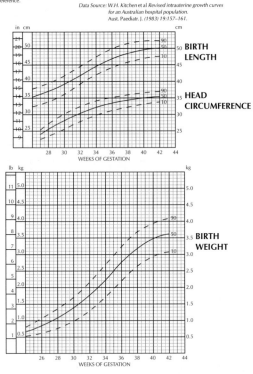

INTRAUTERINE GROWTH CURVES (COMPOSITE MALE/FEMALE)

Measuring techniques: (as for ages 0–36 months—see over page)

Additional Notes: Gestational ages are recorded in completed weeks from the first day of the mother's last menstrual period. Foetal growth is influenced by many factors including age, body weight, height, parity, ethnic origin of the mother and sex of the foetus. Corrections for some of these factors are found in the quoted reference.

*Data Source: W.H. Kitchen et al Revised intrauterine growth curves
for an Australian hospital population.
Aust. Paediatr. J. (1983) 19:157–161.*

Designed by the Department of Endocrinology, The Adelaide Children's Hospital, 1989.

BOYS 0–3 YEARS
LENGTH PERCENTILE CHART

Reproduced with permission of
the Pharmacia Growth Service

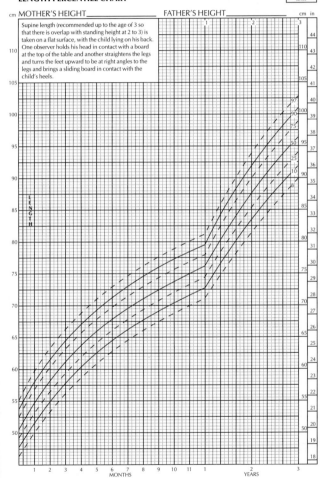

cm MOTHER'S HEIGHT_____ FATHER'S HEIGHT_____ cm in

Supine length (recommended up to the age of 3 so
that there is overlap with standing height at 2 to 3) is
taken on a flat surface, with the child lying on his back.
One observer holds his head in contact with a board
at the top of the table and another straightens the legs
and turns the feet upward to be at right angles to the
legs and brings a sliding board in contact with the
child's heels.

Data Source: Hamill P.V.V.: NCHS growth curves for children. DHEW publication (PHS) 78–1650

BOYS 0–3 YEARS
WEIGHT PERCENTILE CHART

Weight should be taken in the nude, or as near thereto as possible. If a surgical gown or minimum underclothing (vest and pants) is worn, then its estimated weight (about 0.1 kg) must be subtracted before weight is recorded. Weights are conveniently recorded to the last completed 0.1 kg above the age of six months. The bladder should be empty.

DATE	AGE	LENGTH	WEIGHT	HEAD CIRCUM.

SIMPLIFIED CALCULATION OF BODY SURFACE AREA (BSA)

$$BSA\ (m^2) = \sqrt{\frac{Ht\ (cm) \times Wt\ (kg)}{3600}}$$

Ref: Mosteller R.D.
Simplified calculation of body surface area
N.Engl. J.Med. 1987; 317:1098.

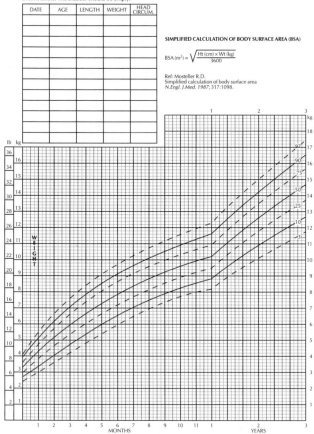

Data Source: Hamill P.V.V.: NCHS growth curves for children. DHEW publication (PHS) 78–1650

HEAD CIRCUMFERENCE
BOYS

Reproduced with permission of
the Pharmacia Growth Service

In utero 28–40 weeks, 0–12 months

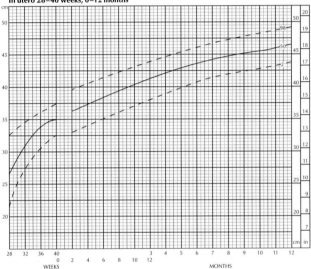

1–3 years

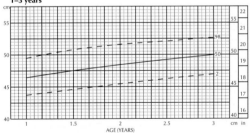

MEASURING TECHNIQUE
HEAD CIRCUMFERENCE

The tape should be placed over the eyebrows,
above the ears and over the most prominent part
of the occiput taking a direct route. A paper tape
is preferable to plastic which stretches unacceptably.
Record to nearest 0.1 cm.

SOURCES
*Head circumference 0–3 years from NSW Health
Commission Publication (Jones DL and Hemphill
W, 1974).*
*Head circumference 28–40 weeks gestation from
Kitchen WH Aust. Paediatr. J. (1983) 19:157–161.*

GIRLS: 2 TO 18 YEARS
HEIGHT PERCENTILE

Reproduced with permission of
the Pharmacia Growth Service

MOTHER'S HEIGHT_____   FATHER'S HEIGHT_____

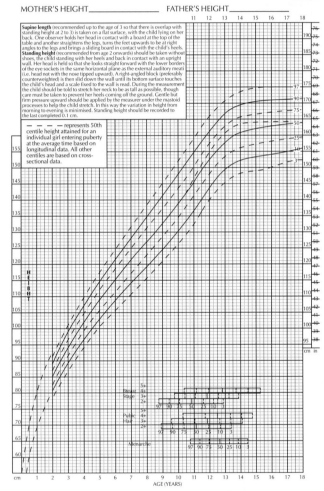

Supine length (recommended up to the age of 3 so that there is overlap with standing height at 2 to 3) is taken on a flat surface, with the child lying on her back. One observer holds her head in contact with a board at the top of the table and another straightens the legs, turns the feet upwards to be at right angles to the legs and brings a sliding board in contact with the child's heels.
Standing height (recommended from age 2 onwards) should be taken without shoes, the child standing with her heels and back in contact with an upright wall. Her head is held so that she looks straight forward with the lower borders of the eye sockets in the same horizontal plane as the external auditory meati (i.e. head not with the nose tipped upward). A right-angled block (preferably counterweighted) is then slid down the wall until its bottom surface touches the child's head and a scale fixed to the wall is read. During the measurement the child should be told to stretch her neck to be as tall as possible, though care must be taken to prevent her heels coming off the ground. Gentle but firm pressure upward should be applied by the measurer under the mastoid processes to help the child stretch. In this way the variation in height from morning to evening is minimised. Standing height should be recorded to the last completed 0.1 cm.

– – – – represents 50th centile height attained for an individual girl entering puberty at the average time based on longitudinal data. All other centiles are based on cross-sectional data.

Source: Adapted from Hamill P.V.V.: NCHS growth curves for children. DHEW publication (PHS) 78–1650

GIRLS: 2 TO 18 YEARS
WEIGHT PERCENTILE

Weight should be taken in the nude, or as near thereto as possible. If a
surgical gown or minimum underclothing (vest and pants) is worn, then its
estimated weight (about 0.1 kg) must be subtracted before weight is recorded.
Weights are conventionally recorded to the last completed 0.1 kg above the
age of six months. The bladder should be empty.

DATE	AGE	HEIGHT	WEIGHT	HEAD CIRCUM.	PUBERTAL STAGES		
					BREAST	PUBIC HAIR	MEN-ARCHE

SIMPLIFIED CALCULATION OF BODY SURFACE AREA (BSA)

$$BSA\ (m^2) = \sqrt{\frac{Ht\ (cm) \times Wt\ (kg)}{3600}}$$

Ref: Mosteller R.D.
Simplified calculation of body surface area
N.Engl. J.Med. 1987; 317:1098.

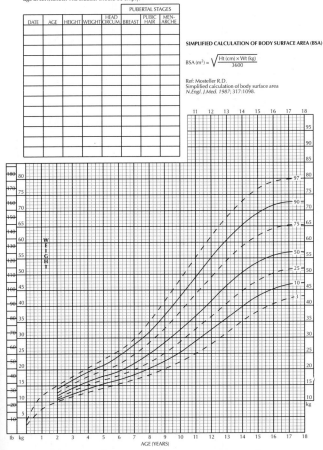

Reproduced with permission of
the Pharmacia Growth Service

HEAD CIRCUMFERENCE, GIRLS

Head Circumference: The tape should be placed over the eyebrows, above
the ears and over the most prominent part of the occiput taking a direct route.
A paper tape is preferable to plastic, which stretches unacceptably under tension.
The maximum measurement should be recorded to the nearest 0.1 cm.

Data Source: 2–5 yr. Jones DL (1973)
NSW Health Comm. Publ.
5–18 yr Nellhaus G. Pediatrics
(1968) 41:106–114

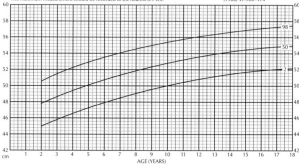

HEIGHT VELOCITY, GIRLS

The standards are appropriate for velocity calculated over a whole year period,
not less, since a smaller period requires wider limits (the 3rd and 97th centiles
for whole year being roughly appropriate for the 10th and 90th centiles over six
months). The yearly velocity should be plotted at the mid-point of a year. The
centiles given in black are appropriate for children of average maturational
tempo, who have their peak velocity at the average age for this event. The red
line is the 50th centile line for the child who is two years early in maturity and
age at peak height velocity, and the blue line refers to a child who is
50th centile in velocity but two years late. The arrows mark the 3rd and
97th centiles at peak velocity for early and late maturers.

Centiles for girls
maturing
at average time

— — — — 97
– – – – – 50
— — — — 3

97 and 3 centiles at peak   ∧
height velocity for   ∨
Early (+2SD) maturers   ▬ ▬ ▬
Late (–2SD) maturers   ▬ ▬ ▬

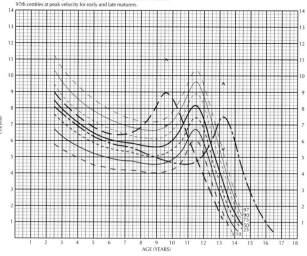

BOYS: 2 TO 18 YEARS
HEIGHT PERCENTILE

Reproduced with permission of
the Pharmacia Growth Service

MOTHER'S HEIGHT_____ FATHER'S HEIGHT_____

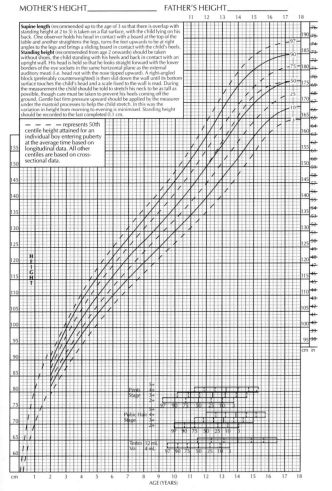

Supine length (recommended up to the age of 3 so that there is overlap with standing height at 2 to 3) is taken on a flat surface, with the child lying on his back. One observer holds his head in contact with a board at the top of the table and another straightens the legs, turns the feet upwards to be at right angles to the legs and brings a sliding board in contact with the child's heels.
Standing height (recommended from age 2 onwards) should be taken without shoes, the child standing with his heels and back in contact with an upright wall. His head is held so that he looks straight forward with the lower borders of the eye sockets in the same horizontal plane as the external auditory meati (i.e. head not with the nose tipped upward). A right-angled block (preferably counterweighted) is then slid down the wall until its bottom surface touches the child's head and a scale fixed to the wall is read. During the measurement the child should be told to stretch his neck to be as tall as possible, though care must be taken to prevent his heels coming off the ground. Gentle but firm pressure upward should be applied by the measurer under the mastoid processes to help the child stretch. In this way the variation in height from morning to evening is minimised. Standing height should be recorded to the last completed 0.1 cm.

— — — — represents 50th centile height attained for an individual boy entering puberty at the average time based on longitudinal data. All other centiles are based on cross-sectional data.

Source: Adapted from Hamill P.V.V.: NCHS growth curves for children. DHEW publication (PHS) 78–1650

BOYS: 2 TO 18 YEARS
WEIGHT PERCENTILE

Reproduced with permission of
the Pharmacia Growth Service

Weight should be taken in the nude, or as near thereto as possible. If a surgical gown or minimum underclothing (vest and pants) is worn, then its estimated weight (about 0.1 kg) must be subtracted before weight is recorded. Weights are conventionally recorded to the last completed 0.1 kg above the age of six months. The bladder should be empty.

| | | | | HEAD | PUBERTAL STAGES | | TESTES | |
| | | | | | | | | |
DATE	AGE	HEIGHT	WEIGHT	CIRCUM.	GENITAL	PUBIC HAIR	R	L

SIMPLIFIED CALCULATION OF BODY SURFACE AREA (BSA)

$$BSA\ (m^2) = \sqrt{\frac{Ht\ (cm) \times Wt\ (kg)}{3600}}$$

Ref: Mosteller R.D.
Simplified calculation of body surface area
N.Engl. J.Med. 1987; 317:1098.

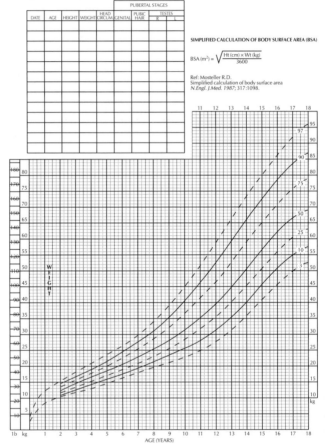

Source: Adapted from Hamill P.V.V.: NCHS growth curves for children. DHEW publication (PHS) 78–1650

HEAD CIRCUMFERENCE, BOYS

Head Circumference: The tape should be placed over the eyebrows, above the ears and over the most prominent part of the occiput taking a direct route. A paper tape is preferable to plastic, which stretches unacceptably under tension. The maximum measurement should be recorded to the nearest 0.1 cm.

Data Source: 2–5 yr. Jones DL (1973) NSW Health Comm. Publ. 5–18 yr Nellhaus G. Pediatrics (1968) 41:106–114

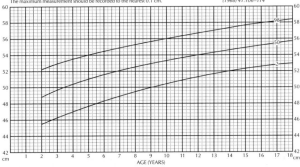

HEIGHT VELOCITY, BOYS

The standards are appropriate for velocity calculated over a whole year period, not less, since a small period requires wider limits (the 3rd and 97th centiles for whole year being roughly appropriate for the 10th and 90th centiles over six months). The yearly velocity should be plotted at the mid-point of a year. The centiles given in black are appropriate to children of average maturational tempo, who have their peak velocity at the average age for this event. The red line is the 50th centile line for the child who is two years early in maturity and age at peak height velocity, and the green line refers to a child who is 50th centile in velocity but two years late. The arrows mark the 3rd and 97th centiles at peak velocity for early and late maturers.

Centiles of whole-year velocity for maturers at average time

97 / 50 / 3

97 and 3 centile at peak height velocity for average maturers
Early (+2SD) maturers
Late (−2SD) maturers

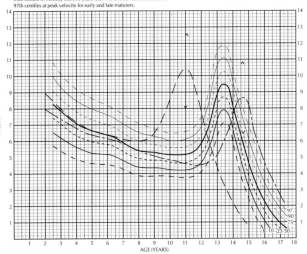

Data Source: Tanner J, Davis PSW, *Journal of Pediatrics* 1985:107

GIRLS 2–18

Reproduced with permission of
the Pharmacia Growth Service

Breast Development

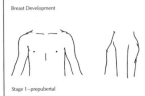

Stage 1–prepubertal

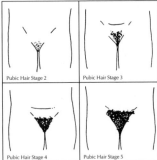

| Pubic Hair Stage 2 | Pubic Hair Stage 3 |
| Pubic Hair Stage 4 | Pubic Hair Stage 5 |

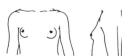

Stage 2–elevation of breasts and papilla

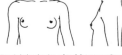

Stage 3–further elevation and areola but no separation of contours

STAGES OF PUBERTY

Ages of attainment of successive stages of pubertal sexual development are given in the height centile chart overpage. The stage Pubic Hair 2+ represents the state of a child who shows the pubic hair appearance stage 2 but not stage 3 (see below). The centiles for age at which this state is normally seen are given, the 97th centile being considered as the early limit, the 3rd centile as the late limit. The child's puberty stages may be plotted at successive ages (Tanner, *Growth at Adolescence*, 2nd Ed., 1962).

Pubic hair:

Stage 1. Pre-adolescent. The vellus over the pubes is not further developed than that over the abdominal wall, i.e. no pubic hair.

Stage 2. Sparse growth of long, slightly pigmented downy hair, straight or slightly curled, chiefly along labia.

Stage 4–areola and papilla form a secondary mound above level of the breast

Stage 3. Considerably darker, coarser and more curled. The hair spreads sparsely over the junction of the pubes.

Stage 4. Hair now adult in type, but area covered is still considerably smaller than in the adult. No spread to the medial surface of thighs.

Stage 5. Adult in quantity and type with distribution of the horizontal (or classically 'feminine') pattern. Spread to medial surface of thighs but not up linea alba or elsewhere above the base of the inverse triangle (spread up linea alba occurs late and is rated stage 6).

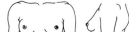

Stage 5–areola recesses to the general contour of the breast

Designed by the Department of Endocrinology, The Adelaide Children's Hospital, 1989.

BOYS 2–18

Reproduced with permission of
the Pharmacia Growth Service

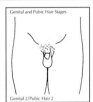

Genital and Pubic Hair Stages

STAGES OF PUBERTY

Ages of attainment of successive stages of pubertal sexual development are
given in the height centile chart overpage. The stage Pubic Hair 2+ represents
the state of a child who shows the pubic hair appearance stage 2 but not stage 3
(see below). The centiles for age at which this state is normally seen are given,
the 97th centile being considered as the early limit, the 3rd centile as the
late limit. The child's puberty stages may be plotted at successive ages (Tanner,
Growth at Adolescence, 2nd Ed., 1962). Testis sizes are judged by comparison
with the Prader orchidometer (Zachmann, Prader, Kind, Haflinger and Budliger,
Helv. Paed. Acta. 29, 61–72, 1974).

Genital (penis) development:
Stage 1. Pre-adolescent, testes, scrotum and penis are of about the same size
and proportion as in early childhood.
Stage 2. Enlargement of scrotum and testes. Skin of scrotum reddens and
changes in texture. Little or no enlargement of penis at this stage.
Stage 3. Enlargement of the penis which occurs at first mainly in length. Further
growth of the testes and scrotum.
Stage 4. Increased size of penis with growth in breadth and development of glans.
Testes and scrotum larger; scrotal skin darkened.
Stage 5. Genitalia adult in size and shape.

Genital 2/Pubic Hair 2

Pubic hair:
Stage 1. Pre-adolescent. The vellus over the pubes is not further developed
than that over the abdominal wall, i.e. no pubic hair.
Stage 2. Sparse growth of long, slightly pigmented downy hair, straight or
slightly curled at the base of the penis.
Stage 3. Considerably darker, coarser and more curled. The hair spreads
sparsely over the junction of the pubes.
Stage 4. Hair now adult in type, but area covered is still considerably smaller
than in the adult. No spread to the medial surface of thighs.
Stage 5. Adult in quantity and type with distribution of the horizontal (or classically
'feminine') pattern. Spread to medial surface of thighs but not up linea
alba or elsewhere above the base of the inverse triangle (spread up
linea alba occurs late and is rated stage 6).

Genital 3/Pubic Hair 3

Stretched Penile Length

Measured from the pubo-penile skin junction to the tip of the glans (Schonfeld
and Beebe, *J. of Urology* 48, 759–777, 1942).

Genital 4/Pubic Hair 4

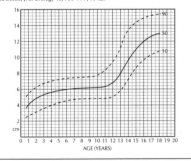

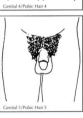

Genital 5/Pubic Hair 5

Designed by the Department of Endocrinology, The Adelaide Children's Hospital, 1989.

APPENDIX 3
ASTHMA MANAGEMENT PLAN

Asthma action plan for _____

Age _____ Date _____

Family doctor _____ Phone _____

Asthma preventive medicine (every day)

| |
| |
| |

When your child is sick

Symptoms:

Give _____ puffs of ventolin via spacer every _____ hours.

When your child is getting worse

The ventolin is needed more than every ____ hours.

Give ___ puffs of ventolin via spacer every _____ hours.

Other: _____

Arrange to see your doctor.

When your child is very sick

If they suffer severe asthma and are:
- so tired that they look like they are going to stop breathing; or
- their lips are turning blue; or
- they can't talk because they are so breathless

CALL THE AMBULANCE ON 000

While waiting, you should stay calm.

Give your child _____ puffs of ventolin (blue) continuously until the ambulance arrives.

APPENDIX 4
ADRENAL CRISIS

Measures to prevent ADRENAL CRISIS

Advice to Parents

VOMITING

Vomiting mildly (1-2 episodes)

↓

Repeat tablets* (triple dose) plus sugar & fluids

↓

Vomits again or becomes sleepy or drowsy

← Yes — Must be seen by doctor and must receive hydrocortisone injection

No → No additional medication. Observe. Glucose & fluids. Next dose as normal.

*Cortisone, Prednisolone or Hydrocortisone (not Florinef)

DIARRHOEA	- Must be seen by a doctor for a hydrocortisone injection	
ILLNESS	- Ill/fever	→ Triple dose until well
		→ Must see a doctor
INJURY (cut or broken bone)		→ Must see a doctor and receive either a triple dose or an injection
SURGERY/ANAESTHETIC		→ Injection of hydrocortisone before surgery
		→ Injection or increase tablets after surgery

Royal Children's Hospital Tel. 9345 5522
Endocrinology Department Tel. 9345 5951
© RCH 1998

APPENDIX 5
PHARMACOPOEIA

Considerable care has been taken to see that the information in this pharmacopoeia is accurate, but the user is advised to check the doses carefully. The authors shall not be responsible for any errors in this publication.

Acetazolamide   2–7.5 mg/kg per dose (adult 100–350 mg) 8 hourly, orally.

Acetylcholine   Adult (NOT/kg): 1%. Inject 0.5–2 mL into the anterior chamber of the eye.

Acetylcysteine   Paracetamol poisoning (regardless of delay): 150 mg/kg in 5% D i.v. over 1 h; then 10 mg/kg per h for 20 h (delay <10 h), 32 h (delay 10–16 h), 72 h (delay >16 h) and longer if still encephalopathic. Monitor serum K^+. Give if paracetamol >1000 µmol/L (150 µg/mL) at 4 h, >500 µmol/mL 8 h, >250 µmol/mL 12 h. Lung disease: 10% solution 0.1 mg/kg per dose (adult 5 mL) 6–12 hourly nebulised or intratracheal. Meconium ileus equivalent: 5 mL/dose (NOT/kg) of 20% solution 8 hourly, orally. CF: 4–8 mg/kg per dose 8 hourly, orally. Eye drops 5% + hypromellose 0.35%: 1–2 drops/eye 6–8 hourly.

Aciclovir   Cutaneous herpes: 5 mg/kg per dose (2–12 weeks), 250 mg/m² per dose (12 weeks–12 years), 5 mg/kg per dose (adult) 8 hourly i.v. over 1 h. Herpes encephalitis, varicella or EB virus: 500 mg/m² per dose (adult 10 mg/kg) 8 hourly i.v. over 1 h; neonate 10 mg/kg per dose i.v. over 1 h daily (<30 weeks' gestation), 18 hourly (30–32 weeks), 12 hourly (first week of life), 8 hourly (2–12 weeks). Genital herpes (NOT/kg): 200 mg/dose oral × 5/day for 10 days, then 200 mg/dose × 2–3/day for 6 months if required. Zoster (NOT/kg): 400 mg/dose (<2 years) or 800 mg/dose (≥2 years) oral × 5/day for 7 days. Cold sores: apply 5% cream × 5/day.

Activated charcoal   Check bowel sounds present: 0.25 g/kg per dose hourly n.g. Laxative: sorbitol 1 g/kg (1.4 mL/kg of 70%) once n.g., may repeat once.

Adenosine 0.10 mg/kg (adult 3 mg) stat rapid i.v. push, increased by 0.05 mg/kg (adult 3 mg) every 2 min to a max of 0.3 mg/kg (adult 18 mg).

Adrenaline Croup: 1% (L isomer) or 2.25% (racemic) 0.05 mL/kg per dose diluted to 4 mL by inhalation; or 1/1000 0.5 mL/kg per dose (max 6 mL) by inhalation. Cardiac arrest: 0.1 mL/kg of 1/10 000 i.v. or intracardiac or via ETT (up to 1 mL/kg per dose if no response). Anaphylaxis: 0.05–0.1 mL/kg per dose of 1/10 000 i.v. Subcutaneous: 0.01 mg/kg (0.01 mL/kg of 1/1000), × three doses 20 min apart if required. Intravenous infusion 0.05–2 µg/kg per min. For 65 kg adult, 5 mg in 50 mL at 2 mL/h is 0.05 µg/kg per min.

Albendazole 20 mg/kg per dose (max 400 mg) once (the usual regimen), 12 hourly for 3 days repeated in 3 weeks (*Strongyloides, cutaneous larva migrans, Taenia, H. nana, O. viverrini, C. sinesis*); 12 hourly for 3–10 days (neurocysticercosis); 12 hourly for three 28-day courses 14 days apart (hydatid).

Albumin 20%: 2–5 mL/kg i.v. 5%: 10–20 mL/kg.

Alginic acid (Gaviscon) <1 year: 1–2 g of powder with feed 4 hourly. 1–12 years: liquid 5–10 mL, or granules 1/2 sachet after meals. >12 years: liquid 10–20 mL, or granules one sachet after meals.

Allopurinol Gout: 2–12 mg/kg per dose (max 600 mg) daily, p.o. Cancer therapy: 2.5–5 mg/kg per dose (max 200 mg) 6 hourly.

Alpha-tocopheryl acetate (1 mg = 1 u Vitamin E) Abetalipoproteinaemia: 100 mg/kg (max 4 g) daily, orally. Cystic fibrosis: 45–200 mg (NOT/kg), p.o. Newborn (high dose, toxicity reported): 10–25 mg/kg daily, i.m. or i.v., 10–100 mg/kg daily, p.o.

Alprostadil (prostaglandin E1, PGE1) 0.01–0.1 µg/kg per min (10–100 ng/kg per min). To maintain PDA with 0.01 µg/kg per min (10 ng/kg per min): <16 kg put 30 µg/kg in 50 mL saline, run at 1 mL/h; >16 kg put 500 µg in 830/wt mL saline, run at 1 mL/h (e.g., 20 kg child, 500 µg in 41.5 mL saline at 1 mL/h). Pulmonary vasodilation with 0.1 µg/kg per min (100 ng/kg per min); put 500 µg in 83/wt mL saline and run at 1 mL/h (5.0 µg/kg per min nitroglyc = 2.0 µg/kg per min nitropr = 0.1 µg/kg per min PGE1 approximately). Erectile dysfunction (adult NOT/kg): 2.5 µg intracavernous injection, increase in 2.5 µg increments if required to a max of 60 µg (max of 3 doses/week).

Alteplase (tissue plasminogen activator) 0.2–0.5 mg/kg per h i.v. for

6–12 h (longer if no response); keep fibrinogen >100 mg/dL (give cryoprecipitate 1 bag/5 kg), give heparin 10 u/kg per h i.v., give fresh frozen plasma (FFP) 10 mL/kg i.v., daily in infants. Local IA infusion: 0.05 mg/kg per h, give FFP 10 mL/kg i.v., daily.

Aluminium acetate, solution 13% (Burrow's lotion) For wet compresses, or daily to molluscum contagiosum.

Aluminium hydroxide 5–50 mg/kg per dose (adult 0.5–1 g) 6–8 hourly, orally. Gel (64 mg/mL) 0.1 mL/kg per dose 6 hourly, p.o.

Aluminium hydroxide 40 mg/mL, magnesium hydroxide 40 mg/mL, simethicone 4 mg/mL (Mylanta) 0.2–0.4 mL/kg per dose (adult 10–20 mL) 4–6 hourly, orally. ICU: 0.5 mL/kg per dose 3 hourly, orally if gastric pH <5.

Amethocaine Gel 4% in methylcellulose (Royal Children's Hospital): 0.5 g to skin, apply occlusive dressing, wait 30–60 min, remove gel. Eye drops 0.5%, 1%: 1–2 drops.

Amikacin Single daily dose i.v. or i.m.: 7.5 mg/kg (<30 weeks gestation), 10 mg/kg (30–35 weeks gestation), 15 mg/kg (first week of life), 22.5 mg/kg (1 week–10 years), 18 mg/kg (>10 years, max 1.5 g). Trough <5 mg/L.

Amiloride 0.2 mg/kg per dose (max 5 mg) 12 hourly, orally.

Aminocaproic acid 100 mg/kg (adult 5 g) stat, then 30 mg/kg per h (max 1.25 g/h) until the bleeding stops (max 18 g/m^2 per day) orally or i.v. Prophylaxis: 70 mg/kg per dose 6 hourly.

Aminophylline (100 mg aminophylline = 80 mg theophylline) Load: 10 mg/kg (max 500 mg) i.v. over 1 h. Maintenance: first week of life—2.5 mg/kg per dose 12 hourly; second week of life—4 mg/kg per dose 12 hourly; 3 weeks–12 months—((0.12 × age in weeks) + 3) mg/kg per dose 8 hourly; 1–9 years—1.1 mg/kg per h (55 mg/kg in 50 mL at 1 mL/h), or 6 mg/kg per dose i.v. over 1 h, 6 hourly; 10–16 years or adult smoker—0.7 mg/kg per h (<35 kg 35 mg/kg in 50 mL at 1 mL/h; >35 kg 25 mg/mL at 0.028 mL/kg per h), or 4 mg/kg per dose i.v. over 1 h, 6 hourly; adult nonsmoker—0.5 mg/kg per h (25 mg/mL at 0.02 mL/kg per h), or 3 mg/kg per dose i.v. over 1 h, 6 hourly; elderly—0.3 mg/kg per h (15 mg/kg in 50 mL at 1 mL/h), or 2 mg/kg per dose i.v. over 1 h, 6 hourly. Monitor theophylline level: 60–80 μmol/L (neonate), 60–110 (asthma) (× 0.18 = μg/mL).

Amiodarone intravenous: 25 μg/kg per min for 4 h, then 5–15 μg/kg per min (max 1.2 g/24 h). Oral: 4 mg/kg per dose (adult 200 mg)

8 hourly 1 week, 12 hourly 1 week, then 12–24 hourly. After starting tablets, taper i.v. infusion over 5 days. Reduce the dose of digoxin and warfarin.

Amitriptyline   Usually 0.5–1 mg/kg per dose (adult 25–50 mg) 8 hourly, p.o. Enuresis: 1–1.5 mg/kg nocte.

Amoxycillin and **clavulanic acid**   Dose as for amoxycillin.

Amoxycillin   10–25 mg/kg per dose (adult 0.25–1 g) 8 hourly i.v., i.m. or p.o. Severe infection: 50 mg/kg per dose (adult 2 g) i.v., 12 hourly (first week of life); 6 hourly (2–4 weeks); 4–6 hourly or constant infusion (>4 weeks).

Amphotericin B   Test dose 0.1 mg/kg i.v. over 1 h, followed immediately by 0.5–1 mg/kg i.v. over 6 h, daily; total dose 30–35 mg/kg over 4–8 weeks. Oral (NOT/kg): 100 mg 6 hourly treatment, 50 mg 6 hourly prophylaxis. Bladder washout: 25 μg/mL. Cream or ointment 3%: apply 6–12 hourly.

Amphotericin, liposomal   1 mg/kg daily, i.v. over 1 h, increase over 2–4 days to 2–3 mg/kg daily. Total dose typically 20–60 mg/kg over 2–4 weeks.

Ampicillin   10–25 mg/kg per dose (adult 0.25–1 g) 6 hourly: i.v., i.m. or p.o. Severe infection: 50 mg/kg per dose (max 2 g) i.v., 12 hourly (first week of life); 6 hourly (2–4 weeks); 3–6 hourly or constant infusion (4+ weeks).

Ampicillin 1 g and **sulbactam 0.5 g**   25–50 mg/kg per dose (adult 1–2 g) of ampicillin 6 hourly, i.m. or i.v. over 30 min.

Amrinone   <4 weeks old: 4 mg/kg i.v. over 1 h, then 3–5 μg/kg per min. >4 weeks: 1–3 mg/kg i.v. over 1 h, then 5–15 μg/kg per min.

Antivenom to Australian jellyfish (box), snakes (black, brown, death adder, sea, taipan and tiger), spiders (funnel-web) and ticks   The dose depends on the amount of venom injected, not size of the patient. Higher doses are needed for multiple bites, severe symptoms or delayed administration. Give adrenaline 0.005 mg/kg (0.005 mL/kg of 1 in 1000) s.c. Initial dose of antivenom is usually 1–2 ampoule diluted 1/10 in Hartmann's solution i.v. over 30 min. Monitor PT, PTT, fibrinogen, platelets. Give repeatedly if symptoms or coagulopathy persist.

Antivenom to black widow spider (USA), red back spider (Australia)   1 ampoule i.m., may repeat in 2 h. Severe envenomation: 2 ampoules diluted 1/10 in Hartmann's solution i.v. over 30 min.

Aprotinin (1 kiu = 140 ng = 0.00056 epu, 1 mg = 7143 kiu)   100 000–1 200 000 kiu/m² over 1 h, then 100 000–300 000 kiu/m² per h i.v. ECMO hge: 10 000 kiu/kg per h i.v.

Arginine hydrochloride   Dose (mg) = BE × wt (kg) × 70 (administer half this) i.v. over 2 h.

Ascorbic acid   Scurvy (NOT/kg): 100 mg/dose 8 hourly, orally for 10 days. Urine acidification: 10–30 mg/kg per dose 6 hourly.

Aspirin   10–15 mg/kg per dose (adult 300–600 mg) 4–6 hourly, orally. Antiplatelet: 2–5 mg/kg daily. Kawasaki: 4 mg/kg daily. Arthritis: 25 mg/kg per dose (max 2 g) 6 hourly for 3 days, then 15–20 mg/kg per dose 6 hourly. Salicylate level (arthritis) 0.7–2.0 mmol/L (× 13.81 = mg/100 mL).

Atenolol   Oral: 1–2 mg/kg per dose (adult 50–100 mg) 12–24 hourly. Intravenously: 0.05 mg/kg (adult 2.5 mg) every 5 min until there is a response (max 4 doses), then 0.1–0.2 mg/kg per dose (adult 5–10 mg) over 10 min, 12–24 hourly.

Atracurium   0.3–0.6 mg/kg stat, then 5–10 μg/kg per min i.v.

Atropine sulphate   0.02 mg/kg (max 0.6 mg) i.v. or i.m., then 0.01 mg/kg per dose, 4–6 hourly. Organophosphate poisoning: 0.05 mg/kg i.v., then 0.02–0.05 mg/kg per dose every 15–60 min until atropinised (continue 12–24 h). Colic: see phenobarbitone.

Azathioprine   25–75 mg/m² (approximately 1–3 mg/kg) daily.

Azithromycin   15 mg/kg (adult 500 mg) day 1, then 7.5 mg/kg (adult 250 mg) days 2–5 oral.

Azlocillin   50 mg/kg per dose (adult 2 g) 8 hourly i.v. Severe infection: 100 mg/kg per dose (adult 5 g) 12 hourly (first week of life), 8 hourly or constant infusion (>2 weeks).

Aztreonam   25 mg/kg per dose (adult 1 g) 8 hourly, i.v. Severe infection: 50 mg/kg per dose (adult 2 g) 12 hourly (first week of life), 8 hourly (2–4 weeks), 6 hourly or constant infusion (>4 weeks).

Bacillus Calmette–Guérin (BCG) suspension, **about 5 × 10⁸ c.f.u./ vial**   Adult: one vial (OncoTICE) or three vials (ImmuCyst) left in bladder for 2 hours each week for 6 weeks, then at 3, 6, 12, 18 and 24 months.

Bacillus Calmette–Guérin (BCG) vaccine (CSL)   Live. Intradermal (1 mg/mL): 0.075 mL (<3 months) or 0.1 mL (>3 months) once. Percutaneous (60 mg/mL suspension): one drop on the skin, inoculated with Heaf apparatus, once.

Bacitracin 400 u/g + neomycin 5 mg/g + polymyxin B 5000 u/g (Neosporin) Ointment or eye ointment: apply × 2–5/day. Powder: apply 6–12 hourly (skin infections), every few days (burns). Eye drops: see gramicidin.

Baclofen 0.1 mg/kg per dose (adult 5 mg) 8 hourly, orally, increase every 3 days to about 0.4 mg/kg per dose (adult 20 mg) 8 hourly, max 0.8 mg/kg per dose (adult 35 mg) 8 hourly. Intrathecal infusion: 2–20 µg/kg (max 1000 µg) per 24 h.

Beclomethasone Rotacap or aerosol (NOT/kg): 100–200 µg (<8 years), 150–500 µg (>8 years) × 2–4/day. Nasal (NOT/kg): aerosol or pump (50 µg/spray): one spray 12 hourly (<12 years), two spray 12 hourly (>12 years).

Benzhexol Initially 0.02 mg/kg per dose (adult 1 mg) 8 hourly, increase to 0.1–0.3 mg/kg per dose (adult 1.5–5 mg) 8 hourly, orally.

Benzocaine, topical 1%–20% Usually applied 4–6 hourly.

Benzoic acid 6% + salicylic acid 3%, ointment (Whitfield's) Apply 12 hourly.

Benztropine mesylate 0.02 mg/kg (adult 1 mg) stat i.m./i.v., may repeat in 15 min 0.02–0.06 mg/kg per dose (adult 1–3 mg) 12–24 hourly, p.o.

Benzyl benzoate, lotion 25% Scabies: apply from neck down after a hot bath, remove in bath after 24 h; repeat after 5 days. Lice: apply to infected region, wash off after 24 h; repeat after 7 days.

Beractant (bovine surfactant, Survanta) 25 mg/mL solution: 4 mL/kg intratracheal four times in 48 h (each dose in four parts: head and body inclined down with head to the right, body down head to left, body up head to the right, body up head to the left).

Betacarotene Porphyria: 1–5 mg/kg (adult 30–300 mg) daily, orally.

Betamethasone 0.01–0.2 mg/kg daily, p.o. Betamethasone has no mineralocorticoid action, 1 mg = 25 mg hydrocortisone in glucocorticoid action. Gel 0.05%; cream, lotion or ointment, 0.02%, 0.05%, 0.1%: apply sparingly 12–24 hourly.

Betamethasone acetate 3 mg/mL with **betamethasone sodium phosphate 3.9 mg/mL (Celestone Chronodose)** Adult: 0.25–2 mL (NOT/kg) i.m., intra-articular, or intralesional injection.

Bethanechol Oral: 0.2–1 mg/kg per dose (adult 10–50 mg) 6–8 hourly. Subcutaneous: 0.05–0.1 mg/kg per dose (adult 2.5–5 mg) 6–8 hourly.

Bicarbonate   Under 5 kg: dose (mmol) = BE × wt/4 slow i.v. Over 5 kg: dose (mmol) = BE × wt/6 slow i.v. These doses correct half the base deficit.

Bisacodyl   NOT/kg: <12 months 2.5 mg p.r., 1–5 years 5 mg p.r. or 5–10 mg p.o., >5 years 10 mg p.r. or 10–20 mg p.o.

Bismuth subcitrate (colloidal)   5 mg/kg per dose (adult 240 mg) 12 hourly, orally 30 min before meals. *H. pylori* (adult, NOT/kg), take 4 doses/day (with meals and at bedtime) orally for 2 weeks: 107.7 mg/dose, tetracycline 500 mg/dose, and metronidazole 200 mg/dose with meals and 400 mg nocte; see also omeprazole.

Blood   4 mL/kg packed cells raises Hb 1 g %. 1 bag = 300 mL.

Botulinum A toxin   NOT/kg: 1.25–2.5 u/site (max 5 u/site) i.m., max total 200 u in 30 days.

Bretylium tosylate   5–10 mg/kg i.v. over 1 h, then 5–30 µg/kg per min.

Bromocriptine   0.025 mg/kg per dose (adult 1.25 mg) 8–12 hourly, increase weekly to 0.05–0.2 mg/kg per dose (adult 2.5–10 mg) 6–12 hourly, p.o. Inhibit lactation (NOT/kg): 2.5 mg/dose 12 hourly for 2 weeks.

Budesonide   Metered dose inhaler (NOT/kg): <12 years: 50–200 µg 6–12 hourly, reducing to 100–200 µg 12 hourly; >12 years: 100–600 µg 6–12 hourly, reducing to 100–400 µg 12 hourly. Nebuliser (NOT/kg): <12 years: 0.5–1 mg 12 hourly, reducing to 0.25–0.5 mg 12 hourly; >12 years: 1–2 mg 12 hourly, reducing to 0.5–1 mg 12 hourly. Croup: 2 mg (NOT/kg) by nebuliser. Nasal spray or aerosol (NOT/kg): 100–200 µg/nostril daily.

Bupivacaine   Maximum dose: 2–3 mg/kg (0.4–0.6 mL/kg of 0.5%). With adrenaline: max dose: 3–4 mg/kg (0.6–0.8 mL/kg of 0.5%). Epidural: 2 mg/kg (0.4 mL/kg 0.5%) stat intra-operation, then 0.25 mg/kg per h (0.2 mL/kg per h 0.125%) post-operation. Epidural in ICU: 25 mL 0.5% + 1000 µg (20 mL) fentanyl + saline to 100 mL at 2–8 mL/h in adult.

Caffeine   1–5 mg/kg per dose (adult 50–250 mg) 4–8 hourly, p.o. or p.r.

Calamine lotion   Usually applied 6–8 hourly.

Calcitonin   Hypercalcaemia: 4 u/kg per dose 12–24 hourly i.m. or s.c., may increase up to 8 u/kg per dose 6–12 hourly. Paget's: 1.5–3 u/kg (max 160 u) × 3/week i.m. or s.c.

Calcium (as carbonate, lactate or phosphate) NOT/kg: <3 years: 100 mg × 2–5/day p.o.; 4–12 years: 300 mg × 2–3/day; >12 years: 1000 mg × 1–2/day.

Calcium carbonate NOT/kg: 840 mg 8–12 hourly, p.o.

Calcium chloride 10% (0.7 mmol/mL Ca) 0.2 mL/kg (max 10 mL) slow i.v. stat. Requirement 2 mL/kg per day. Inotrope: 0.5–2 mmol/kg per day (0.03–0.12 mL/kg per h).

Calcium gluconate 10% (0.22 mmol/mL Ca) 0.5 mL/kg (max 20 mL) slow i.v. stat. Requirement 5 mL/kg per day. Inotrope: 0.5–2 mmol/kg per day (0.1–0.4 mL/kg per h).

Calcium polystyrene sulphonate (Calcium Resonium) 0.3–0.6 g/kg per dose (adult 15–30 g) 6 hourly n.g. (+ lactulose), p.r.

Canrenoate potassium 3–8 mg/kg (adult 150–400 mg) daily, i.v.

Captopril 0.1–1 mg/kg per dose (adult 5–50 mg) 8 hourly, p.o.

Carbamazepine 2 mg/kg per dose (adult 100 mg) 8 hourly, p.o., may increase over 2 weeks to 5–10 mg/kg per dose (adult 250–500 mg) 8 hourly. Level 20–50 μmol/L (× 0.24 = μg/mL) measured Monday, Wednesday and Friday at the Royal Children's Hospital.

Carbenicillin 25–100 mg/kg per dose (adult 1–5 g) 4–6 hourly, i.m. or i.v.

Carbenoxolone sodium Adult (NOT/kg): 20–50 mg, 6 hourly, p.o. Mouth gel 2%, or 2 g granules in 40 mL water, apply 6 hourly.

Carbimazole 0.4 mg/kg per dose (adult 20 mg) 8–12 hourly, p.o. for 2 weeks, then 0.1 mg/kg per dose (adult 5 mg) 8–24 hourly.

Carnitine 20–35 mg/kg per dose (max 1 g) 8 hourly: p.o. or i.v.

Carob bean gum (Carobel Instant) NOT/kg: 1 scoop (1.8 g) in 100 mL water, give 10–20 mL by spoon; or add 1/2 a scoop to every 100–200 mL of milk.

Castor oil Laxative: 1 mL/kg (adult 45 mL) p.o. Purgative: 2 mL/kg (adult 90 mL) p.o.

Cefaclor 10–15 mg/kg per dose (adult 250–500 mg) 8 hourly, p.o. Slow release tab 375 mg (adult, NOT/kg): 1–2 tab 12 hourly, p.o.

Cefotaxime 25 mg/kg per dose (adult 1 g) 12 hourly (<4 weeks), 8 hourly (>4 weeks) i.v. Severe infection: 50 mg/kg per dose (adult 2–3 g) i.v., 12 hourly (preterm), 8 hourly (first week of life), 6 hourly (2–4 weeks), 4–6 hourly or constant infusion (>4 weeks).

Ceftazidime 15–25 mg/kg per dose (adult 0.5–1 g) 8 hourly: i.v. or i.m. Severe infection: 50 mg/kg per dose (max 2 g) 12 hourly (first week of life), 8 hourly (2–4 weeks), 6 hourly or constant infusion (>4 weeks).

Ceftriaxone 25 mg/kg per dose (adult 1 g) 12–24 hourly: i.v., or i.m. (in 1% lignocaine). Severe infection: 50 mg/kg per dose (max 2 g) daily (first week of life), 12 hourly (>2 weeks). Epiglottitis: 100 mg/kg stat, then 50 mg/kg after 24 h. *Haemophilus* or *meningococcus prophylaxis*: 100 mg/kg i.m. in 1% lignocaine once.

Cefuroxime Oral: 10–15 mg/kg per dose (adult 250–500 mg) 12 hourly. Intravenously: 25 mg/kg per dose (adult 1 g) 8 hourly. Severe infection: 50 mg/kg per dose (max 2 g) i.v., 12 hourly (first week of life), 8 hourly (second week), 6 hourly or constant infusion (>2 weeks).

Cephalexin 10–25 mg/kg per dose (adult 0.25–1 g) 6–12 hourly, p.o.

Cephalothin 15–25 mg/kg per dose (adult 0.5–1 g) 6 hourly: i.v. or i.m. Severe infection: 50 mg/kg per dose (max 2 g) i.v.: 4 hourly or constant infusion. Irrigation fluid: 2 g/L (2 mg/mL).

Cephamandole 15–25 mg/kg per dose (adult 0.5–1 g) 6–8 hourly, i.v. over 10 min or i.m. Severe infection: 40 mg/kg per dose (adult 2 g) i.v. over 20 min, 4–6 hourly or constant infusion.

Cephazolin 25 mg/kg (adult 1 g) stat, then 10–15 mg/kg per dose (adult 0.5 g) 6 hourly: i.v. or i.m. Severe infection: 50 mg/kg per dose (adult 2 g) i.v., 4–6 hourly or constant infusion.

Cetirizine 0.2 mg/kg (max 10 mg) p.o. 12 hourly.

Cetylpyridinium + benzocaine, mouth wash (Cepacaine) Apply 3 hourly p.r.n. Do not swallow.

Chloral hydrate Hypnotic: 50 mg/kg (max 2 g) stat (up to 100 mg/kg, max 5 g, in ICU). Sedative: 6 mg/kg per dose 6 hourly, orally.

Chloramphenicol Severe infection: 40 mg/kg (max 2 g) stat, then 25 mg/kg per dose (max 1 g) i.v., i.m. or p.o. First week of life: daily; 2–4 weeks: 12 hourly; 5+ weeks: 8 hourly for 5 days, then 6 hourly. Ensure serum level 20–30 mg/L peak, <15 mg/L trough.

Chlormethiazole Intravenously (edisylate 0.8%): 1–2 mL/kg (8–16 mg/kg) over 15 min, then 0.5–1 mL/kg per h (4–8 mg/kg per h). Oral (capsule 192 mg base): adult 2–4 cap stat (may repeat in 1–2 h), then 1–2 cap, 8 hourly.

Chloroquine Oral: 10 mg/kg (max 600 mg) daily × 3 days. Intramuscularly: 4 mg/kg per dose (max 300 mg) 12 hourly for 3 days. Prophylaxis: 5 mg/kg (adult 300 mg) orally × 1/week. Lupus, rheu arthritis: 12 mg/kg (max 600 mg) daily, reducing to 4–8 mg/kg (max 400 mg) daily, p.o.

Chlorothiazide   5–20 mg/kg per dose (adult 0.25–1 g) 12–24 hourly, p.o., i.v.

Chlorpheniramine maleate   0.1 mg/kg per dose (adult 4 mg) 6–8 hourly, p.o.

Chlorpheniramine maleate 1.25 mg + phenylephrine 2.5 mg in 5 mL syrup   NOT/kg: 1.25–2.5 mL (0–1 years), 2.5–5 mL (2–5 years), 5–10 mL (6–12 years), 10–15 mL (>12 years) 6–8 hourly, p.o.

Chlorpromazine   Oral or p.r.: 0.5–2 mg/kg per dose (max 100 mg) 6–8 hourly; up to 20 mg/kg per dose 8 hourly for psychosis. Slow i.v. or i.m.: 0.25–1 mg/kg per dose (usual max 50 mg) 6–8 hourly.

Chlorpropamide   Adult: initially 125–250 mg (NOT/kg) daily, orally, a max of 500 mg daily.

Chlortetracycline, **cream** or **ointment 3%**   Apply 8–24 hourly.

Cholera vaccine (CSL)   Inactivated. Two doses s.c. 7–28 days apart: 0.1 mL then 0.3 mL (<5 years), 0.3 mL then 0.5 mL (5–9 years), 0.5 mL then 1 mL (>9 years). Boost every 6 months (use first dose).

Cholestyramine   50–150 mg/kg per dose (adult 3–9 g) 6–8 hourly, p.o.

Cimetidine   Oral: 6–8 mg/kg per dose (adult 300–400 mg) 6 hourly, or 16 mg/kg (adult 800 mg) nocte. Intravenously: 10–15 mg/kg per dose (max 200 mg) 12 hourly (newborn), 6 hourly (>4 weeks).

Ciprofloxacin   5–10 mg/kg per dose (adult 250–500 mg) 12 hourly, p.o., 4–7 mg/kg per dose (adult 200–300 mg) 12 hourly, i.v. Severe infection: 15 mg/kg per dose (max 750 mg) 12 hourly, p.o., 8 mg/kg per dose (max 400 mg) 8 hourly, i.v.; higher doses used occasionally. *Meningococcus proph.*: 15 mg/kg (max 750 mg) once orally. Reduce dose of theophylline.

Cisapride   0.1–0.3 mg/kg per dose (adult 5–15 mg) (rarely 0.4 mg/kg per dose, max 20 mg) × 3–4/day p.o.

Clarithromycin   7.5–15 mg/kg per dose (adult 250–500 mg) 12 hourly, p.o. Slow release tab, adult (NOT/kg): 0.5 g or 1 g daily.

Clindamycin   3–6 mg/kg per dose (adult 150–300 mg) 6 hourly, p.o., i.m. or i.v. over 30 min. Severe infection: 10–20 mg/kg per dose (adult 0.5–1 g) 6 hourly, i.v. over 1 h. Acne solution 1%: apply 12 hourly.

Clioquinol, **cream 10 mg/g**, **powder 100%**   Apply 6–12 hourly.

Clobazam   0.1–0.4 mg/kg per dose (adult 10–20 mg) 8–12 hourly, p.o.

Clomiphene   Adult: 50 mg (NOT/kg) daily for 5 days p.o., increase to 100 mg daily for 5 days if no ovulation.

Clomipramine   0.5–1 mg/kg per dose (adult 25–50 mg) 8–12 hourly, p.o.

Clonazepam   0.02 mg/kg per dose (max 0.5 mg) 12 hourly, p.o., slowly increase to 0.05 mg/kg per dose (max 2 mg) 6–12 hourly, p.o. Status (may be repeated), NOT/kg: neonate 0.25 mg (if ventilated), child 0.5 mg, adult 1 mg i.v.

Clonidine   3–5 µg/kg slow i.v., 1–6 µg/kg per dose (adult 50–300 µg) 8–12 hourly, p.o. Migraine: start with 0.5 µg/kg per dose 12 hourly, p.o.

Clotrimazole   Topical: 1% cream or solution 8–12 hourly. Vaginal (NOT/kg): 1% cream or 100 mg tab daily for 6 days, or 2% cream or 500 mg tab daily for 3 days.

Cloxacillin   15 mg/kg per dose (adult 500 mg) 6 hourly, p.o., i.m. or i.v. Severe infection: 25–50 mg/kg per dose (adult 1–2 g) i.v. 12 hourly (first week of life), 8 hourly (2–4 weeks), 4–6 hourly (>4 weeks).

Coal tar, topical   0.5% increase to a max of 10%, applied 6–8 hourly.

Cocaine   Topical: 1–3 mg/kg.

Codeine   Analgesic: 0.5–1 mg/kg per dose 4 hourly oral. Antitussive: 0.25–0.5 mg/kg per dose 6 hourly.

Colchicine   Acute gout: 0.02 mg/kg per dose (adult 1 mg) 2 hourly, p.o. (max 3 doses/day). Chronic use (gout, FMF): 0.01–0.04 mg/kg (adult 0.5–2 mg) daily, p.o.

Colfosceril palmitate (synthetic surfactant, Exosurf Neonatal)   Solution 13.5 mg/mL. Prophylaxis: 5 mL/kg intratracheal over 5 min immediately after birth, and at 12 h and 24 h if still ventilated. Rescue: 5 mL/kg intratracheal over 5 min, repeat in 12 h if still ventilated.

Colistin 3 mg/mL + neomycin 3.3 mg/mL otic   four drops, 8 hourly.

Colistin sulphomethate sodium (1 mg = 12 500, u = 0.625 mg colistin sulphate)   Oral: 30 000–60 000 u/kg per dose (adult 1.5–3 mega u) 8 hourly. Intramuscularly or slow i.v.: 40 000 u/kg per dose (adult 2 000 000 u) 8 hourly, or 3 mg/kg per dose (adult 150 mg) 8 hourly.

Colonic lavage solution   Poisoning: if bowel sounds present, 30 mL/kg per h n.g. for 4–8 h (until the rectal effluent is clear).

Corticotrophin (ACTH)   1 unit/kg (adult 40 u) i.m., daily.

Cortisone acetate   Physiological: 0.2 mg/kg per dose 8 hourly, p.o. Cortisone acetate 1 mg = hydrocortisone 1.25 mg in mineralocorticoid and glucocorticoid action.

Co-trimoxazole (trimethoprim 1 mg + sulphamethoxazole 5 mg)
TMP 1.5–3 mg/kg per dose (adult 80–160 mg) 12 hourly, i.v. over
1 h or p.o. Renal prophylaxis: TMP 2 mg/kg (max 150 mg) daily,
p.o. Pneumocystis: TMP 250 mg/m^2 stat, then 150 mg/m^2 8 hourly
(<11 years) or 12 hourly (>10 years), i.v. over 1 h; in renal failure
dose interval (hour) = serum creatinine (mmol/L) × 135 (max 48 h);
1 h post-infusion serum TMP 5–10 µg/mL, SMX 100–200 µg/mL.
Intravenous infusion: TMP max 1.6 mg/mL in 5% dextrose.

Coumarin   Orally: 1–8 mg/kg (adult 50–400 mg) daily. Cream
100 mg/g: apply 8–12 hourly.

Cromoglycate, sodium   Inhalation (Intal): one cap (20 mg) 6–8 hourly,
2 mL solution (20 mg) 6–8 hourly, aerosol 1–10 mg 6–8 hourly. Eye
drops (2%): 1–2 drops per eye, 4–6 hourly. Oral: 5–10 mg/kg per
dose (max 200 mg) 6 hourly, p.o. Nasal (Rynacrom): insufflator 5 mg
in each nostril, 6 hourly; spray one puff in each nostril, 6 hourly.

Crotamiton, cream or lotion 10%   Apply × 2–3/day.

Cryoprecipitate   Low factor 8: 1 u/kg increase activity 2% (half life
12 h); usual dose 5 mL/kg or 1 bag/4 kg 12 hourly, i.v. for 1–2 infusions (muscle, joint), 3–6 infusions (hip, forearm, retroperitoneal,
oropharynx), 7–14 infusions (intracranial). Low fibrinogen: usual
dose 5 mL/kg or 1 bag/4 kg i.v. A bag is usually 20–30 mL: factor
8 about 5 u/mL and 100 u/bag, fibrinogen about 10 mg/mL and
200 mg/bag.

Cyanocobalamin (Vitamin B12)   20 µg/kg per dose (adult 1000 µg) i.m.,
daily for 7 days and then weekly (treatment), monthly (prophylaxis).
Intravenous treatment is dangerous in megaloblastic anaemia.

Cyclopentolate, eye drops 0.5% or 1%   one drop per eye, repeat after
5 min. Pilocarpine 1% speeds recovery.

Cyclosporin   1–3 µg/kg per min i.v. for 24–48 h, then 5–8 mg/kg per
dose 12 hourly, reducing by 1 mg/kg per dose each month to
3–4 mg/kg per dose p.o. Trough level by Abbott TD × monoclonal
specific assay (× 2.5 = non-specific assay level) on whole blood
(performed Tuesday and Friday at the Royal Children's Hospital):
120–200 ng/mL (marrow), 150–200 ng/mL first 3 months then
100–150 ng/mL (kidney), 100–400 ng/mL (heart and liver).

Cyproheptadine   0.1 mg/kg per dose (adult 4 mg) 8–12 hourly oral.

**Cyproterone acetate + ethinyloestradiol (2 mg/35 µg) × 21 tab,
+ seven inert tab**   Contraception: one tab daily, starting first day
of menstruation.

Cysteamine   0.05 mg/m² per dose 6 hourly, orally. Increase over 6 weeks to 0.33 mg/m² per dose (<50 kg) or 0.5 mg/kg per dose (>50 kg) 6 hourly.

Dalteparin sodium   Proph: 50 u/kg per dose (adult 2500 u) s.c. 1–2 h pre-operation, then daily. Venous thrombosis: 100 u/kg per dose (adult 5000 u) 12 hourly s.c., or i.v. over 12 h. Haemodialysis: 5–10 u/kg stat, then 4–5 u/kg per h i.v. (acute renal failure, anti-Xa 0.2–0.4 u/mL); 30–40 u/kg stat, then 10–15 u/kg per h (chronic renal failure, anti-Xa 0.5–1 u/mL).

Danazol   2–4 mg/kg per dose (adult 100–200 mg) 6–12 hourly, p.o.

Dantrolene   Hyperpyrexia: 1 mg/kg per min until improves (max 10 mg/kg), then 1–2 mg/kg per dose 6 hourly for 1–3 days i.v. or p.o. Spasticity: 0.5–2 mg/kg per dose (adult 25–100 mg) 6 hourly, p.o.

Dapsone   1–2 mg/kg (adult 50–100 mg) daily, p.o. Derm herpet: 1–6 mg/kg (adult 50–300 mg) daily, p.o. See also pyrimethamine.

Desferrioxamine   Antidote: 10–15 mg/kg per h i.v. for 12–24 h (max 6 g/24 h); some also give 5–10 g (NOT/kg) once orally. Thalassaemia (NOT/kg): 500 mg per unit blood; and 5–6 nights/week 1–3 g in 5 mL water s.c. over 10 h, 0.5–1.5 g in 10 mL water s.c. over 5 min.

Desipramine   0.5–1 mg/kg per dose (adult 25–50 mg) 8–12 hourly, p.o.

Desmopressin (DDAVP)   5–10 µg (0.05–0.1 mL) per dose (NOT/kg) 12–24 hourly, nasal. Low Factor VIII: 0.3 µg/kg in 1 mL/kg saline i.v. over 1 h, 12–24 hourly.

Dexamethasone   0.1–0.25 mg/kg per dose 6 hourly: p.o. or i.v. BPD: 0.1 mg/kg per dose 6 hourly for 3 days, then 8 hourly for 3 days, 12 hourly for 3 days, 24 hourly for 3 days, 48 hourly for 7 days. Severe croup: 0.6 mg/kg (max 12 mg) i.m. stat, then prednisolone 1 mg/kg per dose 8–12 hourly, p.o. Eye drops 0.1%: 1–2 drops per eye 3–8 hourly. Dexamethasone has no mineralocorticoid action, but 1 mg = 25 mg hydrocortisone in glucocorticoid action.

Dexamphetamine   0.2 mg/kg (max 10 mg) daily, p.o. Increase to a max of 0.6 mg/kg per dose (max 30 mg) 12 hourly.

Dexchlorpheniramine   0.04 mg/kg per dose (adult 2 mg) 6–8 hourly, p.o.

Diazepam   0.2–0.4 mg/kg (adult 10–20 mg) i.v. or p.r. 0.04–0.2 mg/kg per dose (adult 2–10 mg) 8–12 hourly, p.o. Do not give by i.v. infusion (binds to PVC).

Diazoxide Hypertension: 1–3 mg/kg (max 150 mg) stat by rapid i.v. injection (severe hypotension may occur) repeat once p.r.n., then 2–5 mg/kg per dose, i.v., 6 hourly. Hyperinsulinism: 30–100 mg/m^2 per dose 8 hourly, p.o.

Diclofenac 1 mg/kg per dose (adult 50 mg) 8–12 hourly, p.o. Eye drops 0.1%: pre-operation 1–5 drops over 3 h, postoperation 3 drops stat, then 1 drop, 4–8 hourly. Topical gel: apply 2–4 g, 6–8 hourly.

Dicloxacillin 5–10 mg/kg per dose (adult 250–500 mg) 6 hourly, p.o.: i.m. or i.v. Severe infection: 25–50 mg/kg per dose (max 2 g) i.v., 12 hourly (first week life), 8 hourly (2–4 weeks), 4–6 hourly or constant infusion (>4 weeks).

Digitoxin 4 μg/kg per dose (max 0.2 mg) 12 hourly, orally for 4 days, then 1–6 μg/kg (adult usually 0.15 mg, max 0.3 mg) daily.

Digoxin 15 μg/kg stat and 5 μg/kg after 6 hourly, then 5 μg/kg per dose (max 200 μg i.v., 250 μg p.o.) 12 hourly, slow i.v. or orally. Level 0.5–2.5 nmol/L (× 0.78 = ng/mL).

Digoxin FAB antibodies Intravenously over 30 min. Dose (to the nearest 40 mg) = serum digoxin (nmol/L) × wt (kg) × 0.3, or mg ingested × 55. Give if >0.3 mg/kg ingested, or level >6.4 nmol/L or 5.0 ng/L.

Dihydrocodeine 0.5–1 mg/kg per dose 4–6 hourly, p.o.

Dihydroergotamine mesylate Adult (NOT/kg): 1 mg i.m., s.c. or i.v.; repeat hourly × 2 if needed. Max 6 mg/week.

Diltiazem 1 mg/kg per dose (adult 60 mg) 8 hourly, increase to a max of 3 mg/kg per dose (adult 180 mg) 8 hourly, p.o. Slow release (adult, NOT/kg): 120–240 mg daily, or 90–180 mg 8–12 hourly, p.o.

Diphenhydramine 1–2 mg/kg per dose (adult 50–100 mg) 6–8 hourly, p.o.

Diphtheria + pertussis (acellular) + tetanus vaccine (Infanrix) 0.5 mL i.m. at 2, 4, 6 and 18 months and 4–5 years of age.

Diphtheria + pertussis (whole cell) + tetanus vaccine (Triple Antigen) 0.5 mL i.m. at 2, 4, 6 and 18 months and 4–5 years of age.

Diphtheria + tetanus vaccine, adult (ADT) Inactivated. 0.5 mL i.m. stat, 6 weeks later and 6 months later. Boost every 10 years.

Diphtheria + tetanus vaccine, child <8 years (CDT) Inactivated. 0.5 mL i.m. stat, 6 weeks later and 6 months later. Boost with ADT.

Diphtheria vaccine, adult (CSL) Inactivated. 0.5 mL i.m. stat, 6 weeks later and 6 months later. Boost every 10 years.

Diphtheria vaccine, child <8 years (CSL)   Inactivated. 0.5 mL i.m. stat, 6 weeks later and 6 months later. Boost with adult vaccine.

Dipyridamole   1–2 mg/kg per dose (adult 50–100 mg) 6–8 hourly, p.o.

Disopyramide   Oral: 1.5–4 mg/kg per dose (adult 75–200 mg) 6 hourly. Intravenous: 2 mg/kg (max 150 mg) over 5 min, then 0.4 mg/kg per h (max 800 mg/day). Level 9–15 µmol/L (× 0.3395 = µg/mL).

Disulfiram   Adult (NOT/kg): 500 mg p.o., daily for 1–2 weeks, then 125–500 mg daily.

Dobutamine   Intravenous infusion 1–20 µg/kg per min: for a 65 kg adult 250 mg in 50 mL at 2 mL/h is 2.5 µg/kg per min.

Docusate sodium   NOT/kg: 100 mg (3–10 years), 120–240 mg (>10 years) daily, p.o. Enema (5 mL 18% + 155 mL water): 30 mL (newborn), 60 mL (1–12 months), 60–120 mL (>12 months) p.r.

Docusate sodium 100 mg + bisacodyl 10 mg, suppository   1/2 suppository (<12 months), one suppository (>1 year) when required.

Docusate sodium 50 mg + sennoside 8 mg, tab   >12 years: 1–4 tab at night, p.o.

Domperidone   Oral: 0.2–0.4 mg/kg per dose (adult 10–20 mg) 4–8 hourly. Rectal suppositories: adult (NOT/kg) 30–60 mg 4–8 hourly.

Dopamine   Intravenous infusion 1–20 µg/kg per min: for a 65 kg adult 200 mg in 50 mL at 2 mL/h is 2 µg/kg per min.

Dopexamine   Intravenous infusion 0.5–6 µg/kg per min: for a 65 kg adult 50 mg in 50 mL at 2 mL/h is 0.5 µg/kg per min.

Dornase alpha (deoxyribonuclease I)   NOT/kg: usually 2.5 mg (max 10 mg) inhaled daily (5–21 years), 12–24 hourly (>21 years).

Dothiepin   0.5–1 mg/kg per dose (adult 25–50 mg) 8–12 hourly, p.o.

Doxapram   5 mg/kg i.v. over 1 h, then 0.5–1 mg/kg per h for 1 h (max total dose 400 mg).

Doxycycline   Over 8 years: 2 mg/kg per dose (adult 100 mg) 12 hourly for two doses, then daily.

Droperidol   0.1–0.4 mg/kg per dose (adult 5–20 mg) 4–8 hourly, p.o.; 0.1–0.3 mg/kg per dose (adult 5–15 mg) 4–6 hourly: i.m. or slow i.v. Anti-emetic: postoperation 0.02–0.05 mg/kg per dose (adult 1.25 mg) 4–6 hourly: i.m. or slow i.v.; chemotherapy 0.02–0.1 (adult 1–5 mg) 1–6 hourly.

Econazole   Topical: 1% cream, powder or lotion 8–12 hourly. Vaginal: 75 mg cream or 150 mg ovule twice daily.

Eformoterol   Caps 12 mg (NOT/kg): 1 cap (child) or 1–2 caps (adult) inhaled 12 hourly.

Enalapril   0.2–1 mg/kg (adult 5–40 mg) daily, p.o.

Enoximone   Intravenous: 5–20 µg/kg per min. Oral: 1–3 mg/kg per dose (adult 50–150 mg) 8 hourly.

Ephedrine   0.3–1 mg/kg per dose (adult 15–60 mg) 6–8 hourly, p.o. Nasal (0.25%–1%): 1 drop each nostril 6–8 hourly, for a max of 4 days.

Epoetin alfa, beta   20–50 u/kg × 3/week, increase to a max of 240 u/kg × 1–3/week s.c., i.v. When Hb >10 g %: 20–100 u/kg × 2–3/week.

Epoprostenol (prostacyclin, PGI2)   0.01 µg/kg per min i.v. Pul vasodil: 0.01µg/kg per min epoprost = 5 µg/kg per min nitroglyc = 2 µg/kg per min nitropr = 0.1 µg/kg per min PGE1.

Ergometrine maleate   Adult (NOT/kg): 250–500 µg i.m. or i.v.; 500 µg 8 hourly, p.o., sublingual or p.r.

Ergotamine tartrate   >10 years (NOT/kg): 2 mg sublingual stat, then 1 mg/h (max 6 mg/episode, 10 mg/week). Suppository (1–2 mg): one stat, may repeat once after 1 h.

Erythromycin   Orally or slow i.v. (max 5 mg/kg per h): usually 10 mg/kg per dose (adult 250–500 mg) 6 hourly; severe infection 15–25 mg/kg per dose (adult 0.75–1 g) 6 hourly. Two per cent gel: apply 12 hourly.

Esmolol   0.5 mg/kg over 1 min, then 50 µg/kg per min for 4 min; if there is a poor response repeat 0.5 mg/kg and give 50–200 µg/kg per min for up to 48 h.

Ethacrynic acid   Intravenous: 0.5–1 mg/kg per dose (adult 25–50 mg) 12–24 hourly. Oral: 1–4 mg/kg per dose (adult 50–200 mg) 12–24 hourly.

Ethambutol   25 mg/kg once daily for 8 weeks, then 15 mg/kg daily, p.o. Intermittent: 35 mg/kg × 3/week. Intravenous: 80% oral dose.

Ethamsylate   12.5 mg/kg per dose (max 500 mg) 6 hourly: p.o., i.m. or i.v.

Ethanolamine oleate, solution 5%   Adult: 1.5–5 mL per varix (max 20 mL per treatment).

Ethionamide   TB: 15–20 mg/kg (max 1 g) at night p.o. Leprosy: 5–8 mg/kg (max 375 mg) daily.

Ethosuximide   10 mg/kg (adult 500 mg) daily, orally, increase by 50% each week to a max of 40 mg/kg (adult 2 g) daily.

Etidronate 5–20 mg/kg daily, orally (no food for 2 h before and after dose) for a max of 6 months.

Etomidate 0.3 mg/kg slow i.v.

Factor 8 concentrate (vial 200–250 u), recombinant antihaemophilic factor (rAHF) Joint 20 u/kg, psoas 30 u/kg, cerebral 50 u/kg. Two × dose (u/kg) = % normal activity; e.g. 35 u/kg gives a peak level of 70% normal.

Factor 8 inhibitor bypassing fraction Intravenous infusion—a max of 2 u/kg per min: joint 50 u/kg per dose 12 hourly, mucous membrane 50 u/kg per dose 6 hourly, soft tissue 100 u/kg per dose 12 hourly, cerebral 100 u/kg per dose 6–12 hourly.

Factor 9 complex (factor 2, 9, 10, and some 7) 40–60 iu/kg, then 5–10 iu/kg per dose 12 hourly, i.v. Prophylaxis: 10–20 iu/kg × 1–2/week. Factor 8 antibodies: 75 iu/kg, repeat in 12 h p.r.n.

Famciclovir Zoster: 5 mg/kg (max 250 mg) 8 hourly, orally for 7 days. Genital herpes: 5 mg/kg per dose (max 250 mg) 8 hourly, orally for 5 days, if there is a recurrence 2.5 mg/kg per dose (max 125 mg) 12 hourly for 5 days.

Famotidine 0.5–1 mg/kg per dose (adult 20–40 mg) 12–24 hourly, orally. 0.5 mg/kg per dose (max 20 mg) 12 hourly, slow i.v.

Felodipine 0.05 mg/kg per dose (adult 2.5 mg), increase to 0.2 mg/kg per dose (adult 10 mg) 12 hourly, p.o.

Fenoterol Oral: 0.1 mg/kg per dose 6 hourly. Respiratory solution 1 mg/mL: 0.5 mL/dose diluted to 2 mL 3–6 hourly (mild), 1 mL/dose diluted to 2 mL 1–2 hourly (moderate), undiluted continuous (severe, in ICU). Aerosol (200 μg/puff): 1–2 puffs 4–8 hourly.

Fentanyl 1–4 μg/kg per dose (adult 200 μg) i.m. or i.v.; infuse 2–4 μg/kg per h (<25 kg: 100 μg/kg in 50 mL at 1–2 mL/h, >25 kg: ampoule 50 μg/mL at 0.04–0.08 mL/kg per h). Ventilated: 5–10 μg/kg stat or 50 μg/kg i.v. over 1 h; infuse 5–10 μg/kg per h (ampoule 50 μg/mL at 0.1–0.2 mL/kg per h).

Ferrous salts Prophylaxis 2 mg/kg per day elemental iron p.o., treatment 6 mg/kg per day elemental iron orally. Fumarate 1 mg = 0.33 mg iron. Gluconate 1 mg = 0.12 mg iron; so Fergon (60 mg/mL gluconate) prophylaxis 0.3 mL/kg daily, treatment 1 mL/kg daily, orally. Sulphate (dried) 1 mg = 0.3 mg iron; so Ferro–Gradumet (350 mg dried sulphate) prophylaxis 7 mg/kg (adult 350 mg) daily, treatment 20 mg/kg (adult 1050 mg) daily, p.o.

Filgrastim (granulocyte CSF) Idiopathic or cyclic neutropenia: 5 µg/kg daily, s.c. or i.v. over 30 min. Congenital neutropenia: 12 µg/kg daily, s.c. or i.v. over 1 h. Marrow transplant: 20–30 µg/kg daily, i.v. over 4–24 h, reducing if neutrophils >1 x 10^9 L.

Flecainide 2 mg/kg per dose (max 100 mg) 12 hourly, p.o., i.v. over 30 min; may increase over 2 weeks to a 5 mg/kg per dose (max 200 mg) 12 hourly.

Flucloxacillin 10 mg/kg per dose (adult 250 mg) 6 hourly, p.o., i.m. or i.v. Severe infection: 25–50 mg/kg per dose (adult 1–2 g) i.v., 12 hourly (first week of life), 8 hourly (2–4 weeks), 4–6 hourly or constant infusion (>4 weeks).

Fluconazole 4 mg/kg (adult 200 mg) stat, then 2 mg/kg (adult 100 mg) daily: p.o. or i.v. Severe infection: 8 mg/kg (adult 400 mg) stat, then 4–8 mg/kg (adult 200–400 mg) daily, i.v.

Flucytosine (5-fluorocytosine) 400–1200 mg/m² per dose (max 2 g) 6 hourly: i.v. over 30 min, or p.o. Peak level 25–100 µg/mL, trough <20 µg/mL (× 7.75 = µmol/L).

Fludrocortisone NOT/kg: 0.05–0.2 mg daily, orally. Fludrocortisone 1 mg = hydrocortisone 125 mg in mineralocorticoid activity, 10 mg in glucocorticoid.

Flumazenil 5 µg/kg stat i.v., repeat every 60 s to a max total of 40 µg/kg (max 2 mg), then 2–10 µg/kg per h i.v.

Flunitrazepam Adult (NOT/kg): 0.5–2 mg at night, p.o.

Fluoxetine 0.5 mg/kg (max 20 mg) daily, increase to a max of 1 mg/kg per dose (max 40 mg) 12 hourly, p.o.

Fluticasone Inhaled (NOT/kg): 50–100 µg per dose (child), 100–1000 µg per dose (adult) 12 hourly. 0.05% solution: 1–4 sprays/nostril daily. 0.05% cream: apply sparingly daily.

Fluvastatin 0.4 mg/kg (adult 20 mg) nocte orally, increase to 0.8 mg/kg (adult 40 mg) nocte if required.

Fluvoxamine 2 mg/kg per dose (adult 100 mg) 8–24 hourly, p.o.

Folic acid Treatment: 0.1–0.3 mg/kg (adult 5–15 mg) daily: i.v., i.m. or p.o. Pregnancy: 0.4 mg (NOT/kg) daily.

Folinic acid NOT/kg: 5–15 mg p.o., or 1 mg i.m. or i.v., daily. Rescue starting up to 24 h after methotrexate: 10–15 mg/m² per dose 6 hourly for 36–48 h i.v. Methotrexate toxicity: 100–1000 mg/m² per dose 6 hourly, i.v. Before a fluorouracil dose of 370 mg/m²: 200 mg/m² i.v., daily × 5, repeat every 3–4 weeks.

Follicle stimulating hormone (FSH)   Adult (NOT/kg), monitor urinary oestrogen. Anovulation: usually 75–150 iu i.m., daily for 9–12 days. Superovulation (2 weeks after starting GnRH agonist): 150–225 iu/kg daily, starting day 3 of the cycle.

Foscarnet   20 mg/kg i.v. over 30 min, then 200 mg/kg per day by constant i.v. infusion (less if creatinine >0.11 mmol/L) or 60 mg/kg per dose 8 hourly, i.v. over 2 h. Chronic use: 90–120 mg/kg i.v. over 2 h daily.

Framycetin (Soframycin)   Subconjunctival: 500 mg in 0.5–1 mL water daily × 3 days. Bladder: 500 mg in 50 mL saline 8 hourly × 10 days. Eye/ear 0.5%: 2–3 drops 8 hourly, ointment 8 hourly.

Framycetin 15 mg/g + gramicidin 0.05 mg/g, cream or ointment (Soframycin topical)   Apply 8–12 hourly.

Framycetin 5 mg + gramicidin 0.05 mg + dexamethasone 0.5 mg/mL eye/ear (Sofradex)   2–3 drops 6–8 hourly, ointment 8–12 hourly.

Fresh frozen plasma   Contains all clotting factors. 10–20 mL/kg i.v. One bag is about 230 mL.

Frusemide   Usually 0.5–1 mg/kg per dose (adult 20–40 mg) 6–24 hourly (daily if preterm) i.m., i.v. or p.o. Up to 5 mg/kg per dose in resistant cases. Intravenous infusion: 0.1–1 mg/kg per h.

Fusidic acid   10 mg/kg per dose (adult 500 mg) 8 hourly: p.o. or i.v. over 2–8 h. Peak level 30–200 µmol/L (× 0.52 = µg/mL).

Gabapentin   5–15 mg/kg per dose (adult 300–800 mg) 8–12 hourly, p.o.

Ganciclovir   2.5–5 mg/kg per dose 8–12 hourly, i.v. over 1 h. Chronic use: 5 mg/kg i.v. over 1 h, daily.

Gentamicin   Single daily dose i.v. or i.m.: 2.5 mg/kg (<30 weeks gestation), 3.5 mg/kg (30–35 weeks gestation), 5 mg/kg (first week of life), 7.5 mg/kg (1 week–10 years), 6 mg/kg (>10 years, max 240–360 mg). Trough level <1.0 mg/L, done Monday–Friday at the Royal Children's Hospital.

Glibenclamide   Adult (NOT/kg): initially 2.5 mg daily, p.o., with a max 20 mg daily.

Glucagon   1 u = 1 mg. 0.04 mg/kg (adult 1–2 mg) i.v. or i.m. stat, then 10–50 µg/kg per h (0.5 mg/kg in 50 mL at 1–5 mL/h) i.v.

Glucose   Hypoglycaemia: 1 mL/kg 50% D i.v., then increase the infusion rate. Hyperkalaemia: 0.1 µ/kg insulin + 2 mL/kg 50% D i.v. Neonates: 6 g/kg per day (about 4 mg/kg per min) on day 1, increase to 12 g/kg per day (up to 18 g/kg per day with hypoglycaemia).

Infusion rate (mL/h) = (4.17 × wt × g/kg per day)/% D = (6 × wt × mg/kg per min)/% D. Dose (g/kg per day) = (mL/h × % D)/(4.17 × wt). Dose (mg/kg per min) = (mL/h × % D)/(6.0 × wt). Mg/kg per min = g/kg per day/1.44.

Glucose electrolyte solution   Not dehydrated: one heaped teaspoon of sucrose in a large cup of water (4% sucrose = 2% glucose); do *not* add salt. Dehydrated: one sachet of Gastrolyte in 200 mL water; give frequent small sips, or infuse through a nasogastric tube.

Glutamic acid   10–20 mg/kg (adult 0.5–1 g) p.o. with meals.

Glyceryl trinitrate   Adult (NOT/kg): sublingual tab 0.3–0.9 mg/dose (lasts 30–60 min); sublingual aerosol 0.4–0.8 mg/dose; slow-release buccal tab 1–10 mg 8–12 hourly; transdermal 0.5–5 cm of 2% ointment, or 5–15 mg patch 8–12 hourly. Intravenous infusion 1–10 μg/kg per min: adult 50 mg in 50 mL at 0.8 mL/h is 0.2 μg/kg per min; use polyethylene-lined syringe and tubing (not PVC). Pul vasodil: 5 μg/kg per min nitroglyc = 2 μg/kg per min nitropr = 0.1 μg/kg per min PGE1.

Glycopyrronium   To reduce secretions or to treat bradycardia: 4–8 μg/kg per dose (adult 200–400 μg) 6–8 hourly—i.v. or i.m. With 0.05 mg/kg neostigmine: 10–15 μg/kg i.v. Anticholinergic: 0.02–0.04 mg/kg per dose (max 2 mg) 8 hourly, p.o.

Gramicidin 25 μg/mL + neomycin 2.5 mg/mL + polymyxin B 5000 u/mL (Neosporin)   Eye drops: 1–2 drops/eye every 15–30 min, reducing to 6–12 hourly.

Griseofulvin   10–20 mg/kg (adult 0.5–1 g) daily, p.o.

Griseofulvin (ultramicrosize)   5.5 mg/kg (adult 330 mg) daily, p.o.

***Haemophilus influenzae* type b, vaccines**   Inactivated. <12 months: give diphtheria protein conjugate (HibTITER), or tetanus protein conjugate (Act-HIB) 0.5 mL i.m. at 2, 4, 6 and 15 months; or meningococcal conjugate (Pedvax HIB) 0.5 mL i.m. at 2, 4 and 15 months. If the first dose is at >18 months, give one dose of HibTITER or Pedvax HIB.

Haloperidol   0.01 mg/kg (max 0.5 mg) daily, increase up to 0.1 mg/kg per dose 12 hourly: i.v. or p.o.; up to 2 mg/kg per dose (max 100 mg) 12 hourly used rarely. Acutely disturbed: 0.1–0.2 mg/kg (adult 5–10 mg) i.m. Long-acting decanoate ester: 1–6 mg/kg i.m. every 4 weeks.

Heparin   1 mg = 100 u. Low dose: 75 u/kg i.v. stat, then 10–15 u/kg per h i.v. (500 u/kg in 50 mL at 1 mL/h = 10 u/kg per h). Full dose:

200 u/kg stat, then 15–30 u/kg per h. Extracorporeal circuits: 10–20 u/kg per h prefilter, 2–5 u/kg per h postfilter.

Heparin calcium   Low dose: 75 u/kg per dose s.c. 12 hourly.

Hepatitis A + hepatitis B vaccine (Twinrix)   Inactivated. Adult 1 mL i.m. stat, after 1 month and after 6 months (3 doses). Boost every 5 years.

Hepatitis A vaccine (Havrix)   Inactivated. 0.5 mL (child) or 1 mL (adult) i.m. stat, after 1 month, and after 6–12 months (3 doses). Boost every 5 years.

Hepatitis A vaccine (VAQTA)   Inactivated. 0.5 mL (child) or 1 mL (>17 years) i.m. stat, and after 6–18 months (2 doses).

Hepatitis B vaccine (Engerix-B, HB Vax II)   Inactivated. Engerix-B 10 µg/dose (<10 years), 20 µg (>9 years); Hepatitis B Vax II 2.5 µg/dose (<10 years), 5 µg (10–19 years), 10 µg (>19 years), 40 µg (dialysis) i.m. stat, after 1 month, and after 6 months (3 doses). Boost every 5 years approximately.

Homatropine, eye drops 2%   1–2 drops 4 hourly.

Hydralazine   0.1–0.2 mg/kg (adult 5–10 mg) stat i.v. or i.m., then 4–6 µg/kg per min (adult 200–300 µg/min) i.v. Oral: 0.4 mg/kg per dose (adult 20 mg) 12 hourly, slow increase to 1 mg/kg per dose (usual max 50 mg).

Hydrochloric acid   Use a solution of 150 mmol/L, give i.v. by central line only. Dose (mL) = BE × wt × 2.2 (give half of this). Maximum rate = 1.33 mL/kg per h.

Hydrochlorothiazide   1 mg/kg per dose (adult 50 mg) 12–24 hourly, orally.

Hydrocortisone   Cream or ointment 0.1%, 0.5%, 1%: apply 8–24 hourly. Eye drops 0.5%, 1%: 1–2 drops/eye 2–4 hourly.

Hydrocortisone acetate   Cream or ointment 0.5%: apply 6–12 hourly. Rectal foam 10%: 125 mg/dose (Colifoam). Usually 125 mg 12–24 hourly for 2–3 weeks, then 48 hourly.

Hydrocortisone sodium succinate   2–4 mg/kg per dose 3–6 hourly: i.m. or i.v. Physiological: 0.2 mg/kg per dose 8 hourly: i.m. or i.v.

Hydrogen peroxide 10 volume (3%)   Mouthwash 1 : 2 parts water. Skin or ear disinfectant 1 : 1 part water.

Hydroxocobalamin (Vitamin B12)   20 µg/kg per dose (adult 1000 µg) i.m., daily for 7 days then weekly (treatment), every 2–3 months (prophylaxis). Intravenous treatment is dangerous in megaloblastic anaemia.

Hydroxychloroquine 10 mg/kg (max 600 mg) daily × 3 days p.o. Prophylaxis: 5 mg/kg (max 300 mg) once a week p.o.

Hydroxyzine 0.5–2.0 mg/kg per dose (adult 25–100 mg) 6–8 hourly, p.o.

Hyoscine 0.01 mg/kg per dose (max 0.6 mg) 6 hourly: i.m. or i.v.

Hyoscine butylbromide 0.5 mg/kg per dose (max 40 mg) 6–8 hourly: i.v., i.m. or p.o.

Hyoscine hydrobromide NOT/kg: 0.25 tab (2–7 years), 0.5 tab (7–12 years), 1–2 tab (>12 years) 6–24 hourly, p.o.

Hyoscine transdermal 1.5 mg >10 years: one patch every 72 h.

Ibuprofen 2.5–10 mg/kg per dose (adult 150–600 mg) 6–8 hourly, p.o.

Imipenem/cilastatin 15 mg/kg per dose (adult 500 mg) 6 hourly, i.v. over 30 min. Severe infection: 25 mg/kg per dose i.v. over 1 h (adult 1 g) 12 hourly (first week of life), 8 hourly (2–4 weeks), 6–8 hourly or constant infusion (>4 weeks).

Imipramine 0.5–1.5 mg/kg per dose (adult 25–75 mg) 8 hourly, p.o. Enuresis: 5–6 years 25 mg, 7–10 years 50 mg, >10 years 50–75 mg nocte.

Immunoglobulin, CMV 100–200 mg/kg i.v. over 2 h. Transplant: daily for the first 3 days, weekly × 6, monthly × 6.

Immunoglobulin, diphtheria 250 u i.m. once.

Immunoglobulin, hepatitis B 400 u i.m. within 5 days of needle stick, repeat in 30 days; 100 u i.m. within 24 h of the birth to baby of Hepatitis-B carrier.

Immunoglobulin, lymphocyte (anti-thymocyte immunoglobulin, equine; Atgam) 10 mg/kg daily for 3–5 days i.v. over 4 h in saline.

Immunoglobulin, normal, human Hypogammaglobulinaemia: 10–15 mL/kg of 6% solution (600–900 mg/kg) i.v. over 4 h, then 5–7.5 mL/kg (300–450 mg/kg) monthly; or 0.6 mL/kg of 16% solution (100 mg/kg) every 2–4 weeks i.m. Kawasaki, Guillain–Barre, ITP, myasth gravis, Still's disease: 35 mL/kg of 6% solution (2 g/kg) i.v. over 10 h stat, then if required 15 mL/kg (900 mg/kg) i.v. over 4 h each month. Prevention hepatitis A: 0.1 mL/kg (16 mg/kg) i.m. Prevention measles: 0.2 mL/kg (32 mg/kg) i.m. (repeat next day if immunocompromised).

Immunoglobulin, rabies (Hyperab, Imogam) 20 iu (0.133 mL)/kg i.m. once (1/2 infiltrated around the wound), with rabies vaccine.

Immunoglobulin, respiratory syncytial virus   750 mg/kg every month i.v. (50 mg/mL: 1.5 mL/kg per h for 15 min, 3 mL/kg per h for 15 min, then 6 mL/kg per h).

Immunoglobulin, Rh   1 mL (625 iu, 125 µg) i.m. within 72 h of exposure. Large transfusion: 0.16 mL (100 iu, 20 µg) per mL Rh-positive red cells (maternal serum should be anti-D positive 24–48 h after injection).

Immunoglobulin, tetanus (TIG)   Intramuscular preparation: 250–500 iu (1–2 ampoules). Intravenous preparation: 4000 iu (100 mL) at 0.04 mL/kg per min for 30 min, then 0.075 mL/kg per min.

Immunoglobulin, zoster   Prevention of chickenpox in immuno-compromised, 0.4–1.2 mL/kg (max 6 mL) i.m.

Indomethacin   0.5–1 mg/kg per dose (adult 25–50 mg) 8 hourly (max 6 hourly): p.o. or p.r. PDA: 0.1 mg/kg daily for 6 days p.o. or i.v. in saline over 1 h (0.13 mg/kg daily if >14 days old).

Influenza A and B vaccine (Fluvax, Vaxigrip)   Inactivated. 0.125 mL (<2 years), 0.25 mL (2–6 years), 0.5 mL (>6 years) s.c. stat and 4 weeks later (2 doses). Boost annually (1 dose).

Insulin   Regular insulin: 0.05–0.2 u/kg p.r.n., or 0.1 u/kg per h; later 1 u/10 g dextrose i.v. For hyperkalaemia: 0.1 u/kg insulin and 2 mL/kg 50% dextrose i.v. In TPN: 5–25 u/250 g dextrose. Subcutaneous: insulin lispro onset 10–15 min, peak 1 h, duration 2–5 h; regular insulin onset 30–60 min, peak 4 h, duration 6–8 h; isophane (NPH) insulin onset 2–4 h, peak 4–12 h, duration 18–24 h; zinc (Lente) insulin onset 2–3 h, peak 7–15 h, duration 24 h; crystalline zinc (Ultra-lente) insulin onset 4–6 h, peak 10–30 h, duration 24–36 h; protamine zinc insulin onset 4–8 h, peak 15–20 h, duration 24–36 h.

Interferon alfa-2a, recombinant   1 700 000 u/m² (max 3 000 000 u) s.c. or i.m., daily for 16–24 weeks, then × 3/week.

Interferon alfa-2b, recombinant   Leukaemia: 2 000 000 u/m² s.c. × 3/week. Condylomata: 1 000 000 u into each lesion (max 5) × 3/week for 5 weeks. Hepatitis B: 200 000 u/kg (adult 10 000 000 u) × 3/week s.c., i.m. for 4 months. Hepatitis C: 60 000 u/kg (adult 3 000 000 u) × 3/week, s.c. or i.m. for 24 weeks.

Interferon alfa-n3   Adult: 250 000 u injected into the base of the wart (max 10 doses per session) × 2/week for a max of 8 weeks.

Interferon beta-1a   Adult (MS): 30 µg i.m. once a week.

Interferon beta-1b   Adult (MS): 0.25 mg (8 million iu) s.c. alternate days.

Interferon gamma-1b 1.5 µg/kg per dose (body area ≤0.5 m²) or 50 µg/m² (area >0.5 m²) × 3/week s.c.

Ipecacuanha syrup (total alkaloids 1.4 mg/mL) 1–2 mL/kg (adult 30 mL) stat p.o., n.g.

Ipratropium Respiratory solution (250 µg/mL): 0.25–1 mL diluted to 4 mL 4–6 hourly. Aerosol 20 µg/puff: 2–4 puffs, 6–8 hourly.

Iron dextran, iron polymaltose Fe 50 mg/mL: dose (mL) = 0.05 × wt in kg × (15 – Hb in g %) i.m. (often in divided doses). An i.v. infusion is possible (but dangerous).

Isoniazid 10 mg/kg (max 300 mg) daily: p.o., i.m. or i.v. TB mening-itis: 15–20 mg/kg (max 500 mg) daily.

Isoprenaline Aerosol 80–400 µg/puff: 1–3 puffs 4–8 hourly. Intra-venous infusion <33 kg: 0.3 mg/kg in 50 mL at 1 mL/h = 0.1 µg/kg per min; >33 kg: 0.1 µg/kg per min using 1/5000 (0.2 mg/mL) solution = 0.03 × wt mL/h; for a 65 kg adult 4 mg in 50 mL at 2 mL/h is 0.05 µg/kg per min.

Isosorbide dinitrate Sublingual: 0.1–0.2 mg/kg per dose (max 10 mg) 2 hourly or as needed. Oral: 0.5–1 mg/kg per dose (max 40 mg) 6 hourly or as needed. Slow release tab, adults (NOT/kg): 1–2 tabs daily. Intravenous infusion 0.6–2 µg/kg per min: for a 65 kg adult 50 mg in 50 mL at 2.5 mL/h is 0.5 µg/kg per min.

Isotretinoin Adult: 0.5–1 mg/kg daily, orally for 2–4 weeks, reduc-ing if possible to 0.1–0.2 mg/kg daily for 15–20 weeks. Gel 0.05%: apply sparingly at night.

Ispaghula husk Adult (NOT/kg): 1–2 teaspoonfuls 6–12 hourly, p.o. Half this dose for children.

Itraconazole 2–4 mg/kg per dose (adult 100–200 mg) 12–24 hourly, p.o. after food.

Ivermectin 0.15–0.2 mg/kg (max 12 mg) p.o. every 6–12 months.

Kanamycin Single daily dose i.v. or i.m.: 7.5 mg/kg (<30 weeks gestation), 10 mg/kg (30–35 weeks gestation), 15 mg/kg (first week of life), 22.5 mg/kg (1 week–10 years), 18 mg/kg (>10 years, max 1.5 g). Trough <5 mg/L.

Ketamine 1–2 mg/kg i.v., 5–10 mg/kg i.m. Infusion: anaesthesia 10–20 µg/kg per min, analgesia 4 µg/kg per min.

Ketoconazole Oral: 5 mg/kg per dose (adult 200 mg) 12–24 hourly. Cream 2%: apply 12–24 hourly. Shampoo 2%: wash hair, apply liquid for 5 min, wash off.

Ketoprofen   1–2 mg/kg per dose (adult 50–100 mg) 6–12 hourly (max 4 mg/kg or 200 mg in 24 h): p.o., i.m., p.r. Slow release, adults (NOT/kg): 200 mg daily.

Ketorolac   Oral: 0.2 mg/kg per dose (max 10 mg) 4–6 hourly (max 0.8 mg/kg per day or 40 mg/day). Intramuscular: 0.6 mg/kg (max 30 mg) stat, then 0.2–0.4 mg/kg per dose (max 20 mg) 4–6 hourly for 5 days, then 0.2 mg/kg per dose (max 10 mg) 6 hourly.

Ketotifen   Child >2 years (NOT/kg): 1 mg/dose 12 hourly, p.o. with food. Adult (NOT/kg): 1–2 mg/dose 12 hourly, p.o. with food.

Labetalol   1–2 mg/kg per dose (adult 50–100 mg) 12 hourly, p.o. May increase weekly to a max of 10 mg/kg per dose (max 600 mg) 6 hourly.

Lactulose 50% (Duphalac)   Laxative: 0.5 mL/kg per dose 12–24 hourly, p.o. Hepatic coma: 1 mL/kg per dose hourly until the bowel is cleared, then 6–8 hourly.

Lamotrigine   0.5 mg/kg (adult 25 mg) orally, daily for 2 weeks, then 1 mg/kg (adult 50 mg) daily for 2 weeks, then 1–4 mg/kg per dose (adult 50–200 mg) 12 hourly (double dose if taking carbamaze-pine, phenobarbitone, phenytoin or primidone; halve dose if taking valproate).

Levodopa + benserazide (4 : 1)   Adult (NOT/kg): initially levodopa 100 mg/dose 8 hourly, p.o.; if not controlled, increase weekly by 100 mg/day to a max of 250 mg/dose, 6 hourly.

Levodopa + carbidopa   (250 mg/25 mg   and   100 mg/10 mg   tabs)   Adult (NOT/kg): initially one 100/10 tab, 8 hourly, orally; if not controlled, substitute one 250/25 tab for one 100/25 tab every second day; if not controlled on 250/25 8 hourly, increase by one 250/25 tab every second day to a max of 6–8 tab/day.

Lignocaine   Intravenously 1 mg/kg (0.1 mL/kg of 1%) over 2 min, then 15–50 µg/kg per min: for a 65 kg adult 1 g in 50 mL at 5 mL/h is 25 µg/kg per min. Nerve block: without adrenaline a max of 4 mg/kg (0.4 mL/kg of 1%), with adrenaline 7 mg/kg (0.7 mL/kg of 1%). Topical spray: a max of 3–4 mg/kg (Xylocaine 10% spray pack: about 10 mg/puff). Topical gel 2%, solution 2% and 4%, ointment 5%, dental ointment 10%: apply p.r.n.

Lignocaine 2.5% compound, mouth paint/gel (SM-33)   Apply 3 hourly p.r.n.

Lignocaine 2.5% + prilocaine 2.5%, cream (EMLA)   1.5 g/10 cm² under occlusive dressing for 1–3 h.

Lincomycin   10 mg/kg per dose (max 600 mg) 8 hourly: p.o., i.m. or i.v. over 1 h. Severe infection: up to 20 mg/kg per dose (max 1.2 g) i.v. over 2 h, 6 hourly.

Lindane, cream or lotion 1%   Scabies: apply from the neck down, wash off after 8–12 h. Lice: rub into the hair for 4 min, then wash off; repeat after 24 h (max × 2/week).

Liothyronine (T3)   Oral: 0.2 µg/kg per dose (adult 10 µg) 8 hourly, may increase to 0.4 µg/kg per dose (adult 20 µg) 8 hourly. Intravenously: 0.1–0.4 µg/kg per dose (adult 5–20 µg) 8–12 hourly.

Lipid emulsion 20%   1–3 g/kg per day i.v. (mL/h = g/kg per day × wt × 0.21).

Lisinopril   0.1 mg/kg (adult 5 mg) daily, p.o., may increase over 4–6 weeks to 0.2–0.4 mg/kg (adult 10–20 mg) daily.

Lithium (salts)   5–20 mg/kg per dose 12–24 hourly to maintain trough serum level at 0.8–1.6 mmol/L (>2 mmol/L toxic).

Loperamide   0.05–0.1 mg/kg per dose (max 2 mg) 8–12 hourly, p.o.

Lorazepam   Acute: 0.05–0.2 mg/kg i.v. over 2 min. Chronic: 0.02–0.06 mg/kg per dose (adult 1–3 mg) 8–24 hourly, p.o.

Magnesium chloride   0.48 g/5 mL (1 mmol/mL Mg). 0.4 mmol (0.4 mL)/kg per dose 12 hourly, slow i.v. Myoc infarct (NOT/kg): 5 mmol/h i.v. for 6 h, then 1 mmol/h for 24–48 h.

Magnesium hydroxide   Antacid: 10–40 mg/kg per dose (max 2 g) 6 hourly, p.o. Laxative: 50–100 mg/kg (max 5 g) p.o.

Magnesium sulphate   Deficiency: 50% magnesium sulphate (2 mmol/mL) 0.2 mL/kg per dose (max 10 mL) 12 hourly: i.m., slow i.v. Asthma: 25–40 mg/kg (max 1.2 g) i.v. over 30 min once. Digoxin tachyarrhythmia: 50% magnesium sulphate 0.1 mL/kg (max 5 mL) i.v. over 10 min, then infuse 0.4 mL/kg (max 20 mL) over 6 h, then 0.8 mL/kg (max 40 mL) over 18 h (keep serum Mg 1.5–2.0 mmol/L). Laxative: 0.5 g/kg per dose (max 15 g) as 10% solution 8 hourly for 2 days, p.o. Myoc infarct (NOT/kg): 5 mmol/h i.v. for 6 h, then 1 mmol/h for 24–48 h. Pul ht newborn: aim for 3–4 mmol/L.

Maldison, liquid 0.5%   20 mL to hair, wash off after 12 h.

Mannitol   0.25–0.5 g/kg per dose i.v. (2–4 mL/kg of 12.5%, 1.25–2.5 mL/kg of 20%, 1–2 mL/kg of 25%) 2 hourly p.r.n., provided serum osmolality <320–330 mmol/L.

Measles + mumps + rubella vaccine (MMRII)   Live. >12 months: 0.5 mL s.c.

Measles + mumps vaccine (Rimparix) Live. >12 months: 0.5 mL s.c. once.

Measles vaccine (Attenuvax) Live. >12 months: 0.5 mL s.c. once.

Mebendazole NOT/kg: 100 mg/dose 12 hourly × 3 days. Enterobiasis (NOT/kg): 100 mg once, repeat after 2–4 weeks.

Mebeverine (135 mg tab) Adult (NOT/kg): 1–3 tab daily, p.o.

Mefenamic acid 10 mg/kg per dose (adult 500 mg) 8 hourly, p.o.

Mefloquine 15 mg/kg (adult 750 mg) stat, then 10 mg/kg (adult 500 mg) after 6–8 h. Prophylaxis: 5 mg/kg (adult 250 mg) once a week.

Melatonin Usually 0.1 mg/kg (adult 5 mg) at night, p.o.

Meningococcus group A, C, W135 and Y vaccine (Mencevax ACWY) Inactivated. >2 years: 0.5 mL s.c. Boost 1–3 yearly.

Meropenem 10–20 mg/kg per dose (adult 0.5–1 g) 8 hourly, i.v. over 5–30 min. Severe infection: 20–40 mg/kg per dose (adult 1–2 g) 8 hourly or constant infusion.

Metaraminol Intravenous: 0.01 mg/kg stat (repeat p.r.n.), then 0.1–1 µg/kg per min and titrate dose against BP. Subcutaneous: 0.1 mg/kg.

Methadone Usually 0.1–0.2 mg/kg per dose (adult 5–10 mg) 6–12 hourly: p.o., s.c. or i.m.

Methionine 50 mg/kg per dose (max 2.5 g) p.o., 4 hourly for four doses.

Methotrexate Leukaemia: typically 3.3 mg/m^2 i.v., daily for 4–6 weeks; then 2.5 mg/kg i.v. every 2 weeks, or 30 mg/m^2 p.o. or i.m. × 2/week; higher doses with folinic acid rescue. Intrathecal: 12 mg/m^2 weekly for 2 weeks, then monthly. Adult psoriasis: 0.2–0.5 mg/kg weekly: p.o., i.v. or i.m. until response, then reduce.

Methylcellulose Constipation: 30–60 mg/kg per dose (adult 1.5–3 g) with at least 300 mL fluid 12 hourly, p.o.

Methylene blue 1–4 mg/kg per dose i.v. Septic shock: 0.5 mg/kg over 15 min, i.v., then 0.1–0.25 mg/kg per h.

Methylphenidate Hyperactivity: 0.25 mg/kg daily, p.o., may increase to a max of 2 mg/kg daily. Narcolepsy: 0.1–0.4 mg/kg per dose (max 20 mg) 8 hourly, p.o.

Methylprednisolone Asthma: 0.5–1 mg/kg per dose 6 hourly: p.o., i.v. or i.m. day 1; 12 hourly day 2, then 1 mg/kg daily, reducing to min effective dose. Severe croup: 4 mg/kg i.v. stat, then 1 mg/kg per dose 12 hourly. Severe sepsis before antibiotics (or within 4 h of the first dose): 30 mg/kg i.v. once. Spinal cord injury (within 8 h): 30 mg/kg stat, then 5 mg/kg per h 2 days. Lotion 0.25%: apply sparingly 12–24 hourly. Methylpred 1 mg = hydrocortisone 5 mg in glucocorticoid activity, 0.5 mg in mineralocorticoid.

Methylprednisolone aceponate cream, ointment 0.1% Apply 12–24 hourly.

Methyltestosterone NOT/kg: 2.5–12.5 mg/day buccal.

Methysergide 0.02 mg/kg per dose (max 1 mg) 12 hourly, p.o., increase to a max of 0.04 mg/kg per dose (max 2 mg) 8 hourly, p.o. for 3–6 months.

Metoclopramide 0.12 mg/kg per dose (adult 10–15 mg) 6 hourly: i.v., i.m. or p.o. 0.2–0.4 mg/kg per dose (adult 10–20 mg) 8 hourly p.r.

Metolazone 0.1–0.2 mg/kg (adult 5–10 mg) daily, p.o. Up to 0.5 mg/kg (adult 30 mg) daily, in the short term.

Metoprolol Intravenous: 0.1 mg/kg (adult 5 mg) over 5 min, repeat every 5 min to a max of three doses, then 1–5 µg/kg per min. Oral: 1–2 mg/kg per dose (adult 50–100 mg) 6–12 hourly.

Metronidazole 15 mg/kg stat, then 7.5 mg/kg per dose (max 800 mg) 12 hourly in neonate (first maintenance dose 48 h after load in preterm, 24 h in term baby), 8 hourly (4 + weeks) i.v., p.r. or p.o. Topical gel 0.5%: apply daily. Level 60–300 µmol/mL (× 0.17 µg/mL).

Mianserin 0.2–0.5 mg/kg per dose (adult 10–40 mg) 8 hourly, p.o.

Miconazole 7.5–15 mg/kg per dose (adult 0.6–1.2 g) 8 hourly, i.v. over 1 h. Topical: 2% cream, powder, lotion, tincture or gel 12–24 hourly. Vaginal: 2% cream or 100 mg ovule daily.

Microlax enema <12 months 1.25 mL, 1–2 years 2.5 mL, >2 years 5 mL.

Midazolam Sedation: usually 0.1–0.2 mg/kg i.v. or i.m.; up to 0.5 mg/kg used safely in children. Anaesthesia: 0.5 mg/kg, then 2 µg/kg per min (3 mg/kg in 50 mL at 2 mL/h) i.v.

Milrinone 50 µg/kg i.v. over 10 min, then 0.375–0.75 µg/kg per min (max 1.13 mg/kg per day).

Minocycline Over 8 years: 4 mg/kg (max 200 mg) stat, then 2 mg/kg per dose (max 100 mg) 12 hourly: p.o. or i.v. over 1 h.

Minoxidil 0.1 mg/kg (max 5 mg) daily, increase to a max of 0.5 mg/kg per dose (max 25 mg) 12–24 hourly, p.o. Male baldness: 2% solution 1 mL 12 hourly to a dry scalp.

Mometasone furoate   0.1% cream or ointment: apply daily. 50 µg spray: adult two sprays for each nostril daily.

Morphine   Child or ventilated neonate: 0.1–0.2 mg/kg per dose (adult 5–10 mg) i.v., 0.2 mg/kg per dose (adult 10–20 mg) i.m. (half-life 2–4 h). Infusion: 1 mg/kg in 50 mL 5% D at 0.5–3 mL/h (10–60 µg/kg per h). Patient controlled: 20 µg/kg boluses (1 mL of 1 mg/kg in 50 mL) with 5 min lockout time + (in child) 5 µg/kg per h. Oral: double parenteral dose; slow release, start with 0.6 mg/kg per dose 12 hourly and increase every 48 h if required.

Mumps vaccine (Mumpsvax)   Live. >12 months: 0.5 mL s.c. once. See also measles + mumps + rubella vaccine.

Mupirocin, ointment 2%   Apply 8–12 hourly.

Nalidixic acid   15 mg/kg per dose (adult 1 g) 6 hourly, orally, reducing to 7.5 mg/kg per dose (adult 500 mg) 6 hourly after 2 weeks.

Naloxone   Opiate intoxication (including newborn): 0.1 mg/kg (max 2 mg) stat i.v., i.m., s.c. or intratracheal, then 0.01 mg/kg per h i.v. Postoperative sedation: 0.002 mg/kg per dose repeat every 2 min, then 0.01 mg/kg per h (0.2 µg/kg per min) i.v.

Naltrexone   0.5–1 mg/kg (adult 25–50 mg) daily, p.o.

Naproxen   5–10 mg/kg per dose (adult 250–500 mg) 12–24 hourly, p.o.

Nedocromil   Inhalation: 4 mg/dose (NOT/kg) 6–12 hourly. Eye drops 2%: one drop/eye 6–24 hourly.

Neomycin   12.5–25 mg/kg per dose (adult 0.5–1 g) 6 hourly, p.o. Bladder washout: 40–2000 mg/L.

Neostigmine   Oral: 0.3–0.6 mg/kg per dose 3–4 hourly (max 400 mg/day). Intravenously, i.m.: 0.01–0.05 mg/kg per dose 3–4 hourly (max 20 mg/day). Reverse relaxants: 0.05–0.07 mg/kg per dose i.v.; suggested dilution: neostigmine (2.5 mg/mL) 0.5 mL + atropine (0.6 mg/mL) 0.5 mL + saline 0.5 mL, give 0.1 mL/kg i.v.

Netilmicin   Single daily dose i.v. or i.m.: 2.5 mg/kg (<30 weeks gestation), 3.5 mg/kg (30–35 weeks gestation), 5 mg/kg (first week of life), 7.5 mg/kg (1 week–10 years), 6 mg/kg (>10 years, max 240–360 mg). Trough <1.0 mg/L.

Nicardipine   0.4–0.8 mg/kg per dose (adult 20–40 mg) 8 hourly, p.o.

Nicotine resin chewing gum   NOT/kg: 2–4 mg chewed over 30 min when inclined to smoke; usually need 16–24 mg/day, a max of 60 mg/day.

Nicotine transdermal patches (Nicabate 7 mg, 14 mg, 21 mg; Nicotinell 10 = 17.5 mg, 20 = 35 mg, 30 = 52.5 mg) Adult: if smoked >20 cig./day apply strongest patch daily 3–4 weeks, then medium patch daily 3–4 weeks (initial dose if smoked ≤20 cig./day), then weakest patch daily 3–4 weeks.

Nicotinic acid Hypercholesterolaemia and hypertriglyceridaemia: 5 mg/kg per dose (adult 200 mg) 8 hourly, gradually increase to 20–30 mg/kg per dose (adult 1–2 g) 8 hourly, p.o.

Nifedipine Caps 0.25–0.5 mg/kg (adult 10–20 mg) 6–8 hourly, tabs 0.5–1 mg/kg per dose (adult 20–40 mg) 12 hourly: p.o. or sublingual.

Nimodipine 10–15 μg/kg per h (max 1 mg/h) i.v. for 2 h, then 10–45 μg/kg per h.

Nitrazepam NOT/kg: 1–5 mg/dose 12 hourly. Hypnotic: 2–5 mg.

Nitric oxide 5–40 p.p.m. (up to 80 p.p.m. used occasionally). 0.1 L/min of 1000 p.p.m. added to 10 L/min. Gas gives 10 p.p.m. (NO) = Cylinder (NO) × (1 − (Patient FiO_2/Supply FiO_2)). (NO) = Cylinder (NO) × NO flow/Total flow.

Nitrofurantoin 1.5 mg/kg per dose (adult 100 mg) 6 hourly, p.o. Prophylaxis: 1–2.5 mg/kg at night.

Noradrenaline Intravenous infusion: 0.05–0.5 μg/kg per min.

Norfloxacin 7.5 mg/kg per dose (max 400 mg) 12 hourly, p.o.

Normacol granules 6 months–5 years: 1/2 teaspoon, 12 hourly; 6–10 years: 1 teaspoon 12 hourly; >10 years: 1 teaspoon 8 hourly.

Nortriptyline 0.5–1.5 mg/kg per dose (adult 25–75 mg) 8 hourly, p.o.

Nystatin 500 000 u (1 tab) 6–8 hourly: n.g. or p.o. Neonates: 100 000 u (1 mL) 8 hourly, prophylaxis 50 000 u (0.5 mL), 12 hourly. Topical: 100 000 u/g gel, cream or ointment, 12 hourly. Vaginal: 100 000 u 12–24 hourly.

Omeprazole Usually 0.4–0.8 mg/kg (adult 20–40 mg) daily, p.o. ZE syndrome: 0.4–1 mg/kg (adult 20–60 mg) 12–24 hourly, p.o. Intravenous: 2 mg/kg (max 80 mg) stat, then 1 mg/kg (max 40 mg) 8–12 hourly. *H. pylori*: 0.8 mg/kg per dose (adult 40 mg) daily with metronidazole 8 mg/kg per dose (adult 400 mg) 8 hourly + amoxycillin 10 mg/kg per dose (adult 500 mg) 8 hourly, p.o. for 2 weeks.

Ondansetron Intravenous: 0.1–0.2 mg/kg (usual max 8 mg) over 15 min, then 0.25–0.5 μg/kg per min. Oral: 0.1–0.2 mg/kg per dose (usual max 8 mg) 8–12 hourly.

Oxacillin Oral: 15–30 mg/kg per dose 6 hourly. Severe infection (i.v., i.m.): 40 mg/kg per dose (max 2 g) 12 hourly (first week of life), 8 hourly (second week), 6 hourly or constant infusion (>2 weeks).

Oxandrolone 0.05–0.1 mg/kg per dose (adult 2.5–5 mg) 6–12 hourly, p.o.

Oxazepam 0.2–0.5 mg/kg per dose (adult 10–30 mg) 6–8 hourly, p.o.

Oxycodone 0.1–0.2 mg/kg per dose (adult 5–10 mg) 4–6 hourly, p.o.

Oxytetracycline >8 years (NOT/kg): 250–500 mg per dose 6 hourly, p.o.; or 250–500 mg per dose 6–12 hourly, slow i.v.

Oxytocin Labour (NOT/kg): 1–4 mU/min i.v., may increase to a max of 20 mU/min. Lactation: one spray (4 iu) into each nostril 5 min before the infant feeds.

Packed cells 4 mL/kg raises Hb 1 g %. One bag is about 300 mL.

Pancreatic enzymes With meals (NOT/kg): 1–3 Cotazyme-S Forte cap, 1–5 Pancreas cap oral.

Pancuronium ICU: 0.1–0.15 mg/kg i.v. p.r.n. Theatre: 0.1 mg/kg i.v., then 0.02 mg/kg p.r.n. Infusion: 0.25–0.75 µg/kg per min.

Papaveretum (Omnopon) 0.2 mg/kg per dose i.v., 0.4 mg/kg per dose i.m. (half-life 2–4 h). ICU: 0.3 mg/kg per dose i.v., 0.6 mg/kg per dose i.m.

Papaveretum (20 mg/mL) and hyoscine (0.4 mg/mL) 0.4 mg/kg (P) + 0.008 mg/kg (H) = 0.02 mL/kg per dose i.m.

Paracetamol Oral: 20 mg/kg stat, then 15 mg/kg per dose 4 hourly (max 4 g/day). Rectal: 40 mg/kg stat, then 30 mg/kg per dose 6 hourly (max 5 g/day). In case of an overdose, see acetylcysteine.

Paraffin Liquid: 1 mL/kg (max 45 mL) daily, p.o. Liquid 50% + white soft 50%, ointment: apply 6–12 hourly.

Paraffin, phenolphthalein and agar (Agarol) NOT/kg: 6 months– 2 years—2.5 mL, 3–5 years—2.5–5 mL, >5 years—5 mL 8–24 hourly, p.o.

Paraldehyde Intramuscular: 0.2 mL/kg (adult 10 mL) stat, then 0.1 mL/kg per dose 4–6 hourly. Intravenous: 0.2 mL/kg (adult 10 mL) over 15 min, then 0.02 mL/kg per h (max 1.5 mL/h). Rectal or n.g.: 0.3 mL/kg per dose diluted 1 : 10.

Penicillamine 5–10 mg/kg per dose (adult 250–500 mg) 6 hourly, p.o.

Penicillin, benzathine 1 mg = 1250 u. Usually 20 mg/kg (max 900 mg) i.m., once. Venereal disease: 40 mg/kg (max 1.8 g) i.m., once. *Strep. proph.*: 20 mg/kg (max 900 mg) i.m. 3–4 weekly, or 10 mg/kg i.m. 2 weekly.

Penicillin, benzathine 900 mg + procaine 300 mg in 2 mL   0–2 years: 1/2 vial, 3 years or more: one vial i.m., once.

Penicillin, benzyl (penicillin G, crystalline)   1 mg = 1667 u. 30 mg/kg per dose 6 hourly. Severe infection: 60 mg/kg per dose (max 3 g) i.v. 12 hourly (first week of life), 6 hourly (2–4 weeks), 4 hourly or constant infusion (>4 weeks).

Penicillin, procaine   1 mg = 1000 u. 25–50 mg/kg (max 1.2–2.4 g) 12–24 hourly, i.m. Single dose: 100 mg/kg (max 4.8 g).

Pentamidin   4 mg/kg of base i.v. over 2 h or i.m. daily for 10–14 days (1 mg base = 1.5 mg mesylate = 1.74 mg isethionate).

Pentobarbitone   0.5–1 mg/kg per dose (adult 30–60 mg) 6–8 hourly: p.o., i.m. or slow i.v. Hypnotic: 2–4 mg/kg (adult 100–200 mg).

Permethrin   Cream rinse 1% (head lice): wash hair, apply cream for 10 min, wash off; may repeat in 2 weeks. Cream 5% (scabies): apply to the whole body except the face, wash off after 12–24 h.

Pethidine   0.5–1 mg/kg per dose (adult 25–50 mg) i.v., 0.5–2 mg/kg per dose (adult 25–100 mg) i.m. (half-life 2–4 h). Infusion: 5 mg/kg in 50 mL at 1–3 mL/h (100–300 µg/kg per h).

Pheniramine   0.5–1 mg/kg per dose (adult 25–50 mg) 6 hourly, p.o.

Phenobarbitone   Loading dose in emergency: 20–30 mg/kg i.m. or i.v. over 30 min stat. Ventilated: repeat doses of 10–15 mg/kg up to 100 mg/kg in 24 h (beware hypotension). Usual maintenance: 5 mg/kg (max 300 mg) daily: i.v., i.m. or p.o. Infant colic: 1 mg/kg per dose 4–8 hourly, orally. Level 80–120 µmol/L ($\times$ 0.23 = µg/mL) is performed on Monday, Wednesday and Friday at the Royal Children's Hospital.

Phenoxybenzamine   0.2–1 mg/kg (adult 10–50 mg) 12–24 hourly, orally. Cardiac surgery: 1 mg/kg i.v. over 1 h stat, then 0.5 mg/kg per dose 6–12 hourly, i.v. over 1 h; or p.o.

Phenoxymethylpenicillin (penicillin V)   7.5–15 mg/kg per dose (adult 250–500 mg) 6 hourly, p.o. Proph: 12.5 mg/kg per dose (adult 250 mg) 12 hourly, p.o.

Phentolamine   0.1 mg/kg stat, then 5–50 µg/kg per min i.v.

Phenylephrine   Intravenous: 2–10 µg/kg stat (adult 500 µg), then 1–5 µg/kg per min: for a 65 kg adult, 25 mg in 50 mL at 8 mL/h is 1 µg/kg per min s.c. or i.m.: 0.1–0.2 mg/kg (max 10 mg). Oral: 0.2 mg/kg per dose (max 10 mg) 6–8 hourly. Eye drops (0.12%,

10%): 1–2 drops/eye 6–8 hourly. Nose drops (0.25%, 0.5%): 1–3 drops/sprays per nostril 6–8 hourly.

Phenytoin Loading dose in emergency: 15–20 mg/kg (max 1.5 g) i.v. over 1 h. Maintenance, p.o. or i.v.: 2 mg/kg per dose 12 hourly (preterm); 4 mg/kg per dose 12 hourly (first week of life), 8 hourly (second week), 6 hourly (3 weeks–12 months), 8 hourly (1–2 years), 8–12 hourly (3–12 years); 2 mg/kg per dose (usual max 100 mg) 6–12 hourly >12 years. Level 40–80 µmol/L (× 0.25 = µg/mL), is performed on Monday, Wednesday and Friday at the Royal Children's Hospital.

Pholcodine 0.1–0.2 mg/kg per dose (adult 5–10 mg) 6–12 hourly, p.o.

Phosphate, potassium (1 mmol/mL) 0.1–1 mmol/kg per day (max 20 mmol/day) i.v. infusion.

Phosphate, sodium (500 mg tab) 0.5–1 g (NOT/kg) 8 hourly, p.o.

Physostigmine 0.02 mg/kg (max 1 mg) i.v. every 5 min until there is a response (max 0.1 mg/kg), then 0.5–2.0 µg/kg per min.

Phytomenadione 0.3 mg/kg (max 10 mg), i.m. or i.v. over 1 h. Prophylaxis in neonates (NOT/kg): 1 mg i.m. at birth; or 1 mg p.o. or 0.1 mg i.m. at birth, at 4–7 days, and 3–4 weeks (give half a dose if the weight <1500 g).

Pilocarpine 0.1 mg/kg per dose (adult 5 mg) 4–8 hourly, p.o. Eye drops 0.5%, 1%, 2%, 3%, 4%: 1–2 drops 6–12 hourly.

Pimozide 0.04–0.4 mg/kg (adult 2–20 mg) daily, p.o.

Pine tar, gel, solution 5 mL to baby bath, 15–30 mL to adult bath; soak for 10 min.

Piperacillin 50 mg/kg per dose (adult 2–3 g) i.v. 6–8 hourly (first week of life), 4–6 hourly or constant infusion (>2 weeks).

Piperacillin + tazobactam (1 g/125 mg) Dose as for piperacillin.

Piperazine 75 mg/kg (max 4 g) p.o., daily for 2 days (ascaris), 7 days (pinworm).

Piroxicam 0.2–0.4 mg/kg (adult 10–20 mg) daily, p.o. Gel 5 mg/g: apply 1 g (3 cm) 6–8 hourly for up to 2 weeks.

Pizotifen NOT/kg: 1–3 mg daily, p.o., usually 0.5 mg morning, 1 mg night.

Platelets 10 mL/kg i.v. stat, then daily if necessary. 1 unit is about 60 mL.

Pneumococcus vaccine (Pneumovax 23) Inactivated. >2 years: 0.5 mL s.c. or i.m. once. Boost every 5 years.

Podophyllotoxin, paint 0.5% Apply 12 hourly for 3 days, then none for 4 days; 4-week course.

Polio vaccine, oral (Sabin) Live. Two drops oral at 2, 4 and 6 months. Boost at 5 years, and if going to an epidemic area.

Polio vaccine, SC (Enpovax HDC) Inactivated. 0.5 mL s.c. stat, 8 weeks later, and 8 weeks after that (3 doses). Boost 12 months later, and at school entry.

Poloxamer 10% solution: one drop per month of age (max 25 drops) 8 hourly, p.o.

Poractant alfa (porcine surfactant, Curosurf) Intratracheal: 200 mg/kg stat, then up to four doses of 100 mg/kg, 12 hourly if required.

Potassium The max i.v. dose is 0.4 mmol/kg per h. The max oral dose is 1 mmol/kg per dose (<5 years), 0.5 mmol/kg per dose (>5 years). There is a need of 2–4 mmol/kg per day. 1 g KCl = 13.3 mmol K, 7.5% KCl = 1 mmol/mL.

Pralidoxime 25–50 mg/kg (adult 1–2 g) over 30 min, then up to 10 mg/kg per h (max 12 g/day).

Prazosin 0.005 mg/kg (max 0.25 mg) test dose, then 0.025–0.1 mg/kg per dose (adult 1–5 mg) 6 hourly, p.o.

Prednisolone Asthma: 0.5–1 mg/kg per dose 6 hourly for 24 h, 12 hourly for the next 24 h, then 1 mg/kg daily. Severe croup: 4 mg/kg stat, then 1 mg/kg per dose 8–12 hourly, p.o. Predniso-lone 1 mg = hydrocortisone 0.8 mg in mineralocorticoid action, 4 mg in glucocorticoid. See also methylprednisolone.

Primaquine Usually 0.3 mg/kg (max 15 mg) daily for 14–21 days, orally. Gameteocyte: 0.7 mg/kg (max 45 mg) once.

Primidone 5–15 mg/kg per dose (adult 250–750 mg) 12 hourly, p.o.

Probenicid 25 mg/kg (adult 1 g) stat, then 10 mg/kg per dose (adult 500 mg) 6 hourly, p.o.

Procainamide Intravenous: 0.4 mg/kg per min (adult 20 mg/min) for a max of 25 min, then 20–80 µg/kg per min. Oral: 2–8 mg/kg per dose 4 hourly.

Procaine A max dose of 20 mg/kg (1 mL/kg of 2%).

Prochlorperazine (1 mg base = approx 1.5 mg edisylate, maleate or mesylate) Only use if >10 kg. Intramuscularly or slow i.v.: 0.1–0.2 mg/kg (adult 12.5 mg salt) 6–8 hourly. Orally or p.r.: 0.1–0.4 mg/kg per dose (max 25 mg salt) 6–8 hourly, slow increase to a max of 0.6 mg/kg per dose (max 35 mg salt) 6 hourly in psychosis. Buccal: 0.05–0.1 mg/kg (max 6 mg salt) 12–24 hourly.

Promazine   Oral: 2–4 mg/kg per dose (adult 100–200 mg) 6 hourly. Intramuscular: 0.7 mg/kg per dose (max 50 mg) 6–8 hourly.

Promethazine   Antihistamine, anti-emetic: 0.2–0.5 mg/kg per dose (adult 10–25 mg) 6–8 hourly: i.v., i.m. or p.o. Sedative, hypnotic: 0.5–1.5 mg/kg per dose (adult 25–100 mg).

Propafenone   Oral: 3–5 mg/kg per dose (adult 150–300 mg) 8 hourly. Intravenous: 1–2 mg/kg over 15 min, then 10–20 µg/kg per min.

Propantheline bromide   0.3–0.6 mg/kg per dose (adult 15–30 mg) 6 hourly, p.o.

Propofol   1–3 mg/kg stat, then 4–12 mg/kg per h i.v. Beware acidosis and myocardial depression.

Propranolol   Intravenous: 0.02 mg/kg (adult 1 mg) test dose then 0.1 mg/kg (adult 5 mg) over 10 min (repeat × 1–3 p.r.n.), then 0.1–0.3 mg/kg per dose (adult 5–15 mg) 3 hourly. Oral: 0.2–0.5 mg/kg per dose (adult 10–25 mg) 6–12 hourly, slow increase to a max of 1.5 mg/kg per dose (max 80 mg) 6–12 hourly if required.

Protamine   Intravenous: 1 mg/100 u heparin (or 1 mg per 25 mL pump blood) i.v. stat; subsequent doses of protamine 1 mg/kg (max 50 mg). Heparin 1 mg = 100 u (half-life 1–2 h).

Prothrombinex (factors 2, 9 and 10; 250 u/10 mL)   1 mL/kg slow i.v., daily. There is the risk of thrombosis in acute liver failure.

Pseudoephedrine   1 mg/kg per dose (adult 60 mg) 6 hourly, p.o.

Pumactant (ALEC)   Preterm babies (NOT/kg): disconnect ETT, rapidly inject 100 mg in 1 mL saline via catheter at lower end ETT, flush with 2 mL air; repeat after 1 h and 24 h. Prophylaxis if unintubated: 100 mg into the pharynx.

Pyrantel embonate   10 mg/kg (adult 500 mg) once p.o. Necator: 20 mg/kg (adult 1 g) daily × two doses. Enterobius: 10 mg/kg (adult 500 mg) each 2 weeks × three doses.

Pyrazinamide   20–35 mg/kg per dose (max 3 g) daily, p.o.

Pyridostigmine   1–3 mg/kg per dose (usual max 200 mg) 4–12 hourly, p.o. 180 mg slow release tab (Timespan), adult (NOT/kg): 1–3 tab 12–24 hourly. 1 mg i.v., i.m. or s.c. = 30 mg p.o.

Pyridoxine   With isoniazid (NOT/kg): 5–10 mg daily i.v. or p.o. Neonatal fitting (NOT/kg): 50–100 mg daily: i.v. or p.o. Siderobl anaem: 2–8 mg/kg (max 400 mg) daily: i.v. or p.o.

Pyrimethamine 12.5 mg and dapsone 100 mg (Maloprim)   1–4 years: quarter tab weekly, 5–10 years: half tab, and >10 years: one tab.

Pyrimethamine 25 mg and sulphadoxine 500 mg (Fansidar) <4 years: half tab once, 4–8 years: one tab, 9–14 years: two tabs, and >14 years: three tabs. For prophylaxis: <4 years: quarter tab weekly, 4–8 years: half tab, 9–14 years: three-quarter tab, and >14 years: one tab.

Quinidine, base 10 mg/kg stat, then 5 mg/kg per dose (max 333 mg) 4–6 hourly, p.o. Intravenously: 6.3 mg/kg (10 mg/kg of gluconate) over 2 h, then 0.0125 mg/kg per min. Intramuscularly: 15 mg/kg stat, then 7.5 mg/kg per dose (max 400 mg) 8 hourly. *Note:* 1 mg base = 1.2 mg sulphate = 1.3 mg bisulphate = 1.6 mg gluconate.

Quinine, base Oral: 8.3 mg/kg per dose (max 500 mg) 8 hourly for 7–10 days. Parenteral: 16.7 mg/kg (20 mg/kg of dihydrochloride) i.v. over 4 h or i.m.; then 8.3 mg/kg per dose 8 hourly, i.v. over 2 h or i.m. for 2–3 days; and 8.3 mg/kg per dose 8 hourly, p.o. for 5 days. *Note:* 1 mg base = 1.7 mg bisulphate = 1.2 mg dihydrochloride = 1.2 mg ethyl carbonate = 1.3 mg hydrobromide = 1.2 mg hydrochloride = 1.2 mg sulphate.

Ranitidine Intravenously: 1 mg/kg per dose slowly, 6–8 hourly; or 2 µg/kg per min. Orally: 2 mg/kg per dose (max 150 mg) 12 hourly, or 4 mg/kg (max 300 mg) at night.

Ranitidine bismuth citrate 8 mg/kg per dose (adult 400 mg) 12 hourly, orally; to eradicate *H. pylori*, add an antibiotic.

Reserpine 0.005–0.01 mg/kg per dose (adult 0.25–0.5 mg) 12–24 hourly, p.o.

Ribavirin Inhalation (Viratek nebuliser): 20 mg/mL at 25 mL/h (190 µg/L of gas) for 12–18 h/day for 3–7 days. Oral: 5–15 mg/kg per dose, 8–12 hourly.

Riboflavine NOT/kg: 5–10 mg daily, p.o. Organic acidosis (NOT/kg): 50–200 mg daily—p.o., i.m. or i.v.

Rifampicin 10–15 mg/kg (max 600 mg) daily oral fasting, or i.v. over 3 h (monitor AST). Prophylaxis (meningococcus, haemophilus): 10 mg/kg daily (newborn), 20 mg/kg (max 600 mg) daily (>4 weeks old) p.o. for 4 days (*H. influenzae*) or 2 days (*N. meningitidis*).

Roxithromycin 2.5 mg/kg per dose (adult 150 mg) 12 hourly, p.o. before meals.

Rubella vaccine (Ervevax, Meruvax II) Live. >12 months: 0.5 mL s.c. once. See also measles + mumps + rubella vaccine.

Salbutamol   0.1–0.15 mg/kg per dose (adult 2–4 mg) 6 hourly, p.o. Inhalation—mild: respiratory solution (5 mg/mL, 0.5%) 0.5 mL/dose diluted to 4 mL, or nebule 2.5 mg/2.5 mL 3–6 hourly; moderate: 0.5% solution 1 mL/dose diluted to 4 mL, or nebule 5 mg/2.5 mL 1–2 hourly; severe (in ICU): 0.5% solution undiluted continuous. Aerosol 100 µg/puff: 1–2 puff 4–6 hourly. Rotahaler: 200–400 µg 6–8 hourly. Intramuscularly or s.c.: 10–20 µg/kg per dose (adult 500 µg) 3–6 hourly. Intravenously: child 1–5 µg/kg per min (1 µg/kg per min using 1 mg/mL solution = 0.06 × wt mL/h); adult 5 mg in 50 mL at 4 mL/h is 0.1 µg/kg per min.

Salicylic acid   Cradle cap: 6% solution (Egocappol) 12 hourly, 3–5 days. Plantar warts: 15% solution × 1–2/day, 40% medicated disc 24–48 hourly.

Salmeterol   Aerosol or diskhaler (NOT/kg): 50–100 µg 12 hourly.

Selenium sulphide, 2.5%   Shampoo × 2/week for 2 weeks.

Sennoside   Tab 7.5 mg daily (NOT/kg): 6 months–2 years—half tab, 3–10 years—1–2 tabs, >10 years—2–4 tabs. Granules 22.5 mg/teaspoon, 12–24 hourly (NOT/kg): <6 months—quarter–half teaspoon, 6 months–2 years—half–1 teaspoon, 3–10 years—1–2 teaspoons.

Simvastatin   Initially 0.2 mg/kg (adult 10 mg) daily, may increase every 4 weeks to a max of 1 mg/kg (adult 40 mg) daily, p.o.

Sodium   Deficit: to increase serum Na by 2 mmol/L per h (max safe rate), infusion rate (mL/h) = 8 × wt (kg)/(% saline infused); number of hours of infusion = (140 – serum Na)/2.4 mL/kg of X% saline raises serum Na by X mmol/L. Need 2–6 mmol/kg per day. NaCl MW = 58.45, 1 g NaCl = 17.1 mmol Na, NaCl 20% = 3.4 mmol/mL.

Sodium aurothiomalate   0.25 mg/kg weekly, i.m. Increase to 1 mg/kg (max 50 mg) weekly for 10 weeks, then every 2–6 weeks. After that i.m. every 1–4 weeks.

Sodium benzoate   Neonate: 250 mg/kg over 2 h stat, then 10–20 mg/kg per h i.v.

Sodium nitroprusside   Intravenous infusion 0.5–10 µg/kg per min: for a 65 kg adult, 50 mg in 50 mL at 2 mL/h is 0.5 µg/kg per min. If used for >24 h, the max rate is 4 µg/kg per min. The max total: 70 mg/kg with normal renal function (or sodium thiocyanate <1725 µmol/L, × 0.058 = mg/L). Pul vasodil: 5 µg/kg per min nitroglyc = 2 µg/kg per min nitroprusside = 0.1 µg/kg per min PGE1 approximately.

Sodium polystyrene sulphonate (Resonium)   0.3–0.6 g/kg per dose (adult 15–30 g) 6 hourly n.g. (give lactulose) or p.r.

Sodium valproate   5–15 mg/kg per dose (max 1 g) 8–12 hourly, p.o. Level 0.3–0.7 mmol/L (× 144 = μg/mL).

Sorbolene cream; pure, with 10% glycerin, or with 5% or 10% olive oil or peanut oil   Skin moisturiser, apply p.r.n.

Sotalol   Intravenously: 0.5–2 mg/kg per dose (adult 25–100 mg) over 10 min, 6 hourly. Orally: 1–4 mg/kg per dose (adult 50–200 mg) 8 hourly.

Spironolactone   Orally (NOT/kg): 0–10 kg—6.25 mg/dose 12 hourly, 11–20 kg—12.5 mg/dose 12 hourly, 21–40 kg—25 mg/dose 12 hourly, over 40 kg—25 mg/dose 8 hourly.

Streptokinase (SK)   Short term (myoc infarct): 30 000 u/kg (max 1 500 000 u) i.v. over 60 min, repeat if occlusion recurs <5 days. Long term (DVT, pul emb, art thrombosis): 5000 u/kg (max 250 000 u) i.v. over 30 min, then 2000 u/kg per h (max 100 000 u/h); stop heparin and aspirin, if PTT < × 2 normal at 4 h give extra 10 000 u/kg (max 500 000 u) i.v. over 30 min, stop SK if PTT > × 5 normal then give 1000 u/kg per h. Local infusion: 50 u/kg per h (continue heparin 10–15 u/kg per h). Blocked i.v. cannula: 5000 u/kg in 2 mL in cannula for 2 h then remove, may repeat × 2.

Streptomycin   20–30 mg/kg (max 1 g) i.m., daily.

Sucralfate 1 g tab   NOT/kg: 0–2 years $\frac{1}{4}$ tab 6 hourly, 3–12 years $\frac{1}{2}$ tab 6 hourly, >12 years one tab 6 hourly, p.o.

Sulfadiazine   50 mg/kg per dose (max 2 g) 6 hourly, slow i.v.

Sulindac   4 mg/kg per dose (adult 200 mg) 12 hourly, p.o.

Sulphasalazine   Active disease: 10–15 mg/kg per dose (max 1 g) 6 hourly, p.o. Remission: 5–7.5 mg/kg per dose (max 0.5 g) 6 hourly.

Sumatriptan   Orally: 1–2 mg/kg (adult 50–100 mg) stat, may repeat twice. Subcutaneous: 0.12 mg/kg (max 6 mg) stat, may repeat once after 1 h.

Suxamethonium   Intravenous: neonate 3 mg/kg per dose, child 2 mg/kg per dose, adult 1 mg/kg per dose. Intramuscularly: double i.v. dose.

Tacrolimus (FK506)   Intravenous infusion: 2 mg/m² per day. Orally: 3 mg/m² per dose 12 hourly. Maintain trough plasma level 0.4–1.2 ng/mL, whole blood level 10–20 ng/mL.

Tamoxifen   Adult (NOT/kg): 20 mg daily, increase to 40 mg daily if no response after 1 month.

Teicoplanin 250 mg/m^2 i.v. over 30 min stat, then 125 mg/m^2 i.v. or i.m. daily. Severe infection: 250 mg/m^2 12 hourly × three doses, then 250 mg/m^2 i.v. or i.m., daily.

Temazepam Adult (NOT/kg): 10–30 mg at night, p.o.

Terbutaline Orally: 0.05–0.1 mg/kg per dose (adult 2.5–5 mg) 6 hourly. Subcutaneous: 5–10 µg/kg per dose (adult 0.25–0.5 mg). Intravenously: 5 µg/kg (adult 0.25 mg) stat over 10 min, then 1–10 µg/kg per h. Inhalation—mild: respiratory solution (1%, 10 mg/mL) 0.25 mL/dose diluted to 4 mL 3–6 hourly; moderate: 0.5 mL of 1% diluted to 4 mL, or respule 5 mg/2 mL 1–2 hourly; severe (in ICU): undiluted continuous. Aerosol 250 µg/puff: 1–2 puffs, 4–6 hourly.

Terfenadine 1 mg/kg per dose (adult 60 mg) 12 hourly, p.o.

Testosterone Esters: 100–500 mg (NOT/kg) i.m. every 2–4 weeks. Implant: 8 mg/kg (to nearest 100 mg). Undecanoate: 40–120 mg (NOT/kg) daily, orally. Testosterone level: <16 years 5–10 nmol/L, >16 years 10–30 nmol/L.

Tetanus toxoid (CSL) 0.5 mL i.m. stat, 6 weeks later, and 6 months later. Boost every 10 years, or if contaminated wound. See also diphtheria (+ pertussis) + tetanus vaccines.

Tetracycline Over 8 years (NOT/kg): 250–500 mg/dose 6 hourly, p.o.

Theophylline (80 mg theophylline = 100 mg aminophylline) Loading dose: 8 mg/kg (max 500 mg) p.o. Maintenance: first week of life—2 mg/kg per dose 12 hourly; second week of life—3 mg/kg per dose 12 hourly; 3 weeks–12 months (0.1 × age in weeks) + 3 mg/kg per dose 8 hourly; 1–9 years—4 mg/kg per dose 4–6 hourly, or 10 mg/kg per dose slow release 12 hourly; 10–16 years or adult smoker—3 mg/kg per dose 4–6 hourly, or 7 mg/kg per dose 12 hourly, slow release; adult non-smoker—3 mg/kg per dose 6–8 hourly; elderly—2 mg/kg per dose 6–8 hourly. Monitor serum level: neonate 60–80 umol/L, asthma 60–110 (× 0.18 = µg/mL).

Thiabendazole 25 mg/kg per dose (max 1.5 g) 12 hourly, p.o. for 3 days.

Thiopentone 2–5 mg/kg slowly stat (beware hypotension), then 1–5 mg/kg per h i.v. Level 150–200 µmol/L (× 0.24 = µg/mL).

Thrombin glue 10 000 u thrombin in 9 mL mixed with 1 mL 10% calcium chloride in syringe 1, 10 mL cryoprecipitate in syringe 2: inject into bleeding sites together.

Thrombin, topical 100–2000 u/mL onto bleeding surface.

Thyroxine   Infants: 8–12 µg/kg per day p.o. Adult (NOT/kg): 100–200 µg daily.

Ticarcillin   50 mg/kg per dose (max 3 g) i.v., 6–8 hourly (first week of life); 4–6 hourly or constant infusion (>2 weeks).

Ticarcillin and clavulanic acid   Dose as for ticarcillin.

Tilactase   200 u/drop: 5–15 drops/L added to milk 24 h before use. 3300 u/tab: 1–3 tabs with meals, p.o.

Timolol   0.1 mg/kg per dose (adult 5 mg) 8–12 hourly, increase to a max of 0.3 mg/kg per dose (adult 15 mg) 8 hourly. Eye drops (0.25%, 0.5%): 1 drop/eye 12–24 hourly.

Tinidazole   Giardia: 50 mg/kg (max 2 g) stat, repeat after 48 h. Amoebic dys: 50 mg/kg (max 2 g) daily for 3 days.

Tobramycin   Single daily dose i.v. or i.m.: 2.5 mg/kg (<30 weeks gestation), 3.5 mg/kg (30–35 weeks gestation), 5 mg/kg (first week of life), 7.5 mg/kg (1 week–10 years), 6 mg/kg (>10 years, max 240–360 mg). Trough level <1.0 mg/L, performed Monday–Friday at the Royal Children's Hospital.

Tolazoline   Newborn: 1–2 mg/kg slowly stat (beware hypotension), then 2–6 µg/kg per min (0.12–0.36 mg/kg per h) i.v. *Note*: 1–2 mg/kg per h too much (*Pediatrics* (1986) **77**: 307).

Tolbutamide   Adult (NOT/kg): initially 1 g 12 hourly, p.o., often reducing to 0.5–1 g daily.

Topiramate   1 mg/kg per dose (adult 50 mg) 12–24 hourly, p.o., increase gradually to 4–10 mg/kg per dose (adult 100–500 mg) 12 hourly.

Tranexamic acid   Orally: 15–25 mg/kg per dose (adult 1–1.5 g) 8 hourly. Intravenously: 10–15 mg/kg per dose (adult 0.5–1 g) 8 hourly.

Triamcinolone   Joint, tendon (NOT/kg): 2.5–15 mg stat. Intramuscularly: 0.05–0.2 mg/kg every 1–7 days. Cream or ointment 0.02%, 0.05%: apply sparingly 6–8 hourly. Triamcinolone has no mineralcorticoid action, 1 mg = 5 mg hydrocortisone in glucocorticoid action.

Triamcinolone   0.1% + neomycin   0.25% + gramicidin   0.025% + nystatin 100 000 u/g   Kenacomb cream, ointment: apply 8–12 hourly. Kenacomb otic cream, ointment, drops: apply 8–12 hourly (2–3 drops).

Triazolam   Adult (NOT/kg): 0.125–0.5 mg at night, p.o.

Trifluoperazine   0.02–0.2 mg/kg per dose (adult 1–10 mg, occasionally 20 mg) 12 hourly, p.o.

Trimeprazine Antihistamine: 0.05–0.5 mg/kg per dose (adult 2.5–25 mg) 6 hourly, p.o. Sedation: 0.5–1 mg/kg i.m., 2–4 mg/kg p.o.

Trimethoprim 3–4 mg/kg per dose (usual max 150 mg) 12 hourly, or 6–8 mg/kg (usual max 300 mg) daily: p.o. or i.v.

Trometamol (THAM) mL of 0.3 molar (18 g/500 mL) solution = wt × BE (give 1/2 this) i.v. over 30–60 min.

Typhoid vaccine, oral (Typh-Vax) Live. One cap p.o. on days 1, 3, 5 and (for better immunity) 7. Boost yearly.

Typhoid vaccine, parenteral (CSL) Inactivated. 0.1 mL (<6 years), 0.25 mL (6–12 years), 0.5 mL (>12 years) s.c. stat, and 4 weeks later. Boost every 3 years.

Typhoid vaccine, parenteral, polysaccharide (Typhim Vi) Inactivated. >5 years: 0.5 mL i.m. once. Protects for 3 years or more.

Urea, cream 10% Apply 8–12 hourly.

Urokinase 4000 u/kg i.v. over 10 min, then 4000 u/kg per h for 12 h (start heparin 3–4 h later). Blocked cannula: instill 5000–25 000 u (NOT/kg) in 2–3 mL saline for 2–4 h. Empyema: 2 mL/kg of 1500 u/mL in saline, position head up/down and right side up/down 30 min each, then drain.

Ursodeoxycholic acid 4–8 mg/kg per dose (adult 200–400 mg) 12 hourly, p.o.

Vancomycin 15 mg/kg per dose (max 500 mg) i.v. over 2 h: daily (preterm), 12 hourly (first week of life), 8 hourly (>2 weeks). Oral: 10 mg/kg per dose (adult 500 mg) 6 hourly. Intraventric (NOT/kg): 10 mg per dose 48 hourly. Peak 25–40 mg/L, trough <10 mg/L; performed Monday–Friday at the Royal Children's Hospital.

Varicella vaccine (Varivax) Live. 12 months–12 years: 0.5 mL s.c. once. >12 years: 0.5 mL s.c. stat, and 4–8 weeks later.

Vasopressin Aqueous: put 2–5 u in 1 L fluid, and replace urine output + 10% i.v.; or 2–10 u i.m. or s.c. 8 hourly. Brain death: 0.0003 u/kg per min (1 u/kg in 50 mL at 1 mL/h) + adrenaline 0.1–0.2 µg/kg per min. Oily: 2.5–5 u (NOT/kg) i.m. every 2–4 days. GI hge (aqueous solution): 0.4 u/min i.v. in adult; 0.1 u/min local IA in adult. See desmopressin.

Vecuronium ICU: 0.1 mg/kg p.r.n. Theatre: 0.1 mg/kg stat, then 1–10 µg/kg per min i.v.

Verapamil Intravenously: 0.1–0.2 mg/kg (adult 5–10 mg) over 10 min, then 5 µg/kg per min. Oral: 1–3 mg/kg per dose (adult 80–120 mg) 8–12 hourly.

Vigabatrin Initially 40 mg/kg (adult 2 g) daily, p.o., may increase to 80–100 mg/kg (max 4 g) daily (given in 1–2 doses).

Vitamin A High risk (NOT/kg): 100 000 iu (<8 kg), 200 000 iu (>8 kg) p.o. or i.m. every 4–6 months. Severe measles: 400 000 iu (NOT/kg) once. >10 000 iu daily may be teratogenic.

Vitamin A, B, C, D compound (Pentavite) Neonate 12 drops, 0–6 years 2.5–5 mL, >6 years 5 mL (NOT/kg) daily, p.o.

Vitamin B group Ampoules: i.v. over 30 min. Tab: 1–2/day.

Vitamin D Nutritional rickets: ergocalciferol (D2) 10–250 μg (400–10 000 u) daily (NOT/kg) for 30 days orally; calcifediol (25–OH D3) 1–2 μg/kg daily, p.o. Renal rickets or hypoparathyroidism: calcitriol (1,25–OH D3) start 0.01 μg/kg daily; dihydrotachysterol (1–OH D2) 20 μg/kg per day; ergocalciferol (D2): 50 000–300 000 u/day (NOT/kg).

Vitamin E (Copherol E) Preterm babies (NOT/kg): 40 u (2 drops) daily, p.o. 1 u = 1 mg. See also alpha-tocopheryl.

Vitamins, parenteral MVI-12 (for adult): 5 mL in 1 L i.v. fluid. MVI Paediatric, added to i.v. fluid: 65% of a vial (<3 kg), one vial (3 kg to 11 years).

Vitaprem (RCH) (Pentavite, folate, B12, C) 1 mL daily, p.o.

Warfarin Usually 0.2 mg/kg (adult 10 mg) stat, 0.2 mg/kg (adult 10 mg) next day providing INR <1.3, then 0.05–0.2 mg/kg (adult 2–10 mg) daily, p.o. INR usually 2–2.5 for prophylaxis, 2–3 for treatment. Beware drug interactions.

Whole blood 6 mL/kg raises Hb 1 g %. One bag = 400 mL approximately.

Xylometazoline <6 years: 0.05% one drop or spray 8–12 hourly. 6–12 years: 0.05% 2–3 drops or sprays 8–12 hourly. >12 years: 0.1% 2–3 drops or sprays 6–12 hourly.

Yellow fever vaccine (CSL) Live. >12 months: 0.5 mL s.c. once. Boost every 10 years.

Zidovudine (AZT) Child: 90–180 mg/m^2 per dose (max 150 mg/dose) 6 hourly, p.o.; 8 hourly, i.v. Adult (NOT/kg): usually 200 mg/dose 8 hourly, p.o.; or 150 mg/dose 8 hourly, i.v.

Zinc sulphate Adult (NOT/kg): 50–220 mg 8–24 hourly, p.o.

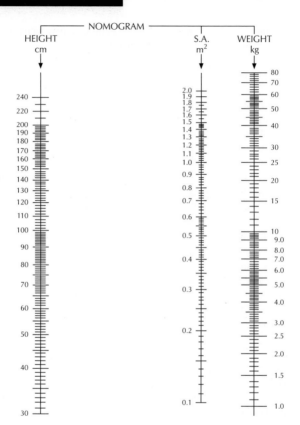

Fig. E1 Nomogram

Table 13

Calculating the composition of drug infusions (50 mL syringe pump)

1 Select the desired drug dosage to be delivered in μg/kg per min.
2 Select the infusion rate of the syringe pump in mL/h (from the centre of the table).
3 Calculate the number of milligrams of the drug to be mixed in a 50 mL syringe. For example, for a 10 kg child, 0.1–2 μg per min, infusion 1–20 mL/h: place 0.3 mg/kg (= 3 mg) in 50 mL.

Drug schematic (nested boxes, associating drugs with concentration columns):

- Noradren
- Dopamine
- Dobutamine
- Morphine
- Tolazoline
- Lignocaine
- Thiopentone
- Glyceryl trinitrate
- Ketamine
- Adrenaline
- isoprenaline
- Nitroprusside — Max hours of infusion: 6 7 8 9 10

Body values are the syringe pump rate in mL/h.

μg/kg per min	0.15 mg/kg in 50 mL	0.3 mg/kg in 50 mL	0.6 mg/kg in 50 mL	1.5 mg/kg in 50 mL	3 mg/kg in 50 mL	6 mg/kg in 50 mL	15 mg/kg in 50 mL	30 mg/kg in 50 mL	60 mg/kg in 50 mL
	mL/h	mL/h	mL/h	mL/h	mL/h	mL/h	mL/h	mL/h	mL/h
0.05	1								
0.1	2	1							
0.2	4	2	1						
0.3	6	3	1.5						
0.4	8	4	2						
0.5	10	5		1					
0.6	12	6	3						
0.7	14	7							
0.8	16	8	4						
0.9	18	9							
1.0	20	10	5	2	1				
1.5		15		3	1.5				
2.0		20	10	4	2	1			
3.0				6	3	1.5			
4.0			20	8	4	2			
5.0				10	5		1		
6.0				12	6	3			
7.0				14	7				
8.0				16	8	4			
9.0				18	9				
10.0				20	10	5	2	1	
12.0					12	6			
14.0					14	7			
15.0					15		3	1.5	
20.0					20	10	4	2	1
25.0							5		
30.0						15	6	3	1.5
40.0						20	8	4	2
50.0							10	5	
100.0							20	10	5
150.0								15	
200.0								20	10

1 mg/kg per h = 16.7 μg/kg per min = 50 mg/kg in 50 mL at 1 mL/h; 1 mg/kg in 50 mL at 1 mL/h: 1 mL/h = 0.2 mg/kg per h = 0.33 μg/kg per min
mg/kg in 50 mL = 3 × dose (μg/kg per min)/rate (mL/h); mg/kg in 50 mL = 50 × dose (mg/kg per h)/rate (mL/h)

ANTIMICROBIAL GUIDELINES

Mike Starr, Mike South and Nigel Curtis

CENTRAL NERVOUS SYSTEM / EYE

Infection	Likely organisms	Initial antimicrobials[1] ( ) = maximum dose	Duration of treatment[2] and other comments	Page
Brain abscess	S. milleri and other streptococci Anaerobes Gram-negatives S. aureus	Flucloxacillin 50 mg/kg (2 g) iv 4H and Cefotaxime 50 mg/kg (2 g) iv 6H and Metronidazole 15 mg/kg (1 g) iv stat, then 7.5 mg/kg (500 mg) iv 8H	3 weeks minimum Penicillin hypersensitivity: substitute Flucloxacillin with Vancomycin 10–15 mg/kg (500 mg) iv 6H	392
...post neurosurgery	As above plus S. epidermidis	As above but substitute Flucloxacillin with Vancomycin 10–15 mg/kg (500 mg) iv 6H		
Encephalitis	Herpes simplex virus Enteroviruses Arboviruses M. pneumoniae	Aciclovir 10 mg/kg iv 8H (age 2 wks–2 yrs) (15–20 mg/kg iv 8H should be considered in neonates) 500 mg/m² iv 8H (age 2 yrs–12 yrs) 10 mg/kg iv 8H (age over 12 yrs)	3 weeks minimum Consider macrolide antibiotic if M. pneumoniae suspected	392
Meningitis				
...over 2 months of age	S. pneumoniae[3] N. meningitidis H. influenzae type b[4]	Cefotaxime 50 mg/kg (2 g) iv 6H	S. pneumoniae 10 days N. meningitidis 7 days H. influenzae type b 7–10 days	388
...over 2 months of age and possibility of penicillin-resistant pneumococci[3]	As above	Cefotaxime 50 mg/kg (2 g) iv 6H and Vancomycin 10–15 mg/kg (500 mg) iv 6H	Penicillin or cephalosporin hypersensitivity: see footnote 5	

Condition	Organisms	Treatment	Notes	Ref
...under 2 months of age	As above plus Group B streptococci E. coli and other Gram-negative coliforms L. monocytogenes	Cefotaxime and Benzylpenicillin and Gentamicin[6] (See doses in 'Septicaemia in neonate' section)	3 weeks minimum See footnote 7 re Gentamicin dosing/monitoring Substitute Benzylpenicillin with Vancomycin if possibility of penicillin-resistant pneumococci[3]	388, 430
...with shunt infection, post-neurosurgery, head trauma or CSF leak	As for over 2 months of age, S. epidermidis, S. aureus, Gram-negative coliforms incl. P. aeruginosa	Vancomycin 10–15 mg/kg (500 mg) iv 6H and Ceftazidime 50 mg/kg (2 g) iv 8H	10 days minimum	389
...contact prophylaxis	N. meningitidis	Rifampicin 10 mg/kg (600 mg) po 12H	2 days (alternatives: see table 26.3)	390
...contact prophylaxis	H. influenzae type b	Rifampicin 20 mg/kg (600 mg) po 24H	4 days (alternatives: see table 26.3)	
Postseptal (orbital) cellulitis	S. aureus H. influenzae spp. S. pneumoniae M. catarrhalis Gram-negatives Anaerobes	Flucloxacillin 50 mg/kg (2 g) iv 4–6H and Cefotaxime 50 mg/kg (2 g) iv 6H	10 days minimum Rule out meningitis Consider adding Metronidazole if not responding	307
Preseptal (periorbital) cellulitis ...mild (outpatient)	Group A streptococci S. aureus H. influenzae spp.[4]	Amoxycillin/clavulanate (400/57 mg per 5 ml) 22.5 mg/kg (875 mg) = 0.3 ml/kg (11 ml) po 12H	7–10 days *Consider adding Cefotaxime if not responding to Flucloxacillin alone	307
...moderate (inpatient)	As above	Flucloxacillin* 50 mg/kg (2 g) iv 6H		
...severe, or under 5 yrs of age and non-Hib immunised	As above plus H. influenzae type b[4]	Flucloxacillin 50 mg/kg (2 g) iv 6H and Cefotaxime 50 mg/kg (2 g) iv 6H	Consider non-infective cause in trivial cases	

CARDIOVASCULAR

Infection	Likely organisms	Initial antimicrobials[1] ( ) = maximum dose	Duration of treatment[2] and other comments	Page
Endocarditis				
...native valve or homograft	Viridans streptococci Other streptococci Enterococcus spp. S. aureus and others	Benzylpenicillin 50 mg/kg (3 g) iv 6H *and* Gentamicin 1 mg/kg (80 mg) iv 8H *and* Flucloxacillin 50 mg/kg (2 g) iv 4–6H	4–6 weeks Gentamicin monitoring may not be required when low dose is used for synergy in this setting	237
...artificial valve or post surgery	As above plus S. epidermidis	Vancomycin 10–15 mg/kg (500 mg) iv 6H *and* Gentamicin 1 mg/kg (80 mg) iv 8H		
Endocarditis prophylaxis				
...low risk and dental or upper respiratory tract procedure	Viridans streptococci S. aureus S. pneumoniae Other Gram-positive cocci Enterococcus spp.	Amoxycillin 50 mg/kg (2 g) Local anaesthetic: give po 1 hr before procedure General anaesthetic: give iv with induction	Penicillin hypersensitivity: substitute Amoxycillin with Clindamycin 20 mg/kg (600 mg) po or iv	
...high risk or procedure involving gastrointestinal or genitourinary tract	As above plus Gram-negative coliforms	Amoxycillin 50 mg/kg (2 g) iv or im *and* Gentamicin 2.5 mg/kg (240 mg) iv or im before procedure, *followed 6 hrs later by* Amoxycillin 25 mg/kg (500 mg) po or iv or im	Penicillin hypersensitivity: substitute Amoxycillin with Vancomycin 20 mg/kg (1 g) iv See footnote 7 re Gentamicin dosing/monitoring	

GASTROINTESTINAL

Infection	Likely organisms	Initial antimicrobials[1] ( ) = maximum dose	Duration of treatment[2] and other comments	Page
Diarrhoea				
...*Salmonella* spp. isolated in infant under 3 months of age or in immunocompromised	*Salmonella* spp.	Cefotaxime 50 mg/kg (2 g) iv 6H	3–5 days Antibiotic treatment is generally unnecessary for most other organisms	395
...antibiotic associated	*C. difficile*	Metronidazole 7.5 mg/kg (400 mg) po 8H	7–10 days	396
Giardiasis	*G. lamblia*	Metronidazole 30 mg/kg (2 g) po daily *or* Tinidazole 50 mg/kg (2 g) po	3 days Single dose	395
Peritonitis or ascending cholangitis	Gram-negative coliforms Anaerobes *Enterococcus* spp.	Benzylpenicillin 50 mg/kg (3 g) iv 6H *and* Gentamicin 7.5 mg/kg (360 mg) iv daily (< 10 yrs) 6 mg/kg (360 mg) iv daily (> 10 yrs) *and* Metronidazole 15 mg/kg (1 g) iv stat, then 7.5 mg/kg (500 mg) iv 8H	Up to 14 days See footnote 7 re Gentamicin dosing/monitoring	523
Threadworm (Pinworm)	*Enterobius vermicularis*	Mebendazole 50 mg po (under 10 kg) 100 mg po (over 10 kg)	Single dose; may need to repeat after 14 days Treat whole family	397

GENITOURINARY

Infection	Likely organisms	Initial antimicrobials[1] ( ) = maximum dose	Duration of treatment[2] and other comments	Page
Urinary tract infection				472
...over 6 months of age and not sick	E. coli P. mirabilis K. oxytoca Other Gram-negatives	Trimethoprim 4 mg/kg (150 mg) po 12H or if syrup is necessary then Co-trimoxazole (Trimethoprim/Sulphamethoxazole 8/40 mg per ml) 0.5 ml/kg (20 ml) po 12H	5 days	
...under 6 months of age or sick or acute pyelonephritis	As above plus Enterococcus spp.	Benzylpenicillin 50 mg/kg (3 g) iv 6H and Gentamicin 7.5 mg/kg (360 mg) iv daily (< 10 yrs) 6 mg/kg (360 mg) iv daily (> 10 yrs) (For infants under 1 month of age, see doses in 'Septicaemia in neonate' section)	5–7 days for UTI 14 days for pyelonephritis See footnote 7 re Gentamicin dosing/monitoring	
...prophylaxis	As above	Trimethoprim 2 mg/kg (150 mg) po daily or if syrup is necessary then Co-trimoxazole (Trimethoprim/Sulphamethoxazole 8/40 mg per ml) 0.25 ml/kg (20 ml) po daily		

RESPIRATORY

Infection	Likely organisms	Initial antimicrobials[1] ( ) = maximum dose	Duration of treatment[2] and other comments	Page
Epiglottitis	*H. influenzae* type b[4]	Ceftriaxone 100 mg/kg (2 g) iv followed by 50 mg/kg (2 g) 24 hrs later	2 doses only	10, 496
Gingivostomatitis ...in immuno- compromised	Herpes simplex virus	Aciclovir 5–10 mg/kg iv 8H (age 2 wks–2 yrs) 250–500 mg/m² iv 8H (age 2 yrs–12 yrs) 5–10 mg/kg iv 8H (age over 12 yrs)	7 days Treatment is only recommended for severe primary disease in the immunocompromised	378
Otitis externa ...acute diffuse	*S. aureus* *S. epidermidis* *P. aeruginosa* *Proteus* spp. *Klebsiella* spp.	Clean ear canal Topical steroid/antibiotic (e.g. Sofradex) drops (± insertion of wick soaked in drops if ear canal oedematous)	7 days	304
...acute localised (furuncle) ± cellulitis	*S. aureus* Group A streptococci	Flucloxacillin 50 mg/kg (2 g) iv 6H	7–10 days	
...failure of first line treatment, high fever or severe persistent pain	As above plus *P. aeruginosa*	Ticarcillin/clavulanate 50 mg/kg (3 g) iv 6H	14 days minimum Consider fungal infection	
Otitis media	Viruses *S. pneumoniae* *M. catarrhalis* *H. influenzae* spp. Group A streptococci	Consider no antibiotics for 48 hrs if over 2 yrs of age *or* Amoxycillin 15 mg/kg (500 mg) po 8H	5 days	300

RESPIRATORY (CONTINUED)

Infection	Likely organisms	Initial antimicrobials[1] ( ) = maximum dose	Duration of treatment[2] and other comments	Page
Pertussis prophylaxis ...household or close contacts	*B. pertussis*	Erythromycin 10 mg/kg (250 mg) po 6H (estolate salt is preferred)	10 days Can be given up to 3 weeks after contact with index case	493
Pneumonia ...mild (outpatient)	Viruses *S. pneumoniae* *H. influenzae* spp.	Amoxycillin 15 mg/kg (500 mg) po 8H	7–10 days Consider admission for all children under 1 yr of age	499
...moderate (inpatient)	As above	Benzylpenicillin 50 mg/kg (3 g) iv 6H		
...mild or moderate where *M. pneumoniae* is suspected (especially over 5 yrs of age)	As above plus *M. pneumoniae*	Roxithromycin 2.5–4 mg/kg (150 mg) po 12H	10 days	
...severe systemic toxicity or pneumatocoele or large pleural effusion	As above plus *S. aureus* Group A streptococci Gram-negatives	Flucloxacillin 50 mg/kg (2 g) iv 4–6H *and* Cefotaxime 50 mg/kg (2 g) iv 6H *and* consider Roxithromycin as above	10 days minimum	
Tonsillitis	Viruses Group A streptococci *A. haemolyticum*	Consider no antibiotics *or* Phenoxymethylpenicillin (Penicillin V) 250 mg po 12H (age under 10 yrs) 500 mg po 12H (age over 10 yrs)	10 days	304

SEPTICAEMIA

Infection	Likely organisms	Initial antimicrobials[1] ( ) = maximum dose	Duration of treatment[2] and other comments	Page
Septicaemia with unknown CSF	*S. pneumoniae* *N. meningitidis* *S. aureus* Group A streptococci Gram-negatives	Flucloxacillin 50 mg/kg (2 g) iv 4H *and* Cefotaxime 50 mg/kg (2 g) iv 6H	See notes below	8
Septicaemia with normal CSF	As above	Flucloxacillin 50 mg/kg (2 g) iv 4H *and* Gentamicin 7.5 mg/kg (360 mg) iv daily (< 10 yrs) 6 mg/kg (360 mg) iv daily (> 10 yrs)	Consider adding Clindamycin 10 mg/kg (600 mg) iv 6H if suspect Gram-positive toxic shock syndrome Duration depends on culture results	8, 363
...in non-Hib immunised	As above plus *H. influenzae* type b[4]	Flucloxacillin 50 mg/kg (2 g) iv 4H *and* Cefotaxime 50 mg/kg (2 g) iv 6H	See footnote 7 re Gentamicin dosing/monitoring	
...in neutropenic patient	As above plus *Enterococcus* spp. *P. aeruginosa*	Piperacillin 50 mg/kg (3 g) iv 6H *and* Gentamicin 7.5 mg/kg (360 mg) iv daily (< 10 yrs) 6 mg/kg (360 mg) iv daily (> 10 yrs)	Consult local protocols and also consider anaerobic and fungal infection in neutropenic patients	
...in neutropenic patient with potential line infection	As above plus Gram-positive cocci incl. *S. epidermidis*	Piperacillin 50 mg/kg (3 g) iv 6H *and* Gentamicin 7.5 mg/kg (360 mg) iv daily (< 10 yrs) 6 mg/kg (360 mg) iv daily (> 10 yrs) *and* Vancomycin 10–15 mg/kg (500 mg) iv 6H		

SEPTICAEMIA (IN NEONATE)

Infection	Likely organisms	Initial antimicrobials[1] () = maximum dose	Duration of treatment[2] and other comments	Page
Septicaemia in neonate				
...community-acquired infection	Group B streptococci E. coli and other Gram-negative coliforms L. monocytogenes H. influenzae spp.[4] plus those listed above for 'Septicaemia with unknown CSF'	Benzylpenicillin 50 mg/kg iv 12H (first week of life) 6H (1–4 weeks of age) 4H (over 4 week of ages) and Gentamicin 2.5 mg/kg iv 12H (first week of life) 8H (over 1 week of age)	Consider adding Flucloxacillin if infection with S. aureus suspected Duration depends on culture results See footnote 7 re Gentamicin dosing/monitoring Premature neonates require special dosing consideration	430
...if meningitis suspected	As above	Benzylpenicillin and Gentamicin[6] as above plus Cefotaxime 50 mg/kg iv 12H (first week of life) 6H (over 1 week of age)		
...if abdominal source suspected	As above plus Anaerobes	Benzylpenicillin and Gentamicin as above plus Metronidazole 15 mg/kg iv stat, then 7.5 mg/kg iv 12H		

SKIN/SOFT TISSUE/BONE

Infection	Likely organisms	Initial antimicrobials[1] () = maximum dose	Duration of treatment[2] and other comments	Page
Adenitis	S. aureus Group A streptococci Oral anaerobes	Flucloxacillin 50 mg/kg (2 g) iv 6H	10–14 days	373
Bites (animal/human)	Viridans streptococci S. aureus Group A streptococci Oral anaerobes E. corrodens Pasteurella spp. (cat and dog) C. canimorsus (dog)	Amoxycillin/clavulanate (400/57 mg per 5 ml) 22.5 mg/kg (875 mg) ≈ 0.3 ml/kg (11 ml) po 12H	3–5 days for prophylaxis 7–14 days for treatment Check tetanus immunisation status and consider risk of hepatitis B and C, and HIV	49
...if severe, penetrating injuries, esp. involving joints or tendons	As above	Cefotaxime 50 mg/kg (2 g) iv 6H and Metronidazole 7.5 mg/kg (400/500 mg) po/iv 8H		
Cellulitis				
...mild (outpatient)	Group A streptococci S. aureus	Flucloxacillin 25 mg/kg (500 mg) po 6H	5–10 days	261
...moderate/severe (inpatient)	As above	Flucloxacillin 50 mg/kg (2 g) iv 6H	Consider adding Clindamycin 10 mg/kg (600 mg) iv 6H if rapid progression suggestive of necrotising fasciitis	
...if facial cellulitis in child under 5 yrs of age and non-Hib immunised	As above plus S. pneumoniae H. influenzae spp.[4]	Flucloxacillin 50 mg/kg (2 g) iv 6H and Cefotaxime 50 mg/kg (2 g) iv 6H		

SKIN/SOFT TISSUE/BONE (CONTINUED)

Infection	Likely organisms	Initial antimicrobials[1] ( ) = maximum dose	Duration of treatment[2] and other comments	Page
Head lice	Pediculus humanus var. capitis	1% Permethrin liquid or cream rinse	One application; may need to repeat after one week	269
Impetigo	Group A streptococci S. aureus	Mupirocin 2% ointment 8H if localised or Flucloxacillin 15 mg/kg (500 mg) po 6H	5–10 days	248
Osteomyelitis	S. aureus Group A streptococci S. pneumoniae	Flucloxacillin 50 mg/kg (2 g) iv 4–6H	3–4 weeks for uncomplicated cases	468
...if under 5 yrs of age and non-Hib immunised	As above plus H. influenzae type b[4]	Flucloxacillin 50 mg/kg (2 g) iv 4–6H and Cefotaxime 50 mg/kg (2 g) iv 6H		
...in patient with sickle cell anaemia	As above plus Salmonella spp.	Flucloxacillin 50 mg/kg (2 g) iv 4–6H and Cefotaxime 50 mg/kg (2 g) iv 6H		
...with penetrating foot injury	As above plus P. aeruginosa	Ceftazidime 50 mg/kg (2 g) iv 8H and Gentamicin 7.5 mg/kg (360 mg) iv daily (< 10 yrs) 6 mg/kg (360 mg) iv daily (> 10 yrs)	Surgical intervention important See footnote 7 re Gentamicin dosing/monitoring	
Scabies	Sarcoptes scabiei	5% Permethrin	One application; may need to repeat after 14 days Treat whole family	252
Septic arthritis	As for osteomyelitis	As for osteomyelitis	2–3 weeks for uncomplicated cases	468
Shingles	Varicella zoster virus	Aciclovir 10 mg/kg iv 8H (age 2 wks–2 yrs) 500 mg/m² iv 8H (age 2 yrs–12 yrs) 10 mg/kg iv 8H (age over 12 yrs) and Aciclovir ointment to eye 5 times/day	7 days	383
...in immunocompromised or involving eye			Shingles in immunocompetent children does not generally require treatment	

NOTES TO ANTIMICROBIAL GUIDELINES

These guidelines have been developed to assist doctors with their choice of initial empiric treatment. The choice of antimicrobial, dose and frequency of administration for continuing treatment may require adjustment according to the clinical situation. The recommendations are not intended to be proscriptive and alternative regimens may also be appropriate.

1 Antimicrobial choice

- Antibiotics should be changed to narrow spectrum agents once sensitivities are known.

- Dose adjustments may be necessary for neonates, and for children with renal or hepatic impairment.

- Alternative antimicrobial regimens may be more appropriate for neonates, immunocompromised patients or others with a special infection risk (e.g. cystic fibrosis, sickle cell anaemia).

- Resistance to antimicrobials is an increasing problem worldwide. Of particular concern is the increasing incidence of penicillin-resistant pneumococci (see footnote 3). It is important to take into account local resistance patterns when using these guidelines.

- Cefotaxime can usually be substituted by:
  Ceftriaxone 100 mg/kg (4 g) iv daily or 50 mg/kg (2 g) iv 12H

2 Duration of treatment

Duration of treatment is given as a guide only and may vary with the clinical situation. 'Step down' from intravenous to oral treatment is appropriate in many cases. Durations given generally refer to the total intravenous and oral treatment.

3 Penicillin-resistant pneumococci

The prevalence of invasive strains that are highly resistant to penicillin or cephalosporins in Melbourne in 1999 is low. Cefotaxime remains the drug of first choice for the empiric treatment of meningitis. The prevalence of resistant strains is being monitored and this recommendation may change. Penicillin remains the drug of first choice for the empiric treatment of suspected pneumococcal pneumonia and other non-CNS infections, regardless of susceptibility. High doses of penicillin overcome resistance in this setting and should be used for confirmed non-CNS infection caused by penicillin-resistant pneumococci.

4 Invasive H. influenzae type b disease

Since the introduction of *H. influenzae* type b (Hib) immunisation, there has been a dramatic decline in the incidence of invasive disease. However, in children with potential invasive disease, who are not fully immunised against Hib, therapy should include cover against Hib.

5 Treatment of meningitis in patients with penicillin or cephalosporin hypersensitivity

In patients with a history of severe (anaphylactic) penicillin hypersensitivity, avoid cephalosporins: use Chloramphenicol 25 mg/kg (1 g) iv 6H and Vancomycin 10–15 mg/kg (500 mg) iv 6H.

6 Empiric treatment of neonatal meningitis

Gentamicin is recommended in this setting to provide double Gram-negative cover, and for synergy with benzylpenicillin against *Listeria monocytogenes* and group B streptococci.

7 Gentamicin dosing/monitoring

Once-daily administration of gentamicin is safe and effective for most patients. Certain patients, such as neonates and those with cystic fibrosis, endocarditis or renal failure, may require special dosing consideration.

The regimen for monitoring gentamicin levels is different for once-daily and 8, 12 or 18H dosing, and depends on renal function:

Once-daily dosing

- Normal renal function—if the patient is to have more than 3 doses, the trough level (predose) should be checked before the third dose and then every 3 days (target level <1 mg/L).

- Abnormal renal function—trough levels may need to be checked earlier and more frequently (target level <1 mg/L).

- Renal failure—levels should be checked post-dose at 2, 12 and 24 hours, and adjusted accordingly. The results should be discussed with a specialist familiar with therapeutic drug monitoring.

8, 12 and 18 hourly dosing

- The trough level should be checked before the fourth dose and peak level 1 hour after the start of the fourth dose (target trough <2 mg/L, target peak 5–10 mg/L).

- Levels should be repeated every 3 days, or more frequently if levels are inappropriate or if renal function is abnormal.

INDEX

Bold denotes figures or table

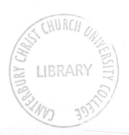